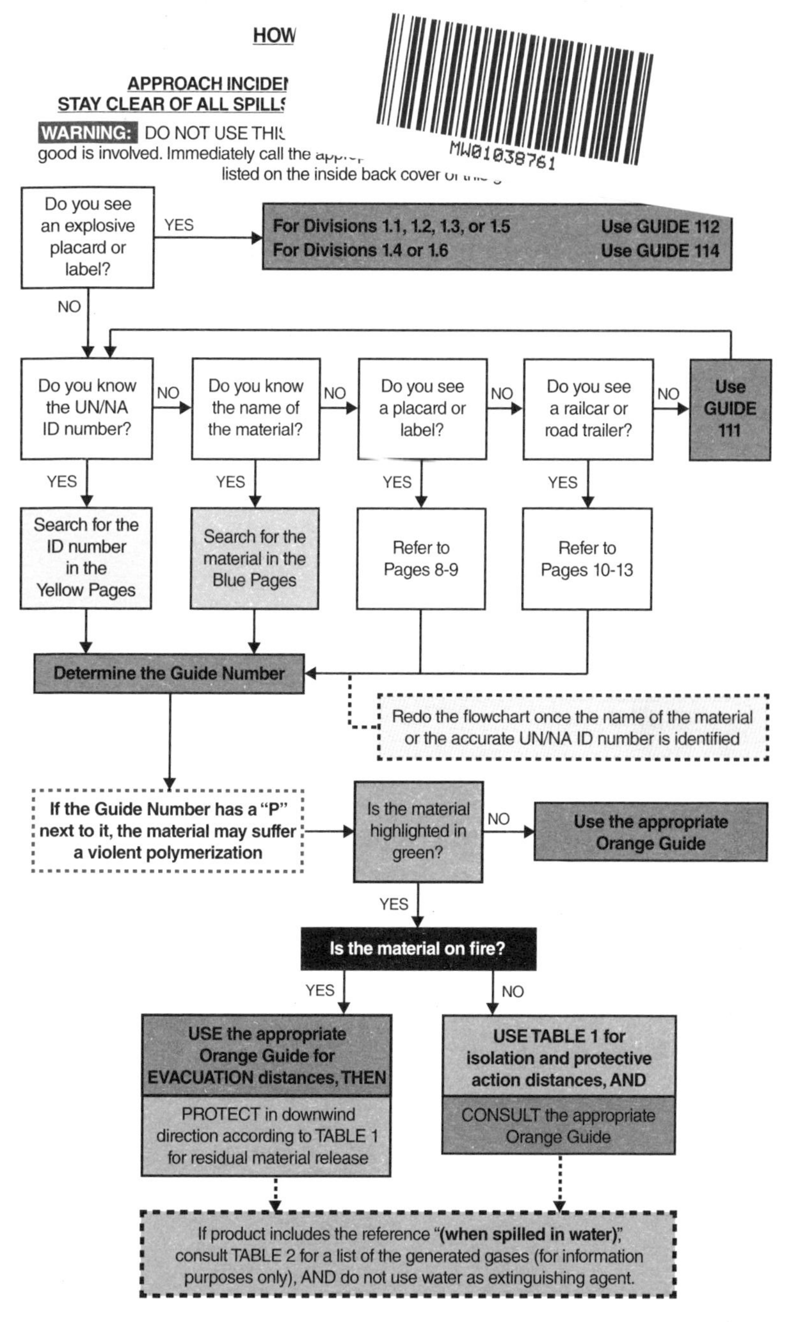

HOW
APPROACH INCIDE
STAY CLEAR OF ALL SPILLS
WARNING: DO NOT USE THIS
good is involved. Immediately call the
listed on the inside back cover
MW01038761
Do you see an explosive placard or label?
YES
For Divisions 1.1, 1.2, 1.3, or 1.5 Use GUIDE 112
For Divisions 1.4 or 1.6 Use GUIDE 114
NO
Do you know the UN/NA ID number?
NO
Do you know the name of the material?
NO
Do you see a placard or label?
NO
Do you see a railcar or road trailer?
NO
Use GUIDE 111
YES
Search for the ID number in the Yellow Pages
YES
Search for the material in the Blue Pages
YES
Refer to Pages 8-9
YES
Refer to Pages 10-13
Determine the Guide Number
Redo the flowchart once the name of the material or the accurate UN/NA ID number is identified
If the Guide Number has a "P" next to it, the material may suffer a violent polymerization
Is the material highlighted in green?
NO
Use the appropriate Orange Guide
YES
Is the material on fire?
YES
NO
USE the appropriate Orange Guide for EVACUATION distances, THEN
PROTECT in downwind direction according to TABLE 1 for residual material release
USE TABLE 1 for isolation and protective action distances, AND
CONSULT the appropriate Orange Guide
If product includes the reference "(when spilled in water)", consult TABLE 2 for a list of the generated gases (for information purposes only), AND do not use water as extinguishing agent.

**BEFORE AN EMERGENCY - BECOME FAMILIAR WITH THIS GUIDEBOOK!**

First responders must be trained in the use of this guidebook.

## LOCAL EMERGENCY TELEPHONE NUMBERS

**Please populate this page with emergency telephone numbers for local assistance:**

### HAZMAT CONTRACTORS

### RAIL COMPANIES

### FEDERAL/STATE/PROVINCIAL AGENCIES

### OTHERS

## SAFETY PRECAUTIONS

## RESIST RUSHING IN!

**APPROACH CAUTIOUSLY FROM *UPWIND, UPHILL* OR *UPSTREAM*:**

- Stay clear of ***Vapor, Fumes, Smoke* and *Spills***
- Keep vehicle at a safe distance from the scene

**SECURE THE SCENE:**

- Isolate the area and protect yourself and others

**IDENTIFY THE HAZARDS USING ANY OF THE FOLLOWING:**

- Placards
- Container labels
- Shipping documents
- Rail Car and Road Trailer Identification Chart
- Material Safety Data Sheets (MSDS)
- Knowledge of persons on scene
- Consult applicable guide page

**SESS THE SITUATION:**

- Is there a fire, a spill or a leak?
- What are the weather conditions?
- What is the terrain like?
- Who/what is at risk: people, property or the environment?
- What actions should be taken – evacuation, shelter in-place or dike?
- What resources (human and equipment) are required?
- What can be done immediately?

**HELP:**

- dvise your headquarters to notify responsible agencies and call for assistance from ualified personnel

**D:**

- er only when wearing appropriate protective gear
- cue attempts and protecting property must be weighed against you becoming of the problem
- blish a command post and lines of communication
- nually reassess the situation and modify response accordingly
- der safety of people in the immediate area first, including your own safety

Do not assume that gases or vapors are harmless because of lack of a ss gases or vapors may be harmful. Use **CAUTION** when handling empty ause they may still present hazards until they are cleaned and purged of

## TABLE OF CONTENTS




AS

OBTAIN

RESPON

ABOVE ALL

smell – odorl

containers be

all residues.

Page 4

## NOTIFICATION AND REQUEST FOR TECHNICAL INFORMATION

Follow the steps outlined in your organization's standard operating procedures and/or local emergency response plan for obtaining qualified assistance. Generally, the notification sequence and requests for technical information beyond what is available in this guidebook should occur in the following order:

1. **NOTIFY YOUR ORGANIZATION/AGENCY**
   - Based on information provided, this will set in motion a series of events
   - Actions may range from dispatching additional trained personnel to the scene, to activating the local emergency response plan
   - Ensure that local fire and police departments have been notified

2. **CALL THE EMERGENCY RESPONSE TELEPHONE NUMBER ON THE SHIPPING DOCUMENT**
   - If shipping paper is not available, use guidance under next section "**NATIONAL ASSISTANCE**"

3. **NATIONAL ASSISTANCE**
   - Contact the appropriate emergency response agency listed on the inside back cover of this guidebook
   - Provide as much information about the hazardous material and the nature of the incident
   - The agency will provide immediate advice on handling the early stages of the incident
   - The agency will also contact the shipper or manufacturer of the material for more detailed information if necessary
   - The agency will request on-scene assistance when necessary

4. **PROVIDE AS MUCH OF THE FOLLOWING INFORMATION AS POSSIBLE:**
   - Your name, call-back telephone number, fax number
   - Location and nature of problem (spill, fire, etc.)
   - Name and identification number of material(s) involved
   - Shipper/consignee/point-of-origin
   - Carrier name, rail car or truck number
   - Container type and size
   - Quantity of material transported/released
   - Local conditions (weather, terrain)
   - Proximity to schools, hospitals, waterways, etc.
   - Injuries and exposures
   - Local emergency services that have been notified

## HAZARD CLASSIFICATION SYSTEM

The hazard class of dangerous goods is indicated either by its class (or division) number or name. Placards are used to identify the class or division of a material. The hazard class or division number must be displayed in the lower corner of a placard and is required for both primary and subsidiary hazard classes and divisions, if applicable. For other than Class 7 placards, text indicating a hazard (for example, "CORROSIVE") is not required. Text is shown only in the U.S. The hazard class or division number and subsidiary hazard classes or division numbers placed in parentheses (when applicable), must appear on the shipping document after each proper shipping name.

**Class 1 - Explosives**

| | |
|---|---|
| Division 1.1 | Explosives which have a mass explosion hazard |
| Division 1.2 | Explosives which have a projection hazard but not a mass explosion hazard |
| Division 1.3 | Explosives which have a fire hazard and either a minor blast hazard or a minor projection hazard or both, but not a mass explosion hazard |
| Division 1.4 | Explosives which present no significant blast hazard |
| Division 1.5 | Very insensitive explosives with a mass explosion hazard |
| Division 1.6 | Extremely insensitive articles which do not have a mass explosion hazard |

**Class 2 - Gases**

| | |
|---|---|
| Division 2.1 | Flammable gases |
| Division 2.2 | Non-flammable, non-toxic* gases |
| Division 2.3 | Toxic* gases |

**Class 3 - Flammable liquids (and Combustible liquids** [U.S.]**)**

**Class 4 - Flammable solids; Substances liable to spontaneous combustion; Substances which, on contact with water, emit flammable gases**

| | |
|---|---|
| Division 4.1 | Flammable solids, self-reactive substances and solid desensitized explosives |
| Division 4.2 | Substances liable to spontaneous combustion |
| Division 4.3 | Substances which in contact with water emit flammable gases |

**Class 5 - Oxidizing substances and Organic peroxides**

| | |
|---|---|
| Division 5.1 | Oxidizing substances |
| Division 5.2 | Organic peroxides |

**Class 6 - Toxic* substances and Infectious substances**

| | |
|---|---|
| Division 6.1 | Toxic*substances |
| Division 6.2 | Infectious substances |

**Class 7 - Radioactive materials**

**Class 8 - Corrosive substances**

**Class 9 - Miscellaneous dangerous goods/hazardous materials and articles**

* The words "poison" or "poisonous" are synonymous with the word "toxic".

## INTRODUCTION TO THE TABLE OF MARKINGS, LABELS AND PLACARDS

**USE THIS TABLE ONLY WHEN THE ID NUMBER OR PROPER SHIPPING NAME IS NOT AVAILABLE.**

The next two pages display the placards used on transport vehicles carrying dangerous goods with the applicable reference GUIDE circled. Follow these steps:

1. **Approach scene from upwind, uphill or upstream at a safe distance to safely identify and/or read the placard or orange panel. Use binoculars if available.**
2. **Match the vehicle placard(s) with one of the placards displayed on the next two pages.**
3. **Consult the circled guide number associated with the placard. Use that guide information for now. For example:**
   - Use GUIDE 127 for a FLAMMABLE (Class 3) placard
   - Use GUIDE 153 for a CORROSIVE (Class 8) placard
   - Use GUIDE 111 when the DANGER/DANGEROUS placard is displayed or the nature of the spilled, leaking or burning material is not known. Also use this GUIDE when the presence of dangerous goods is suspected but no placards can be seen.

   If multiple placards point to more than one guide, initially use the most conservative guide (i.e., the guide requiring the greatest degree of protective actions).
4. **Guides associated with the placards provide the most significant risk and/or hazard information.**
5. **When specific information, such as ID number or proper shipping name, becomes available, the more specific Guide recommended for that material must be consulted.**
6. **A single asterisk (*) on orange placards represent an explosive's compatibility group letter. The asterisk must be replaced with the appropriate compatibility group letter. Refer to the Glossary (page 376).**
7. **Double asterisks (**) on orange placards represent the division of the explosive. The double asterisks must be replaced with the appropriate division number.**

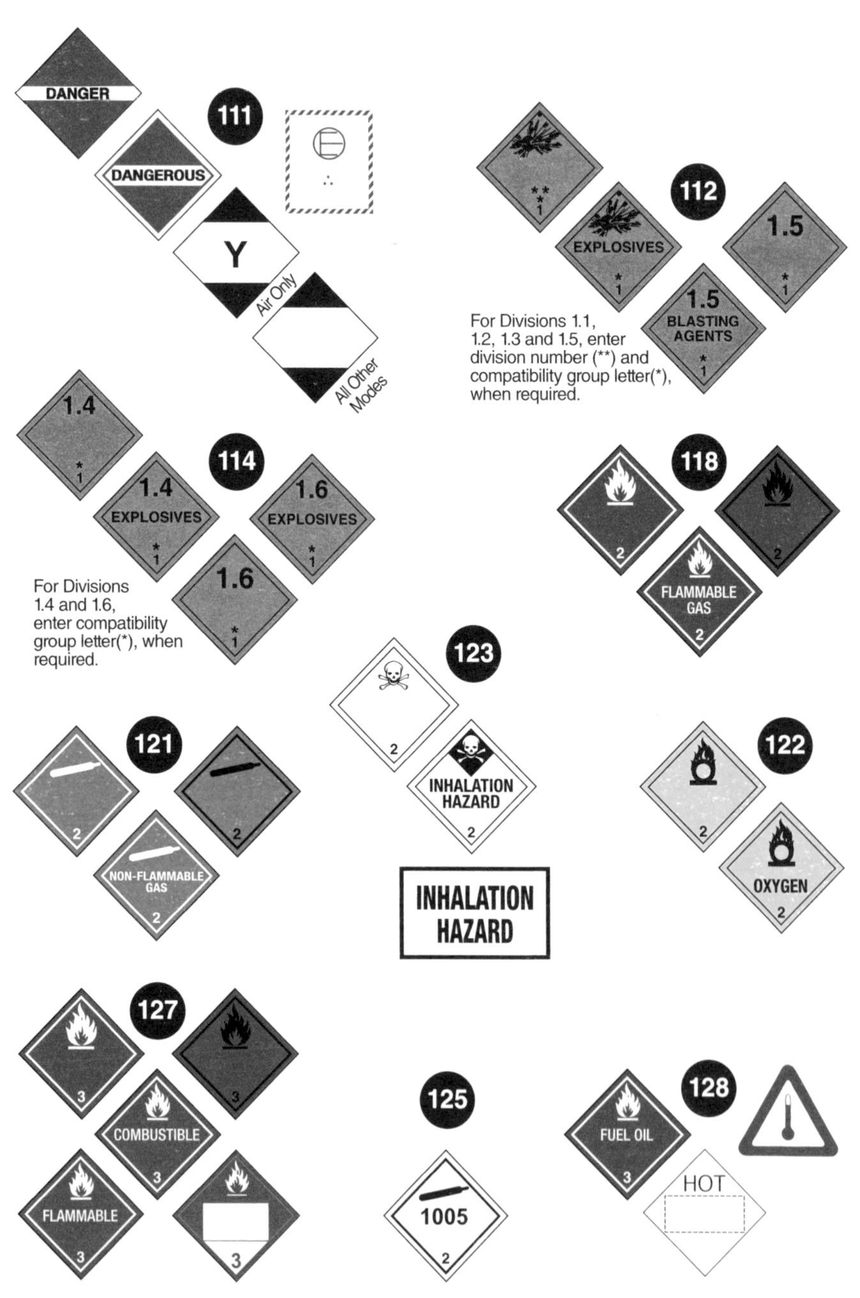

DANGER
111
DANGEROUS
Y
Air Only
All Other Modes
112
EXPLOSIVES
1.5
1.5
BLASTING AGENTS
For Divisions 1.1, 1.2, 1.3 and 1.5, enter division number (**) and compatibility group letter(*), when required.
1.4
114
1.4
EXPLOSIVES
1.6
EXPLOSIVES
1.6
For Divisions 1.4 and 1.6, enter compatibility group letter(*), when required.
118
FLAMMABLE GAS
123
INHALATION HAZARD
121
NON-FLAMMABLE GAS
122
OXYGEN
INHALATION HAZARD
127
COMBUSTIBLE
FLAMMABLE
125
1005
128
FUEL OIL
HOT

**AND INITIAL RESPONSE GUIDE TO USE ON-SCENE**

USING THE SHIPPING DOCUMENT, NUMBERED PLACARD, OR ORANGE PANEL NUMBER

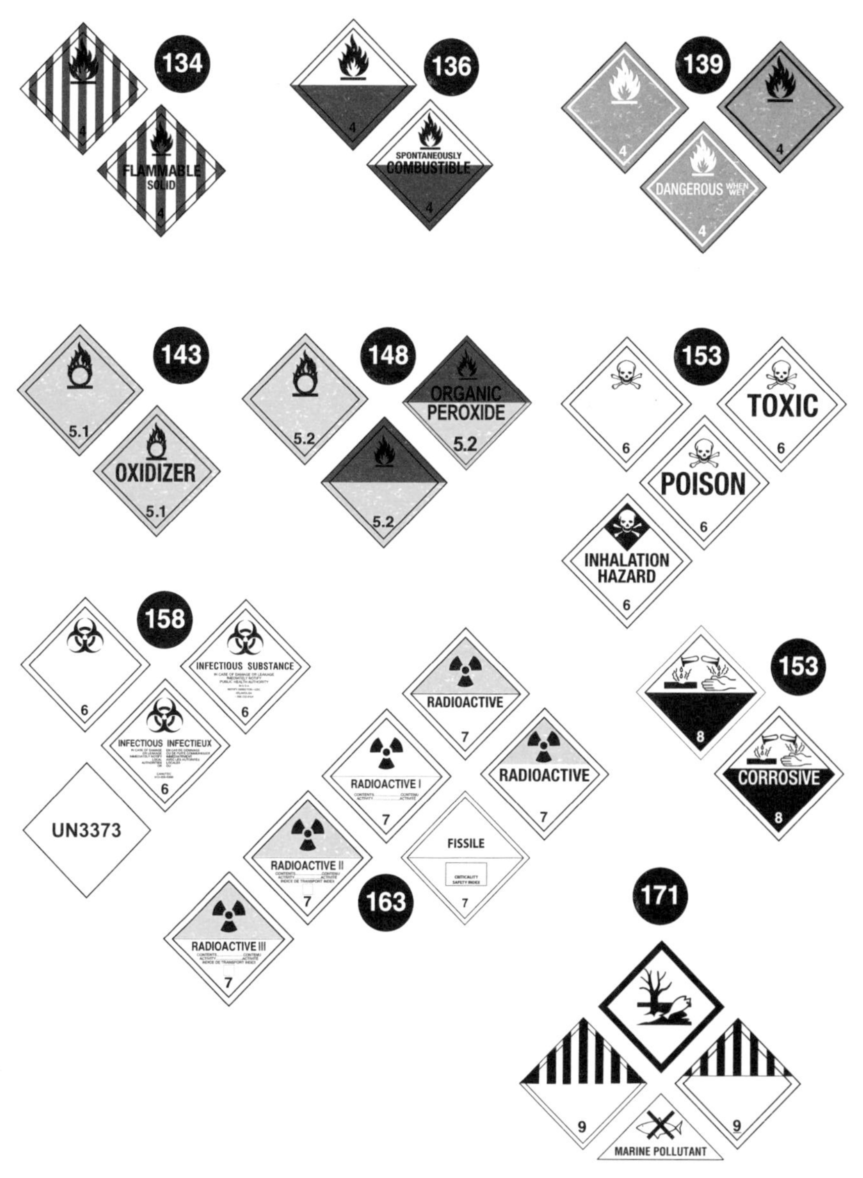

# RAIL CAR IDENTIFICATION CHART*

## 117 Pressure tank car

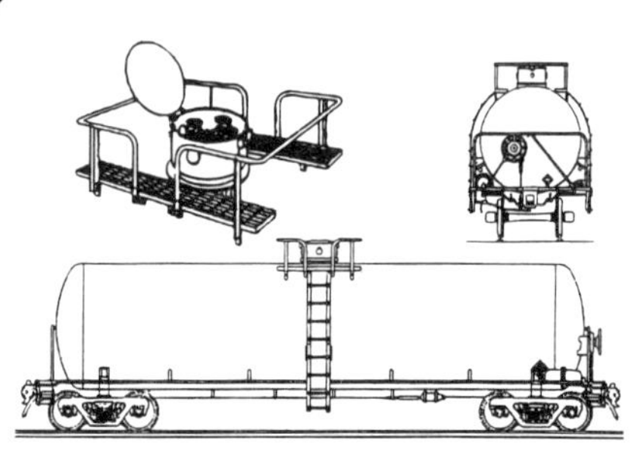

- For flammable, non-flammable, toxic and/or liquefied compressed gases
- Protective housing
- No bottom fittings
- Pressures usually above 40 psi

## 131 General service tank car (low pressure)

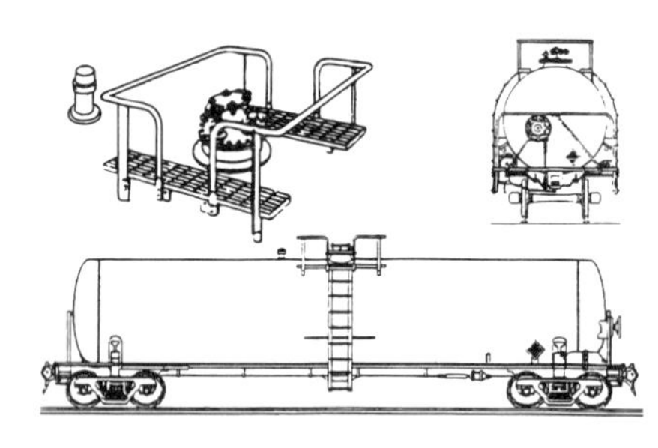

- For variety of hazardous and non-hazardous materials
- Fittings and valves normally visible at the top of the tank
- Some may have bottom outlet valve
- Pressures usually below 25 psi

## 128 Low pressure tank car (TC117, DOT117)

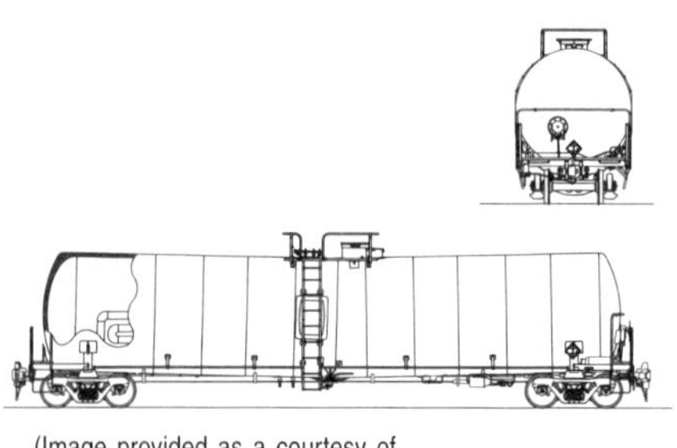

(Image provided as a courtesy of The Greenbrier Companies, Inc.)

- For flammable liquids (e.g., Petroleum crude oil, ethanol)
- Protective housing separate from manway
- Bottom outlet valve
- Pressures usually below 25 psi

# RAIL CAR IDENTIFICATION CHART*

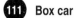

## 111 Box car

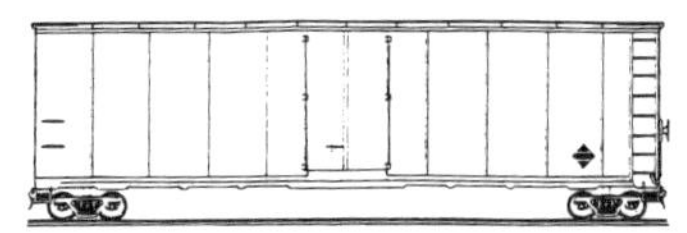

- For general freight that carry bulk or non-bulk packages
- May transport hazardous materials in small packages or "tote bins"
- Single or double sliding door

## 140 Hopper car

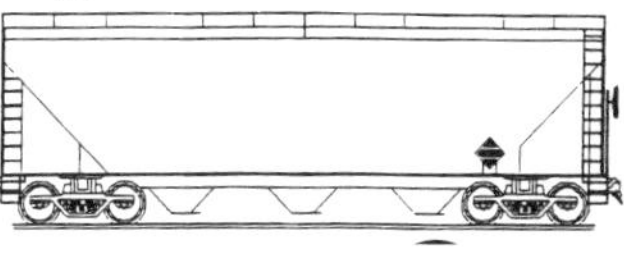

- For bulk commodities and bulk cargo (e.g., coal, ore, cement and solid granular materials)
- Bulk lading discharged by gravity through the hopper bottom doors when doors opened

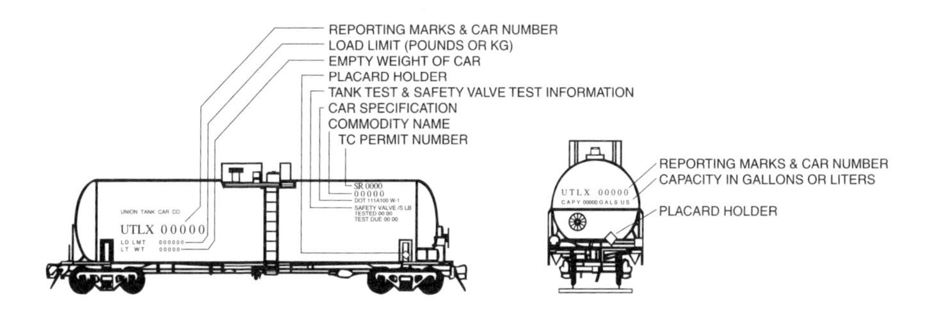


**CAUTION:** Emergency response personnel must be aware that rail tank cars vary widely in construction, fittings and purpose. Tank cars could transport products that may be solids, liquids or gases. The products may be under pressure. It is essential that products be identified by consulting shipping documents or train consist or contacting dispatch centers before emergency response is initiated.

The information stenciled on the sides or ends of tank cars, as illustrated above, may be used to identify the product utilizing:

a. the commodity name shown; or
b. the other information shown, especially reporting marks and car number which, when supplied to a dispatch center, will facilitate the identification of the product.

* **The recommended guides should be considered as last resort if the material cannot be identified by any other means.**

# ROAD TRAILER IDENTIFICATION CHART*

**WARNING:** Road trailers may be jacketed, the cross-section may look different than shown and external ring stiffeners would be invisible.

**NOTE:** An emergency shut-off valve is commonly found at the front of the tank, near the driver door.

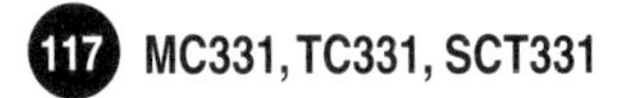

## 117 MC331, TC331, SCT331

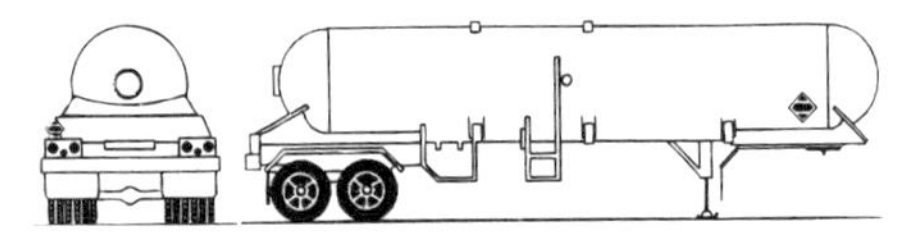

- For liquefied compressed gases (e.g., LPG, ammonia)
- Rounded heads
- Design pressure between 100-500 psi**

## 117 MC338, TC338, SCT338, TC341, CGA341

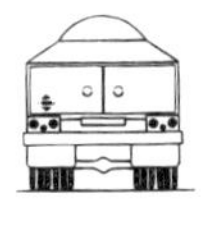

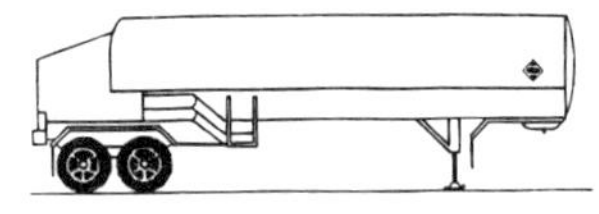

- For refrigerated liquefied gases (cryogenic liquids)
- Similar to a "giant thermo-bottle"
- Fitting compartments located in a cabinet at the rear of the tank
- MAWP between 25-500 psi**

## 131 DOT406, TC406, SCT306, MC306, TC306

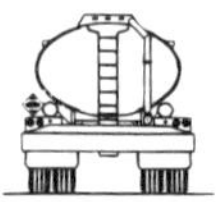

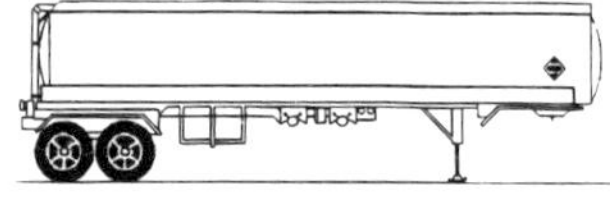

- For flammable liquids (e.g., gasoline, diesel)
- Elliptical cross-section
- Rollover protection at the top
- Bottom outlet valves
- MAWP between 3-15 psi**

## 112 TC423

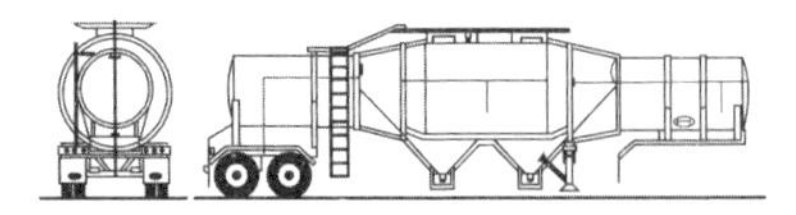

- For emulsion and water-gel explosives
- Hopper-style configuration
- MAWP between 5-15 psi**

## 137 DOT407, TC407, SCT307, MC307, TC307

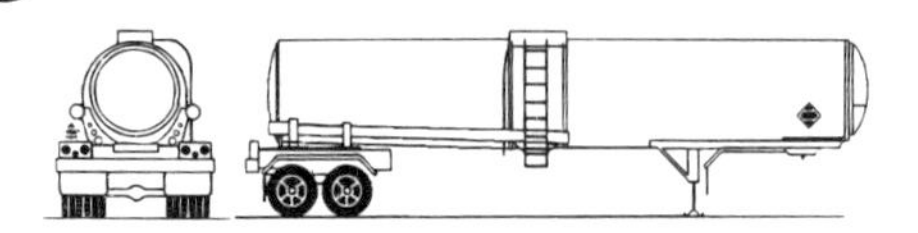

- For toxic, corrosive, and flammable liquids
- Circular cross-section
- May have external ring stiffeners
- MAWP of at least 25 psi**

## ROAD TRAILER IDENTIFICATION CHART*

### 137 DOT412, TC412, SCT312, MC312, TC312

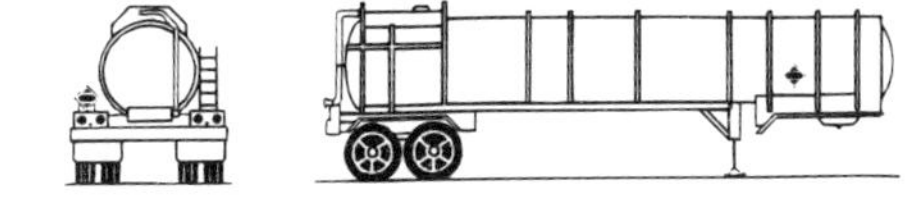

- Usually for corrosive liquids
- Circular cross-section
- External ring stiffeners
- Tank diameter is relatively small
- MAWP of at least 15 psi**

### 137 Compressed Gas/Tube Trailer

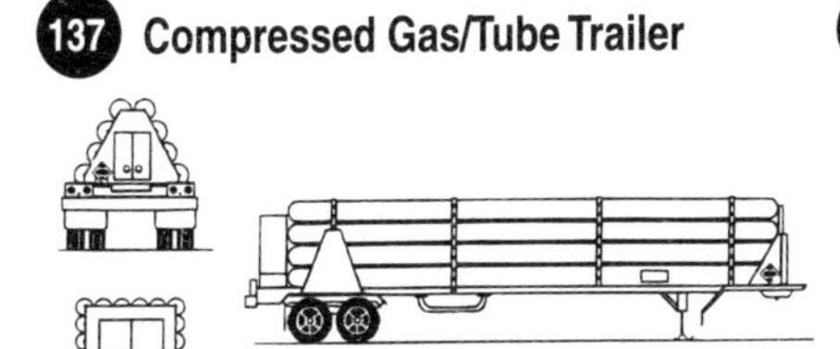

### 111 Mixed Cargo

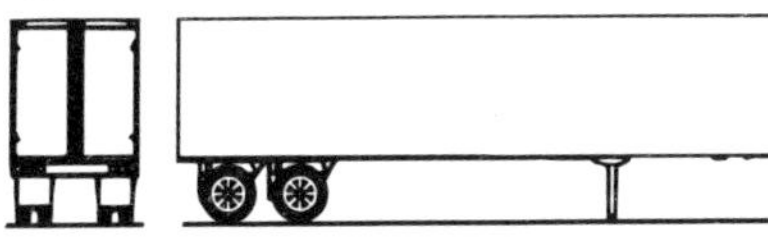

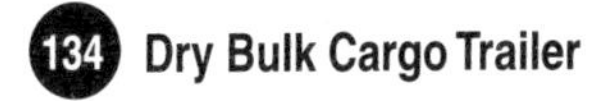

### 134 Dry Bulk Cargo Trailer

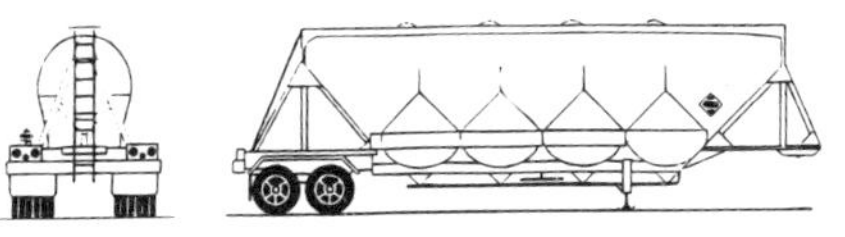

### 117 Intermodal Tank

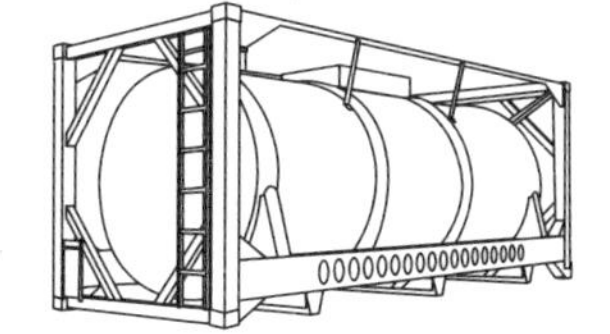

### 137 Vacuum Tanker

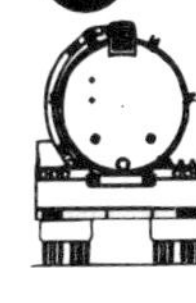

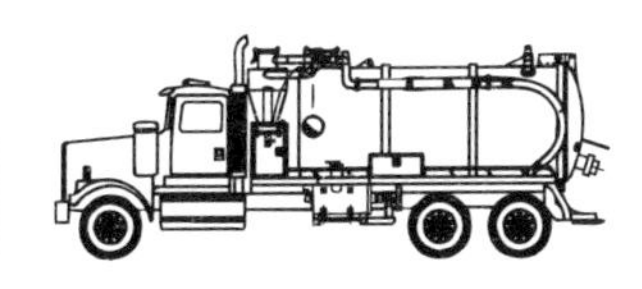

**CAUTION:** This chart depicts only the most general shapes of road trailers. Emergency response personnel must be aware that there are many variations of road trailers, not illustrated above, that are used for shipping chemical products. The suggested guides are for the most hazardous products that may be transported in these trailer types.

* **The recommended guides should be considered as last resort if the material cannot be identified by any other means.**

** **MAWP: Maximum Allowable Working Pressure.**

## GLOBALLY HARMONIZED SYSTEM OF CLASSIFICATION AND LABELING OF CHEMICALS (GHS)

**(May be found on means of containment during transport)**

The Globally Harmonized System of Classification and Labeling of Chemicals (GHS) is an international guideline published by the United Nations. The GHS aims to harmonize the classification and labeling systems for all sectors involved in the life cycle of a chemical (production, storage, transport, workplace use, consumer use and presence in the environment).

The GHS has nine symbols used to convey specific physical, health and environmental hazard information. These symbols are part of a pictogram that is diamond shaped and includes the GHS symbol in black on a white background with a red frame. The pictogram is part of the GHS label, which also includes the following information:

- **Signal word**
- **Hazard statement**
- **Precautionary statements**
- **Product identifier**
- **Supplier identification**

GHS pictograms are similar in shape to transport labels; however, transport labels have backgrounds of different colors.

The elements of the GHS that address signal words and hazard statements are not expected to be adopted in the transport sector. For substances and mixtures covered by the UN Recommendations on the Transport of Dangerous Goods, Model Regulations, the transport labels for physical hazards will have precedence. In transport, a GHS pictogram for the same (or lesser) hazard as the one reflected by the transport label or placard should not be present, but it could exist on the package.

**Examples of GHS labeling:**

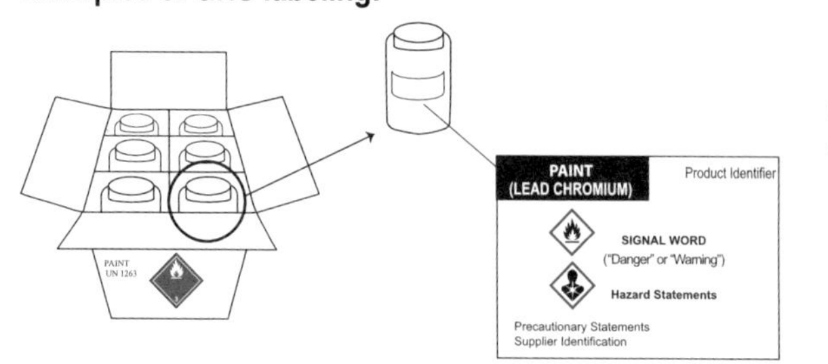




**Outer Packaging:** Box with flammable liquid transport label

**Inner Packaging:** Plastic bottle with GHS hazard warning label

**Single Packaging:** 200 L (55 US gallons) drum with a flammable liquid transport label combined with GHS hazard warning label

In some cases, such as on drums or international bulk containers (IBCs), which must address information for all sectors, the GHS label may be found in addition to the required transport labels and placards. Both types of labels (GHS and transport) will differ in a way that will make them easy to identify during an emergency.

| GHS Pictograms | Physical hazards | GHS Pictograms | Health and Environmental hazards |
|---|---|---|---|
| | Explosive;<br>Self-reactive;<br>Organic peroxide | | Skin corrosion;<br>Serious eye damage |
| | Flammable;<br>Pyrophoric;<br>Self-reactive;<br>Organic peroxide;<br>Self-heating;<br>Emits flammable gases when in contact with water | | Acute toxicity (harmful);<br>Skin sensitizer;<br>Irritant (skin and eye);<br>Narcotic effect;<br>Respiratory tract irritant;<br>Hazardous to ozone layer (environment) |
| | Oxidizer | | Respiratory sensitizer;<br>Mutagen;<br>Carcinogen;<br>Reproductive toxicity;<br>Target organ toxicity;<br>Aspiration hazard |
| | Gas under pressure | | Hazardous to aquatic environment |
| | Corrosive to metals | | Acute toxicity (fatal or toxic) |

## HAZARD IDENTIFICATION NUMBERS DISPLAYED ON SOME INTERMODAL CONTAINERS

Hazard identification numbers, utilized under European and some South American regulations, may be found in the top half of an orange panel on some intermodal bulk containers. The United Nations 4-digit identification number is in the bottom half of the orange panel.

The hazard identification number in the top half of the orange panel consists of two or three digits. In general, the digits indicate the following hazards:

- **2 -** Emission of gas due to pressure or chemical reaction
- **3 -** Flammability of liquids (vapors) and gases or self-heating liquid
- **4 -** Flammability of solids or self-heating solid
- **5 -** Oxidizing (fire-intensifying) effect
- **6 -** Toxicity or risk of infection
- **7 -** Radioactivity
- **8 -** Corrosivity
- **9 -** Risk of spontaneous violent reaction

**NOTE:** The risk of spontaneous violent reaction within the meaning of digit 9 includes the possibility, due to the nature of a substance, of a risk of explosion, disintegration and polymerization reaction followed by the release of considerable heat or flammable and/or toxic gases.

- Doubling of a digit indicates an intensification of that particular hazard (i.e., 33, 66, 88).
- Where the hazard associated with a substance can be adequately indicated by a single digit, the digit is followed by a zero (i.e., 30, 40, 50).
- A hazard identification number prefixed by the letter "X" indicates that the substance will react dangerously with water (i.e., X88).

## HAZARD IDENTIFICATION NUMBERS DISPLAYED ON SOME INTERMODAL CONTAINERS

The hazard identification numbers listed below have the following meanings:

| | |
|---|---|
| 20 | Asphyxiant gas or gas with no subsidiary risk |
| 22 | Refrigerated liquefied gas, asphyxiant |
| 223 | Refrigerated liquefied gas, flammable |
| 225 | Refrigerated liquefied gas, oxidizing (fire-intensifying) |
| 23 | Flammable gas |
| 238 | Gas, flammable corrosive |
| 239 | Flammable gas which can spontaneously lead to violent reaction |
| 25 | Oxidizing (fire-intensifying) gas |
| 26 | Toxic gas |
| 263 | Toxic gas, flammable |
| 265 | Toxic gas, oxidizing (fire-intensifying) |
| 268 | Toxic gas, corrosive |
| 28 | Gas, corrosive |
| 30 | Flammable liquid (flash-point between 23°C and 60°C, inclusive), or flammable liquid or solid in the molten state with a flash point above 60°C, heated to a temperature equal to or above its flash point, or self-heating liquid |
| 323 | Flammable liquid which reacts with water, emitting flammable gases |
| X323 | Flammable liquid which reacts dangerously with water, emitting flammable gases |
| 33 | Highly flammable liquid (flash-point below 23°C) |
| 333 | Pyrophoric liquid |
| X333 | Pyrophoric liquid which reacts dangerously with water |
| 336 | Highly flammable liquid, toxic |
| 338 | Highly flammable liquid, corrosive |
| X338 | Highly flammable liquid, corrosive, which reacts dangerously with water |
| 339 | Highly flammable liquid which can spontaneously lead to violent reaction |
| 36 | Flammable liquid (flash-point between 23°C and 60°C, inclusive), slightly toxic, or self-heating liquid, toxic |
| 362 | Flammable liquid, toxic, which reacts with water, emitting flammable gas |
| X362 | Flammable liquid, toxic, which reacts dangerously with water, emitting flammable gases |
| 368 | Flammable liquid, toxic, corrosive |
| 38 | Flammable liquid (flash-point between 23°C and 60°C, inclusive), slightly corrosive or self-heating liquid, corrosive |
| 382 | Flammable liquid, corrosive, which reacts with water, emitting flammable gases |
| X382 | Flammable liquid, corrosive, which reacts dangerously with water, emitting flammable gases |
| 39 | Flammable liquid, which can spontaneously lead to violent reaction |
| 40 | Flammable solid, or self-reactive substance, or self-heating substance |

| | |
|---|---|
| 423 | Solid which reacts with water, emitting flammable gases, or flammable solid which reacts with water, emitting flammable gases, or self-heating solid which reacts with water, emitting flammable gases |
| X423 | Solid which reacts dangerously with water, emitting flammable gases, or flammable solid which reacts dangerously with water, emitting flammable gases, or self-heating solid which reacts dangerously with water, emitting flammable gases |
| 43 | Spontaneously flammable (pyrophoric) solid |
| X432 | Spontaneously flammable (pyrophoric) solid which reacts dangerously with water, emitting flammable gases |
| 44 | Flammable solid, in the molten state at an elevated temperature |
| 446 | Flammable solid, toxic, in the molten state at an elevated temperature |
| 46 | Flammable or self-heating solid, toxic |
| 462 | Toxic solid which reacts with water, emitting flammable gases |
| X462 | Solid which reacts dangerously with water, emitting toxic gases |
| 48 | Flammable or self-heating solid, corrosive |
| 482 | Corrosive solid which reacts with water, emitting flammable gases |
| X482 | Solid which reacts dangerously with water, emitting corrosive gases |
| 50 | Oxidizing (fire-intensifying) substance |
| 539 | Flammable organic peroxide |
| 55 | Strongly oxidizing (fire-intensifying) substance |
| 556 | Strongly oxidizing (fire-intensifying) substance, toxic |
| 558 | Strongly oxidizing (fire-intensifying) substance, corrosive |
| 559 | Strongly oxidizing (fire-intensifying) substance which can spontaneously lead to violent reaction |
| 56 | Oxidizing substance (fire-intensifying), toxic |
| 568 | Oxidizing substance (fire-intensifying), toxic, corrosive |
| 58 | Oxidizing substance (fire-intensifying), corrosive |
| 59 | Oxidizing substance (fire-intensifying) which can spontaneously lead to violent reaction |
| 60 | Toxic or slightly toxic substance |
| 606 | Infectious substance |
| 623 | Toxic liquid, which reacts with water, emitting flammable gases |
| 63 | Toxic substance, flammable (flash-point between 23°C and 60°C, inclusive) |
| 638 | Toxic substance, flammable, (flash-point between 23°C and 60°C, inclusive), corrosive |
| 639 | Toxic substance, flammable, (flash-point not above 60°C) which can spontaneously lead to violent reaction |
| 64 | Toxic solid, flammable or self-heating |
| 642 | Toxic solid which reacts with water, emitting flammable gases |
| 65 | Toxic substance, oxidizing (fire-intensifying) |

## HAZARD IDENTIFICATION NUMBERS DISPLAYED ON SOME INTERMODAL CONTAINERS

| | |
|---|---|
| 66 | Highly toxic substance |
| 663 | Highly toxic substance, flammable (flash-point not above 60°C) |
| 664 | Highly toxic solid, flammable or self-heating |
| 665 | Highly toxic substance, oxidizing (fire-intensifying) |
| 668 | Highly toxic substance, corrosive |
| X668 | Highly toxic substance, corrosive, which reacts dangerously with water |
| 669 | Highly toxic substance which can spontaneously lead to violent reaction |
| 68 | Toxic substance, corrosive |
| 69 | Toxic or slightly toxic substance which can spontaneously lead to violent reaction |
| 70 | Radioactive material |
| 78 | Radioactive material, corrosive |
| 80 | Corrosive or slightly corrosive substance |
| X80 | Corrosive or slightly corrosive substance which reacts dangerously with water |
| 823 | Corrosive liquid which reacts with water, emitting flammable gases |
| 83 | Corrosive or slightly corrosive substance, flammable (flash-point between 23°C and 60°C, inclusive) |
| X83 | Corrosive or slightly corrosive substance, flammable (flash-point between 23°C and 60°C, inclusive), which reacts dangerously with water |
| 839 | Corrosive or slightly corrosive substance, flammable (flash-point between 23°C and 60°C, inclusive), which can spontaneously lead to violent reaction |
| X839 | Corrosive or slightly corrosive substance, flammable (flash-point between 23°C and 60°C, inclusive), which can spontaneously lead to violent reaction and which reacts dangerously with water |
| 84 | Corrosive solid, flammable or self-heating |
| 842 | Corrosive solid which reacts with water, emitting flammable gases |
| 85 | Corrosive or slightly corrosive substance, oxidizing (fire-intensifying) |
| 856 | Corrosive or slightly corrosive substance, oxidizing (fire-intensifying) and toxic |
| 86 | Corrosive or slightly corrosive substance, toxic |
| 88 | Highly corrosive substance |
| X88 | Highly corrosive substance which reacts dangerously with water |
| 883 | Highly corrosive substance, flammable (flash-point between 23°C and 60°C, inclusive) |
| 884 | Highly corrosive solid, flammable or self-heating |
| 885 | Highly corrosive substance, oxidizing (fire-intensifying) |
| 886 | Highly corrosive substance, toxic |
| X886 | Highly corrosive substance, toxic, which reacts dangerously with water |
| 89 | Corrosive or slightly corrosive substance which can spontaneously lead to violent reaction |
| 90 | Environmentally hazardous substance; miscellaneous dangerous substances |
| 99 | Miscellaneous dangerous substance carried at an elevated temperature |

# PIPELINE TRANSPORTATION

In North America, hazardous materials are commonly transported through millions of miles of pipelines and related structures. Products transported include natural gas, natural gas liquids, crude oil, gasoline, diesel fuel, anhydrous ammonia, carbon dioxide, jet fuel, and other commodities. Although most pipelines are buried, often there are above-ground structures and markers indicating the presence of pipelines. First responders should be aware of the pipelines in their jurisdictions, the products they transport, and the operators responsible for those pipelines. Proactive relationships can be beneficial in the safe and effective management of pipeline emergencies.

## Types of Pipelines

### Natural Gas Pipelines

#### Natural Gas Transmission Pipelines

Large-diameter, steel pipelines transport flammable natural gas (toxic and non-toxic) at very high pressures ranging from 200 to 1,500 psi*. Natural gas in transmission pipelines is odorless — generally *not odorized* with mercaptan (the "rotten egg" smell); however, natural gas containing hydrogen sulfide ($H_2S$) *will* have a distinct "rotten egg" odor.

#### Natural Gas Distribution Pipelines

Natural gas is delivered directly to customers via distribution pipelines. These pipelines are typically smaller-diameter, lower-pressure pipelines constructed of steel, plastic, or cast iron. Natural gas in distribution pipelines *is odorized* with mercaptan (the "rotten egg" smell).

#### Natural Gas-Gathering and Natural Gas Well Production Pipelines

Natural gas-gathering/well production pipelines collect "raw" natural gas from wellheads and transport the product to gas-processing and/or gas-treating plants. These gathering pipelines carry natural gas mixed with some quantity of gas liquids, water, and, in some areas, contaminants such as toxic hydrogen sulfide ($H_2S$). Natural gas in these pipelines is *not odorized* with mercaptan (the "rotten egg" smell); however, natural gas that contains hydrogen sulfide ($H_2S$) will have a distinct "rotten egg" odor.

### Liquid Petroleum and Hazardous Liquids Pipelines

#### Liquid Petroleum Pipelines

Crude oil, refined petroleum products, and hazardous liquids often are transported by pipelines and include gasoline, jet fuels, diesel fuel, home heating oils, carbon dioxide, anhydrous ammonia, and other hazardous liquids.

Many liquid petroleum pipelines transport different types of liquid petroleum in the same pipeline. To do so, the pipeline operator sends different products in "batches." For example, an operator could send gasoline for several hours, and then switch to jet fuels, before switching to diesel fuel.

* Data from http://naturalgas.org/naturalgas/transport/

### Other Hazardous Liquids Pipelines

Some liquid pipelines transport highly volatile liquids that rapidly change from liquid to gaseous when released from a pressurized pipeline. Examples of these types of liquids include carbon dioxide, anhydrous ammonia, propane, and others.

## <u>Pipeline Markers</u>

Since pipelines are usually buried underground, pipeline markers are used to indicate their presence in an area along the pipeline route. Of the three types of pipelines typically buried underground — distribution, gathering, and transmission — only transmission pipelines are marked with the following above-ground markers used to indicate their route.

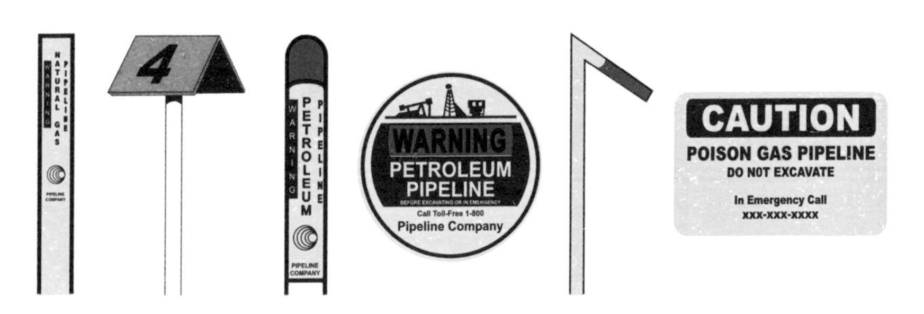


Markers warn that a transmission pipeline is located in the area, identify the product transported in the line, and provide the name and telephone number of the pipeline operator to call. Markers and warning signs are located at frequent intervals along natural gas and liquid transmission pipeline rights-of-way, and are located at prominent points such as where pipelines intersect streets, highways, railways, or waterways.

*Pipeline markers only indicate the presence of a pipeline—they do not indicate the exact location of the pipeline.* Pipeline locations within a right-of-way may vary along its length and there may be multiple pipelines located in the same right-of-way.

NOTE:

- Markers for pipelines transporting materials containing dangerous levels of hydrogen sulfide ($H_2S$) may have markers that say: "Sour" or "Poison."
- Natural gas distribution pipelines are not marked with above-ground signs.
- Gathering/production pipelines are often not marked with above-ground signs.

## Pipeline Structures (Above Ground)

| | |
|---|---|
| **Natural Gas Transmission Pipelines:** | Compressor stations, valves, metering stations. |
| **Natural Gas Distribution Pipelines:** | Regulator stations, customer meters and regulators, valve box covers. |
| **Natural Gas Gathering/Well Production Pipelines:** | Compressor stations, valves, metering stations, wellheads, piping, manifolds. |
| **Petroleum and Hazardous Liquids Pipelines:** | Storage tanks, valves, pump stations, loading racks. |

## Indications of Pipeline Leaks and Ruptures

Pipeline releases can range from relatively minor leaks to catastrophic ruptures. It is important to remember that gases and liquids behave differently once they are released from a pipeline. Generally, the following could be indications of a pipeline leak or rupture:

- Hissing, roaring, or explosive sound
- Flames appearing from the ground or water (perhaps very large flames)
- Vapor cloud/fog/mist
- Dirt/debris/water blowing out of the ground
- Liquids bubbling up from the ground or bubbling in water
- Distinctive, unusually strong odor of rotten eggs, skunk, or petroleum
- Discolored/dead vegetation or discolored snow above a pipeline right-of-way
- Oil slick or sheen on flowing/standing water

## General Considerations for Responding to a Pipeline Emergency

- **Safety First!** Your safety and the safety of the community you protect is top priority. Remember to approach a pipeline incident from upwind, uphill, and upstream while using air monitoring equipment to detect for the presence of explosive and/or toxic levels of hazardous materials.
  - **Always** wear proper personal protective equipment. Be prepared for a flash fire. Use shielding to protect first responders in the event of an explosion. Use respiratory protection.
  - **Never** operate pipeline valves (except in coordination with the pipeline operator); this could make the incident worse and put you and others in danger.
  - **Never** attempt to extinguish a pipeline fire before supply is shut off; this could result in the accumulation of a large flammable/explosive vapor cloud or liquid pool that could make the incident worse and put you and others in danger.
  - **Do not** enter a vapor cloud in an attempt to identify the product(s) involved.
- **Secure the site** and determine a plan to evacuate or shelter-in-place. Work with other responders to deny entry to an area.
- **Identify the product and the operator.** If safe to do so, you may be able to identify the product based on its characteristics or other external clues. Look for pipeline markers indicating the product, operator of the pipeline, and their emergency contact information. Pipelines transport many different types of products, including gases, liquids, and highly volatile liquids that are in a liquid state inside the pipeline but in a gaseous state if released from the pipeline. The vapor density of gases determines if they rise or sink in air. Viscosity and specific gravity also are important characteristics of hazardous liquids to consider. Identification of the product also will help you determine the appropriate distance for isolation of the affected area.
- **Notify the pipeline operator** using the emergency contact information on the pipeline marker or other contact information you may have received from the pipeline operator. The pipeline operator will be a resource to you in the response.
- **Establish a command post.** Implement the Incident Command Structure, as needed, and be prepared to implement a Unified Command as additional stakeholders and resources arrive.

## Other Important Considerations

- If no flames are present, do not introduce ignition sources such as open flames, running vehicles, or electrical equipment (cell phones, pagers, two-way radios, lights, garage door openers, fans, door bells, etc.).
- Abandon any equipment used in or near the area of the pipeline release.
- If there is no risk to your safety or the safety of others, move far enough away from any noise coming from the pipeline to allow for normal conversation.
- Pipelines often are close to other public utilities, railroads, and highways; these can be impacted by pipeline releases or may be potential ignition sources.
- Natural gas can migrate underground from the source of a release to other areas via the path of least resistance (including through sewers, water lines, and geologic formations).

## Considerations for Establishing Protective Action Distances

- Type of product
  - If you know the material involved, identify the three-digit guide number by looking up the name in the alphabetical list (blue-bordered pages), then using the three-digit guide number, consult the recommendations in the assigned guide.
- Pressure and diameter of pipe (the pipeline operator can tell you this if you don't already know it)
- Timing of valve closure by the pipeline operator (quickly for automated valves; longer for manually operated valves)
- Dissipation time of the product in the pipeline once valves are closed
- Ability to conduct atmospheric monitoring and/or air sampling
- Weather (wind direction, etc.)
- Local variables such as topography, population density, demographics, and fire suppression methods available
- Nearby building construction material/density
- Natural and man-made barriers (such as highways, railroads, rivers, etc.)

## U.S. Pipeline Resources

U.S. Pipeline Locations: The National Pipeline Mapping System (NPMS) *http://www.npms.phmsa.dot.gov* indicates the general locations of hazardous liquids and natural gas transmission pipelines found within the U.S. The pipelines depicted in the NPMS are within 500 feet of their actual locations. Emergency responders may apply for an NPMS web viewer account that will allow access to more detailed information than is available to the general public. The NPMS does not contain gathering/production or natural gas distribution pipelines.

U.S. Pipeline Emergency Response Training: Where appropriate, reference Pipeline Emergencies training materials, produced by PHMSA and the National Association of State Fire Marshals (NASFM). This training guide is available at *http://www.pipelineemergencies.com* and *http://nasfm-training.org/pipeline* and offers a thorough overview of U.S. pipeline operations and emergency response considerations. Your state or jurisdiction also may provide training on how to handle the response to a pipeline incident.

Other Resources:

Pipeline Association for Public Awareness *http://www.pipelineawareness.org/*

U.S. DOT, Pipeline and Hazardous Materials Safety Administration *http://phmsa.dot.gov/pipeline*

Pipeline 101 *http://pipeline101.com/*

## Canadian Pipeline Resources

Canadian Pipeline Locations: The Canadian Energy Pipeline Association (CEPA) provides the general locations of natural gas and liquid pipelines found within Canada.

http://www.cepa.com/library/maps

## GREEN HIGHLIGHTED ENTRIES IN YELLOW PAGES

For entries highlighted in green follow these steps:

- **IF THERE IS NO FIRE**:
  - Go directly to **Table 1** (green-bordered pages)
  - Look up the ID number and name of material
  - Identify initial isolation and protective action distances

- **IF A FIRE IS INVOLVED**:
  - Also consult the assigned orange guide
  - If applicable, apply the evacuation information shown under PUBLIC SAFETY

**Note 1:** If the name in **Table 1** is shown with ***"(when spilled in water)"***, these materials produce large amounts of Toxic Inhalation Hazard (TIH) (PIH in the US) gases when spilled in water. Some Water Reactive materials are also TIH materials themselves (e.g., Bromine trifluoride (UN1746), Thionyl chloride (UN1836), etc.). In these instances, two entries are provided in **Table 1** for land-based and water-based spills. If the Water Reactive material **is NOT** a TIH and this material **is NOT** spilled in water, **Table 1** and **Table 2 do NOT** apply and safety distances will be found within the appropriate orange guide.

**Note 2:** **Explosives** are not individually listed by their ID number because in an emergency situation, the response will be based only on the division of the explosive, not on the individual explosive.

**For divisions 1.1, 1.2, 1.3 and 1.5, refer to GUIDE 112.**

**For divisions 1.4 and 1.6, refer to GUIDE 114.**

| ID No. | Guide No. | Name of Material |
|---|---|---|
| —— | **112** | Ammonium nitrate-fuel oil mixtures |
| —— | **158** | Biological agents |
| —— | **112** | Blasting agent, n.o.s. |
| —— | **112** | Explosives, division 1.1, 1.2, 1.3 or 1.5 |
| —— | **114** | Explosives, division 1.4 or 1.6 |
| —— | **153** | Toxins |
| 1001 | **116** | Acetylene, dissolved |
| 1002 | **122** | Air, compressed |
| 1003 | **122** | Air, refrigerated liquid (cryogenic liquid) |
| 1003 | **122** | Air, refrigerated liquid (cryogenic liquid), non-pressurized |
| 1005 | **125** | Ammonia, anhydrous |
| 1005 | **125** | Anhydrous ammonia |
| 1006 | **121** | Argon |
| 1006 | **121** | Argon, compressed |
| 1008 | **125** | Boron trifluoride |
| 1008 | **125** | Boron trifluoride, compressed |
| 1009 | **126** | Bromotrifluoromethane |
| 1009 | **126** | Refrigerant gas R-13B1 |
| 1010 | **116P** | Butadienes, stabilized |
| 1010 | **116P** | Butadienes and hydrocarbon mixture, stabilized |
| 1010 | **116P** | Hydrocarbon and butadienes mixture, stabilized |
| 1011 | **115** | Butane |
| 1012 | **115** | Butylene |
| 1013 | **120** | Carbon dioxide |
| 1013 | **120** | Carbon dioxide, compressed |
| 1014 | **122** | Carbon dioxide and Oxygen mixture, compressed |
| 1014 | **122** | Oxygen and Carbon dioxide mixture, compressed |
| 1015 | **126** | Carbon dioxide and Nitrous oxide mixture |
| 1015 | **126** | Nitrous oxide and Carbon dioxide mixture |
| 1016 | **119** | Carbon monoxide |
| 1016 | **119** | Carbon monoxide, compressed |
| 1017 | **124** | Chlorine |
| 1018 | **126** | Chlorodifluoromethane |
| 1018 | **126** | Refrigerant gas R-22 |
| 1020 | **126** | Chloropentafluoroethane |
| 1020 | **126** | Refrigerant gas R-115 |
| 1021 | **126** | 1-Chloro-1,2,2,2-tetrafluoroethane |
| 1021 | **126** | Refrigerant gas R-124 |
| 1022 | **126** | Chlorotrifluoromethane |
| 1022 | **126** | Refrigerant gas R-13 |
| 1023 | **119** | Coal gas |
| 1023 | **119** | Coal gas, compressed |
| 1026 | **119** | Cyanogen |
| 1027 | **115** | Cyclopropane |
| 1028 | **126** | Dichlorodifluoromethane |
| 1028 | **126** | Refrigerant gas R-12 |
| 1029 | **126** | Dichlorofluoromethane |
| 1029 | **126** | Refrigerant gas R-21 |
| 1030 | **115** | 1,1-Difluoroethane |
| 1030 | **115** | Refrigerant gas R-152a |
| 1032 | **118** | Dimethylamine, anhydrous |
| 1033 | **115** | Dimethyl ether |
| 1035 | **115** | Ethane |
| 1035 | **115** | Ethane, compressed |
| 1036 | **118** | Ethylamine |

| ID No. | Guide No. | Name of Material |
|---|---|---|
| 1037 | **115** | Ethyl chloride |
| 1038 | **115** | Ethylene, refrigerated liquid (cryogenic liquid) |
| 1039 | **115** | Ethyl methyl ether |
| 1039 | **115** | Methyl ethyl ether |
| 1040 | **119P** | Ethylene oxide |
| 1040 | **119P** | Ethylene oxide with Nitrogen |
| 1041 | **115** | Carbon dioxide and Ethylene oxide mixture, with more than 9% but not more than 87% Ethylene oxide |
| 1041 | **115** | Ethylene oxide and Carbon dioxide mixture, with more than 9% but not more than 87% Ethylene oxide |
| 1043 | **125** | Fertilizer, ammoniating solution, with free Ammonia |
| 1044 | **126** | Fire extinguishers with compressed gas |
| 1044 | **126** | Fire extinguishers with liquefied gas |
| 1045 | **124** | Fluorine |
| 1045 | **124** | Fluorine, compressed |
| 1046 | **121** | Helium |
| 1046 | **121** | Helium, compressed |
| 1048 | **125** | Hydrogen bromide, anhydrous |
| 1049 | **115** | Hydrogen |
| 1049 | **115** | Hydrogen, compressed |
| 1050 | **125** | Hydrogen chloride, anhydrous |
| 1051 | **117** | AC |
| 1051 | **117** | Hydrocyanic acid, aqueous solutions, with more than 20% Hydrogen cyanide |
| 1051 | **117** | Hydrogen cyanide, anhydrous, stabilized |
| 1051 | **117** | Hydrogen cyanide, stabilized |
| 1052 | **125** | Hydrogen fluoride, anhydrous |
| 1053 | **117** | Hydrogen sulfide |
| 1053 | **117** | Hydrogen sulphide |
| 1055 | **115** | Isobutylene |
| 1056 | **121** | Krypton |
| 1056 | **121** | Krypton, compressed |
| 1057 | **115** | Lighter refills (cigarettes) (flammable gas) |
| 1057 | **115** | Lighters (cigarettes) (flammable gas) |
| 1057 | **128** | Lighters, non-pressurized, containing flammable liquid |
| 1058 | **120** | Liquefied gases, non-flammable, charged with Nitrogen, Carbon dioxide or Air |
| 1060 | **116P** | Methylacetylene and Propadiene mixture, stabilized |
| 1060 | **116P** | Propadiene and Methylacetylene mixture, stabilized |
| 1061 | **118** | Methylamine, anhydrous |
| 1062 | **123** | Methyl bromide |
| 1063 | **115** | Methyl chloride |
| 1063 | **115** | Refrigerant gas R-40 |
| 1064 | **117** | Methyl mercaptan |
| 1065 | **121** | Neon |
| 1065 | **121** | Neon, compressed |
| 1066 | **121** | Nitrogen |
| 1066 | **121** | Nitrogen, compressed |
| 1067 | **124** | Dinitrogen tetroxide |
| 1067 | **124** | Nitrogen dioxide |
| 1069 | **125** | Nitrosyl chloride |
| 1070 | **122** | Nitrous oxide |

| ID No. | Guide No. | Name of Material |
|---|---|---|
| 1070 | **122** | Nitrous oxide, compressed |
| 1071 | **119** | Oil gas |
| 1071 | **119** | Oil gas, compressed |
| 1072 | **122** | Oxygen |
| 1072 | **122** | Oxygen, compressed |
| 1073 | **122** | Oxygen, refrigerated liquid (cryogenic liquid) |
| 1075 | **115** | Butane |
| 1075 | **115** | Butylene |
| 1075 | **115** | Isobutane |
| 1075 | **115** | Isobutylene |
| 1075 | **115** | Liquefied petroleum gas |
| 1075 | **115** | LPG |
| 1075 | **115** | Petroleum gases, liquefied |
| 1075 | **115** | Propane |
| 1075 | **115** | Propylene |
| 1076 | **125** | CG |
| 1076 | **125** | DP |
| 1076 | **125** | Phosgene |
| 1077 | **115** | Propylene |
| 1078 | **126** | Dispersant gas, n.o.s. |
| 1078 | **126** | Refrigerant gas, n.o.s. |
| 1079 | **125** | Sulfur dioxide |
| 1079 | **125** | Sulphur dioxide |
| 1080 | **126** | Sulfur hexafluoride |
| 1080 | **126** | Sulphur hexafluoride |
| 1081 | **116P** | Tetrafluoroethylene, stabilized |
| 1082 | **119P** | Refrigerant gas R-1113 |
| 1082 | **119P** | Trifluorochloroethylene, stabilized |
| 1083 | **118** | Trimethylamine, anhydrous |
| 1085 | **116P** | Vinyl bromide, stabilized |
| 1086 | **116P** | Vinyl chloride, stabilized |
| 1087 | **116P** | Vinyl methyl ether, stabilized |
| 1088 | **127** | Acetal |
| 1089 | **129P** | Acetaldehyde |
| 1090 | **127** | Acetone |
| 1091 | **127** | Acetone oils |
| 1092 | **131P** | Acrolein, stabilized |
| 1093 | **131P** | Acrylonitrile, stabilized |
| 1098 | **131** | Allyl alcohol |
| 1099 | **131** | Allyl bromide |
| 1100 | **131** | Allyl chloride |
| 1104 | **129** | Amyl acetates |
| 1105 | **129** | Pentanols |
| 1106 | **132** | Amylamine |
| 1107 | **129** | Amyl chloride |
| 1108 | **128** | n-Amylene |
| 1108 | **128** | 1-Pentene |
| 1109 | **129** | Amyl formates |
| 1110 | **127** | n-Amyl methyl ketone |
| 1110 | **127** | Methyl amyl ketone |
| 1111 | **130** | Amyl mercaptan |
| 1112 | **140** | Amyl nitrate |
| 1113 | **129** | Amyl nitrite |
| 1114 | **130** | Benzene |
| 1120 | **129** | Butanols |
| 1123 | **129** | Butyl acetates |
| 1125 | **132** | n-Butylamine |
| 1126 | **130** | 1-Bromobutane |
| 1126 | **130** | n-Butyl bromide |
| 1127 | **130** | n-Butyl chloride |
| 1127 | **130** | Chlorobutanes |

| ID No. | Guide No. | Name of Material |
|---|---|---|
| 1128 | **129** | n-Butyl formate |
| 1129 | **129** | Butyraldehyde |
| 1130 | **128** | Camphor oil |
| 1131 | **131** | Carbon bisulfide |
| 1131 | **131** | Carbon bisulphide |
| 1131 | **131** | Carbon disulfide |
| 1131 | **131** | Carbon disulphide |
| 1133 | **128** | Adhesives (flammable) |
| 1134 | **130** | Chlorobenzene |
| 1135 | **131** | Ethylene chlorohydrin |
| 1136 | **128** | Coal tar distillates, flammable |
| 1139 | **127** | Coating solution |
| 1143 | **131P** | Crotonaldehyde |
| 1143 | **131P** | Crotonaldehyde, stabilized |
| 1144 | **128** | Crotonylene |
| 1145 | **128** | Cyclohexane |
| 1146 | **128** | Cyclopentane |
| 1147 | **130** | Decahydronaphthalene |
| 1148 | **129** | Diacetone alcohol |
| 1149 | **128** | Butyl ethers |
| 1149 | **128** | Dibutyl ethers |
| 1150 | **130P** | 1,2-Dichloroethylene |
| 1152 | **130** | Dichloropentanes |
| 1153 | **127** | Ethylene glycol diethyl ether |
| 1154 | **132** | Diethylamine |
| 1155 | **127** | Diethyl ether |
| 1155 | **127** | Ethyl ether |
| 1156 | **127** | Diethyl ketone |
| 1157 | **128** | Diisobutyl ketone |
| 1158 | **132** | Diisopropylamine |
| 1159 | **127** | Diisopropyl ether |
| 1160 | **132** | Dimethylamine, aqueous solution |
| 1160 | **132** | Dimethylamine, solution |
| 1161 | **129** | Dimethyl carbonate |
| 1162 | **155** | Dimethyldichlorosilane |
| 1163 | **131** | 1,1-Dimethylhydrazine |
| 1163 | **131** | Dimethylhydrazine, unsymmetrical |
| 1164 | **130** | Dimethyl sulfide |
| 1164 | **130** | Dimethyl sulphide |
| 1165 | **127** | Dioxane |
| 1166 | **127** | Dioxolane |
| 1167 | **128P** | Divinyl ether, stabilized |
| 1169 | **127** | Extracts, aromatic, liquid |
| 1170 | **127** | Ethanol |
| 1170 | **127** | Ethanol, solution |
| 1170 | **127** | Ethyl alcohol |
| 1170 | **127** | Ethyl alcohol, solution |
| 1171 | **127** | Ethylene glycol monoethyl ether |
| 1172 | **129** | Ethylene glycol monoethyl ether acetate |
| 1173 | **129** | Ethyl acetate |
| 1175 | **130** | Ethylbenzene |
| 1176 | **129** | Ethyl borate |
| 1177 | **130** | 2-Ethylbutyl acetate |
| 1177 | **130** | Ethylbutyl acetate |
| 1178 | **130** | 2-Ethylbutyraldehyde |
| 1179 | **127** | Ethyl butyl ether |
| 1180 | **130** | Ethyl butyrate |
| 1181 | **155** | Ethyl chloroacetate |
| 1182 | **155** | Ethyl chloroformate |
| 1183 | **139** | Ethyldichlorosilane |

| ID No. | Guide No. | Name of Material |
|---|---|---|
| 1184 | **131** | Ethylene dichloride |
| 1185 | **131P** | Ethyleneimine, stabilized |
| 1188 | **127** | Ethylene glycol monomethyl ether |
| 1189 | **129** | Ethylene glycol monomethyl ether acetate |
| 1190 | **129** | Ethyl formate |
| 1191 | **129** | Ethylhexaldehydes |
| 1191 | **129** | Octyl aldehydes |
| 1192 | **129** | Ethyl lactate |
| 1193 | **127** | Ethyl methyl ketone |
| 1193 | **127** | Methyl ethyl ketone |
| 1194 | **131** | Ethyl nitrite, solution |
| 1195 | **129** | Ethyl propionate |
| 1196 | **155** | Ethyltrichlorosilane |
| 1197 | **127** | Extracts, flavoring, liquid |
| 1197 | **127** | Extracts, flavouring, liquid |
| 1198 | **132** | Formaldehyde, solution, flammable |
| 1198 | **132** | Formalin (flammable) |
| 1199 | **132P** | Furaldehydes |
| 1199 | **132P** | Furfural |
| 1199 | **132P** | Furfuraldehydes |
| 1201 | **127** | Fusel oil |
| 1202 | **128** | Diesel fuel |
| 1202 | **128** | Fuel oil |
| 1202 | **128** | Gas oil |
| 1202 | **128** | Heating oil, light |
| 1203 | **128** | Gasohol |
| 1203 | **128** | Gasoline |
| 1203 | **128** | Motor spirit |
| 1203 | **128** | Petrol |
| 1204 | **127** | Nitroglycerin, solution in alcohol, with not more than 1% Nitroglycerin |
| 1206 | **128** | Heptanes |
| 1207 | **130** | Hexaldehyde |
| 1208 | **128** | Hexanes |
| 1208 | **128** | Neohexane |
| 1210 | **129** | Ink, printer's, flammable |
| 1210 | **129** | Printing ink, flammable |
| 1210 | **129** | Printing ink related material |
| 1212 | **129** | Isobutanol |
| 1212 | **129** | Isobutyl alcohol |
| 1213 | **129** | Isobutyl acetate |
| 1214 | **132** | Isobutylamine |
| 1216 | **128** | Isooctenes |
| 1218 | **130P** | Isoprene, stabilized |
| 1219 | **129** | Isopropanol |
| 1219 | **129** | Isopropyl alcohol |
| 1220 | **129** | Isopropyl acetate |
| 1221 | **132** | Isopropylamine |
| 1222 | **130** | Isopropyl nitrate |
| 1223 | **128** | Kerosene |
| 1224 | **127** | Ketones, liquid, n.o.s. |
| 1228 | **131** | Mercaptan mixture, liquid, flammable, poisonous, n.o.s. |
| 1228 | **131** | Mercaptan mixture, liquid, flammable, toxic, n.o.s. |
| 1228 | **131** | Mercaptans, liquid, flammable, poisonous, n.o.s. |
| 1228 | **131** | Mercaptans, liquid, flammable, toxic, n.o.s. |
| 1229 | **129** | Mesityl oxide |
| 1230 | **131** | Methanol |
| 1230 | **131** | Methyl alcohol |

| ID No. | Guide No. | Name of Material |
|---|---|---|
| 1231 | **129** | Methyl acetate |
| 1233 | **130** | Methylamyl acetate |
| 1234 | **127** | Methylal |
| 1235 | **132** | Methylamine, aqueous solution |
| 1237 | **129** | Methyl butyrate |
| 1238 | **155** | Methyl chloroformate |
| 1239 | **131** | Methyl chloromethyl ether |
| 1242 | **139** | Methyldichlorosilane |
| 1243 | **129** | Methyl formate |
| 1244 | **131** | Methylhydrazine |
| 1245 | **127** | Methyl isobutyl ketone |
| 1246 | **127P** | Methyl isopropenyl ketone, stabilized |
| 1247 | **129P** | Methyl methacrylate monomer, stabilized |
| 1248 | **129** | Methyl propionate |
| 1249 | **127** | Methyl propyl ketone |
| 1250 | **155** | Methyltrichlorosilane |
| 1251 | **131P** | Methyl vinyl ketone, stabilized |
| 1259 | **131** | Nickel carbonyl |
| 1261 | **129** | Nitromethane |
| 1262 | **128** | Isooctane |
| 1262 | **128** | Octanes |
| 1263 | **128** | Paint (flammable) |
| 1263 | **128** | Paint related material (flammable) |
| 1264 | **129** | Paraldehyde |
| 1265 | **128** | Isopentane |
| 1265 | **128** | Pentanes |
| 1266 | **127** | Perfumery products, with flammable solvents |
| 1267 | **128** | Petroleum crude oil |
| 1268 | **128** | Petroleum distillates, n.o.s. |
| 1268 | **128** | Petroleum products, n.o.s. |
| 1270 | **128** | Oil, petroleum |
| 1270 | **128** | Petroleum oil |
| 1272 | **129** | Pine oil |
| 1274 | **129** | n-Propanol |
| 1274 | **129** | Propyl alcohol, normal |
| 1275 | **129** | Propionaldehyde |
| 1276 | **129** | n-Propyl acetate |
| 1277 | **132** | Propylamine |
| 1278 | **129** | 1-Chloropropane |
| 1278 | **129** | Propyl chloride |
| 1279 | **130** | 1,2-Dichloropropane |
| 1280 | **127P** | Propylene oxide |
| 1281 | **129** | Propyl formates |
| 1282 | **129** | Pyridine |
| 1286 | **127** | Rosin oil |
| 1287 | **127** | Rubber solution |
| 1288 | **128** | Shale oil |
| 1289 | **132** | Sodium methylate, solution in alcohol |
| 1292 | **129** | Ethyl silicate |
| 1292 | **129** | Tetraethyl silicate |
| 1293 | **127** | Tinctures, medicinal |
| 1294 | **130** | Toluene |
| 1295 | **139** | Trichlorosilane |
| 1296 | **132** | Triethylamine |
| 1297 | **132** | Trimethylamine, aqueous solution |
| 1298 | **155** | Trimethylchlorosilane |
| 1299 | **128** | Turpentine |
| 1300 | **128** | Turpentine substitute |
| 1301 | **129P** | Vinyl acetate, stabilized |

| ID No. | Guide No. | Name of Material |
|---|---|---|
| 1302 | **127P** | Vinyl ethyl ether, stabilized |
| 1303 | **130P** | Vinylidene chloride, stabilized |
| 1304 | **127P** | Vinyl isobutyl ether, stabilized |
| 1305 | **155P** | Vinyltrichlorosilane |
| 1305 | **155P** | Vinyltrichlorosilane, stabilized |
| 1306 | **129** | Wood preservatives, liquid |
| 1307 | **130** | Xylenes |
| 1308 | **170** | Zirconium suspended in a flammable liquid |
| 1308 | **170** | Zirconium suspended in a liquid (flammable) |
| 1309 | **170** | Aluminum powder, coated |
| 1310 | **113** | Ammonium picrate, wetted with not less than 10% water |
| 1312 | **133** | Borneol |
| 1313 | **133** | Calcium resinate |
| 1314 | **133** | Calcium resinate, fused |
| 1318 | **133** | Cobalt resinate, precipitated |
| 1320 | **113** | Dinitrophenol, wetted with not less than 15% water |
| 1321 | **113** | Dinitrophenolates, wetted with not less than 15% water |
| 1322 | **113** | Dinitroresorcinol, wetted with not less than 15% water |
| 1323 | **170** | Ferrocerium |
| 1324 | **133** | Films, nitrocellulose base |
| 1325 | **133** | Flammable solid, organic, n.o.s. |
| 1325 | **133** | Fusee (rail or highway) |
| 1326 | **170** | Hafnium powder, wetted with not less than 25% water |
| 1327 | **133** | Bhusa, wet, damp or contaminated with oil |
| 1327 | **133** | Hay, wet, damp or contaminated with oil |
| 1327 | **133** | Straw, wet, damp or contaminated with oil |
| 1328 | **133** | Hexamethylenetetramine |
| 1330 | **133** | Manganese resinate |
| 1331 | **133** | Matches, "strike anywhere" |
| 1332 | **133** | Metaldehyde |
| 1333 | **170** | Cerium, slabs, ingots or rods |
| 1334 | **133** | Naphthalene, crude |
| 1334 | **133** | Naphthalene, refined |
| 1336 | **113** | Nitroguanidine, wetted with not less than 20% water |
| 1336 | **113** | Picrite, wetted with not less than 20% water |
| 1337 | **113** | Nitrostarch, wetted with not less than 20% water |
| 1338 | **133** | Phosphorus, amorphous |
| 1338 | **133** | Red phosphorus |
| 1339 | **139** | Phosphorus heptasulfide, free from yellow and white Phosphorus |
| 1339 | **139** | Phosphorus heptasulphide, free from yellow and white Phosphorus |
| 1340 | **139** | Phosphorus pentasulfide, free from yellow and white Phosphorus |
| 1340 | **139** | Phosphorus pentasulphide, free from yellow and white Phosphorus |
| 1341 | **139** | Phosphorus sesquisulfide, free from yellow and white Phosphorus |
| 1341 | **139** | Phosphorus sesquisulphide, free from yellow and white Phosphorus |
| 1343 | **139** | Phosphorus trisulfide, free from yellow and white Phosphorus |

| ID No. | Guide No. | Name of Material |
|---|---|---|
| 1343 | **139** | Phosphorus trisulphide, free from yellow and white Phosphorus |
| 1344 | **113** | Picric acid, wetted with not less than 30% water |
| 1344 | **113** | Trinitrophenol, wetted with not less than 30% water |
| 1345 | **133** | Rubber scrap, powdered or granulated |
| 1345 | **133** | Rubber shoddy, powdered or granulated |
| 1346 | **170** | Silicon powder, amorphous |
| 1347 | **113** | Silver picrate, wetted with not less than 30% water |
| 1348 | **113** | Sodium dinitro-o-cresolate, wetted with not less than 15% water |
| 1349 | **113** | Sodium picramate, wetted with not less than 20% water |
| 1350 | **133** | Sulfur |
| 1350 | **133** | Sulphur |
| 1352 | **170** | Titanium powder, wetted with not less than 25% water |
| 1353 | **133** | Fabrics impregnated with weakly nitrated Nitrocellulose, n.o.s. |
| 1353 | **133** | Fibers impregnated with weakly nitrated Nitrocellulose, n.o.s. |
| 1353 | **133** | Fibres impregnated with weakly nitrated Nitrocellulose, n.o.s. |
| 1354 | **113** | Trinitrobenzene, wetted with not less than 30% water |
| 1355 | **113** | Trinitrobenzoic acid, wetted with not less than 30% water |
| 1356 | **113** | TNT, wetted with not less than 30% water |
| 1356 | **113** | Trinitrotoluene, wetted with not less than 30% water |

| ID No. | Guide No. | Name of Material |
|---|---|---|
| 1357 | **113** | Urea nitrate, wetted with not less than 20% water |
| 1358 | **170** | Zirconium powder, wetted with not less than 25% water |
| 1360 | **139** | Calcium phosphide |
| 1361 | **133** | Carbon, animal or vegetable origin |
| 1361 | **133** | Charcoal |
| 1362 | **133** | Carbon, activated |
| 1363 | **135** | Copra |
| 1364 | **133** | Cotton waste, oily |
| 1365 | **133** | Cotton |
| 1365 | **133** | Cotton, wet |
| 1366 | **135** | Diethylzinc |
| 1369 | **135** | p-Nitrosodimethylaniline |
| 1370 | **135** | Dimethylzinc |
| 1372 | **133** | Fibers, animal or vegetable, burnt, wet or damp |
| 1372 | **133** | Fibres, animal or vegetable, burnt, wet or damp |
| 1373 | **133** | Fabrics, animal or vegetable or synthetic, n.o.s. with oil |
| 1373 | **133** | Fibers, animal or vegetable or synthetic, n.o.s. with oil |
| 1373 | **133** | Fibres, animal or vegetable or synthetic, n.o.s. with oil |
| 1374 | **133** | Fish meal, unstabilized |
| 1374 | **133** | Fish scrap, unstabilized |
| 1376 | **135** | Iron oxide, spent |
| 1376 | **135** | Iron sponge, spent |
| 1378 | **170** | Metal catalyst, wetted |
| 1379 | **133** | Paper, unsaturated oil treated |
| 1380 | **135** | Pentaborane |
| 1381 | **136** | Phosphorus, white, dry or under water or in solution |

| ID No. | Guide No. | Name of Material |
|---|---|---|
| 1381 | **136** | Phosphorus, yellow, dry or under water or in solution |
| 1381 | **136** | White phosphorus, dry |
| 1381 | **136** | White phosphorus, in solution |
| 1381 | **136** | White phosphorus, under water |
| 1381 | **136** | Yellow phosphorus, dry |
| 1381 | **136** | Yellow phosphorus, in solution |
| 1381 | **136** | Yellow phosphorus, under water |
| 1382 | **135** | Potassium sulfide, anhydrous |
| 1382 | **135** | Potassium sulfide, with less than 30% water of crystallization |
| 1382 | **135** | Potassium sulphide, anhydrous |
| 1382 | **135** | Potassium sulphide, with less than 30% water of crystallization |
| 1383 | **135** | Aluminum powder, pyrophoric |
| 1383 | **135** | Pyrophoric alloy, n.o.s. |
| 1383 | **135** | Pyrophoric metal, n.o.s. |
| 1384 | **135** | Sodium dithionite |
| 1384 | **135** | Sodium hydrosulfite |
| 1384 | **135** | Sodium hydrosulphite |
| 1385 | **135** | Sodium sulfide, anhydrous |
| 1385 | **135** | Sodium sulfide, with less than 30% water of crystallization |
| 1385 | **135** | Sodium sulphide, anhydrous |
| 1385 | **135** | Sodium sulphide, with less than 30% water of crystallization |
| 1386 | **135** | Seed cake, with more than 1.5% oil and not more than 11% moisture |
| 1387 | **133** | Wool waste, wet |
| 1389 | **138** | Alkali metal amalgam |
| 1389 | **138** | Alkali metal amalgam, liquid |
| 1390 | **139** | Alkali metal amides |
| 1391 | **138** | Alkali metal dispersion |
| 1391 | **138** | Alkaline earth metal dispersion |
| 1392 | **138** | Alkaline earth metal amalgam |
| 1392 | **138** | Alkaline earth metal amalgam, liquid |
| 1393 | **138** | Alkaline earth metal alloy, n.o.s. |
| 1394 | **138** | Aluminum carbide |
| 1395 | **139** | Aluminum ferrosilicon powder |
| 1396 | **138** | Aluminum powder, uncoated |
| 1397 | **139** | Aluminum phosphide |
| 1398 | **138** | Aluminum silicon powder, uncoated |
| 1400 | **138** | Barium |
| 1401 | **138** | Calcium |
| 1402 | **138** | Calcium carbide |
| 1403 | **138** | Calcium cyanamide, with more than 0.1% Calcium carbide |
| 1404 | **138** | Calcium hydride |
| 1405 | **138** | Calcium silicide |
| 1407 | **138** | Caesium |
| 1407 | **138** | Cesium |
| 1408 | **139** | Ferrosilicon |
| 1409 | **138** | Metal hydrides, water-reactive, n.o.s. |
| 1410 | **138** | Lithium aluminum hydride |
| 1411 | **138** | Lithium aluminum hydride, ethereal |
| 1413 | **138** | Lithium borohydride |
| 1414 | **138** | Lithium hydride |
| 1415 | **138** | Lithium |
| 1417 | **138** | Lithium silicon |
| 1418 | **138** | Magnesium alloys powder |
| 1418 | **138** | Magnesium powder |

| ID No. | Guide No. | Name of Material |
|---|---|---|
| 1419 | **139** | Magnesium aluminum phosphide |
| 1420 | **138** | Potassium, metal alloys |
| 1420 | **138** | Potassium, metal alloys, liquid |
| 1421 | **138** | Alkali metal alloy, liquid, n.o.s. |
| 1422 | **138** | Potassium sodium alloys |
| 1422 | **138** | Potassium sodium alloys, liquid |
| 1422 | **138** | Sodium potassium alloys |
| 1422 | **138** | Sodium potassium alloys, liquid |
| 1423 | **138** | Rubidium |
| 1423 | **138** | Rubidium metal |
| 1426 | **138** | Sodium borohydride |
| 1427 | **138** | Sodium hydride |
| 1428 | **138** | Sodium |
| 1431 | **138** | Sodium methylate |
| 1431 | **138** | Sodium methylate, dry |
| 1432 | **139** | Sodium phosphide |
| 1433 | **139** | Stannic phosphides |
| 1435 | **138** | Zinc ashes |
| 1435 | **138** | Zinc dross |
| 1435 | **138** | Zinc residue |
| 1435 | **138** | Zinc skimmings |
| 1436 | **138** | Zinc dust |
| 1436 | **138** | Zinc powder |
| 1437 | **138** | Zirconium hydride |
| 1438 | **140** | Aluminum nitrate |
| 1439 | **141** | Ammonium dichromate |
| 1442 | **143** | Ammonium perchlorate |
| 1444 | **140** | Ammonium persulfate |
| 1444 | **140** | Ammonium persulphate |
| 1445 | **141** | Barium chlorate |
| 1445 | **141** | Barium chlorate, solid |
| 1446 | **141** | Barium nitrate |
| 1447 | **141** | Barium perchlorate |
| 1447 | **141** | Barium perchlorate, solid |
| 1448 | **141** | Barium permanganate |
| 1449 | **141** | Barium peroxide |
| 1450 | **141** | Bromates, inorganic, n.o.s. |
| 1451 | **140** | Caesium nitrate |
| 1451 | **140** | Cesium nitrate |
| 1452 | **140** | Calcium chlorate |
| 1453 | **140** | Calcium chlorite |
| 1454 | **140** | Calcium nitrate |
| 1455 | **140** | Calcium perchlorate |
| 1456 | **140** | Calcium permanganate |
| 1457 | **140** | Calcium peroxide |
| 1458 | **140** | Borate and Chlorate mixture |
| 1458 | **140** | Chlorate and Borate mixture |
| 1459 | **140** | Chlorate and Magnesium chloride mixture |
| 1459 | **140** | Chlorate and Magnesium chloride mixture, solid |
| 1459 | **140** | Magnesium chloride and Chlorate mixture |
| 1459 | **140** | Magnesium chloride and Chlorate mixture, solid |
| 1461 | **140** | Chlorates, inorganic, n.o.s. |
| 1462 | **143** | Chlorites, inorganic, n.o.s. |
| 1463 | **141** | Chromium trioxide, anhydrous |
| 1465 | **140** | Didymium nitrate |
| 1466 | **140** | Ferric nitrate |
| 1467 | **143** | Guanidine nitrate |
| 1469 | **141** | Lead nitrate |
| 1470 | **141** | Lead perchlorate |

| ID No. | Guide No. | Name of Material |
|---|---|---|
| 1470 | **141** | Lead perchlorate, solid |
| 1471 | **140** | Lithium hypochlorite, dry |
| 1471 | **140** | Lithium hypochlorite mixture |
| 1471 | **140** | Lithium hypochlorite mixtures, dry |
| 1472 | **143** | Lithium peroxide |
| 1473 | **140** | Magnesium bromate |
| 1474 | **140** | Magnesium nitrate |
| 1475 | **140** | Magnesium perchlorate |
| 1476 | **140** | Magnesium peroxide |
| 1477 | **140** | Nitrates, inorganic, n.o.s. |
| 1479 | **140** | Oxidizing solid, n.o.s. |
| 1481 | **140** | Perchlorates, inorganic, n.o.s. |
| 1482 | **140** | Permanganates, inorganic, n.o.s. |
| 1483 | **140** | Peroxides, inorganic, n.o.s. |
| 1484 | **140** | Potassium bromate |
| 1485 | **140** | Potassium chlorate |
| 1486 | **140** | Potassium nitrate |
| 1487 | **140** | Potassium nitrate and Sodium nitrite mixture |
| 1487 | **140** | Sodium nitrite and Potassium nitrate mixture |
| 1488 | **140** | Potassium nitrite |
| 1489 | **140** | Potassium perchlorate |
| 1490 | **140** | Potassium permanganate |
| 1491 | **144** | Potassium peroxide |
| 1492 | **140** | Potassium persulfate |
| 1492 | **140** | Potassium persulphate |
| 1493 | **140** | Silver nitrate |
| 1494 | **141** | Sodium bromate |
| 1495 | **140** | Sodium chlorate |
| 1496 | **143** | Sodium chlorite |
| 1498 | **140** | Sodium nitrate |
| 1499 | **140** | Potassium nitrate and Sodium nitrate mixture |
| 1499 | **140** | Sodium nitrate and Potassium nitrate mixture |
| 1500 | **140** | Sodium nitrite |
| 1502 | **140** | Sodium perchlorate |
| 1503 | **140** | Sodium permanganate |
| 1504 | **144** | Sodium peroxide |
| 1505 | **140** | Sodium persulfate |
| 1505 | **140** | Sodium persulphate |
| 1506 | **143** | Strontium chlorate |
| 1507 | **140** | Strontium nitrate |
| 1508 | **140** | Strontium perchlorate |
| 1509 | **143** | Strontium peroxide |
| 1510 | **143** | Tetranitromethane |
| 1511 | **140** | Urea hydrogen peroxide |
| 1512 | **140** | Zinc ammonium nitrite |
| 1513 | **140** | Zinc chlorate |
| 1514 | **140** | Zinc nitrate |
| 1515 | **140** | Zinc permanganate |
| 1516 | **143** | Zinc peroxide |
| 1517 | **113** | Zirconium picramate, wetted with not less than 20% water |
| 1541 | **155** | Acetone cyanohydrin, stabilized |
| 1544 | **151** | Alkaloids, solid, n.o.s. (poisonous) |
| 1544 | **151** | Alkaloid salts, solid, n.o.s. (poisonous) |
| 1545 | **155** | Allyl isothiocyanate, stabilized |
| 1546 | **151** | Ammonium arsenate |
| 1547 | **153** | Aniline |
| 1548 | **153** | Aniline hydrochloride |

| ID No. | Guide No. | Name of Material |
|---|---|---|
| 1549 | **157** | Antimony compound, inorganic, solid, n.o.s. |
| 1550 | **151** | Antimony lactate |
| 1551 | **151** | Antimony potassium tartrate |
| 1553 | **154** | Arsenic acid, liquid |
| 1554 | **154** | Arsenic acid, solid |
| 1555 | **151** | Arsenic bromide |
| 1556 | **152** | Arsenic compound, liquid, n.o.s. |
| 1556 | **152** | Arsenic compound, liquid, n.o.s., inorganic |
| 1556 | **152** | MD |
| 1556 | **152** | Methyldichloroarsine |
| 1556 | **152** | PD |
| 1557 | **152** | Arsenic compound, solid, n.o.s. |
| 1557 | **152** | Arsenic compound, solid, n.o.s., inorganic |
| 1558 | **152** | Arsenic |
| 1559 | **151** | Arsenic pentoxide |
| 1560 | **157** | Arsenic chloride |
| 1560 | **157** | Arsenic trichloride |
| 1561 | **151** | Arsenic trioxide |
| 1562 | **152** | Arsenical dust |
| 1564 | **154** | Barium compound, n.o.s. |
| 1565 | **157** | Barium cyanide |
| 1566 | **154** | Beryllium compound, n.o.s. |
| 1567 | **134** | Beryllium powder |
| 1569 | **131** | Bromoacetone |
| 1570 | **152** | Brucine |
| 1571 | **113** | Barium azide, wetted with not less than 50% water |
| 1572 | **151** | Cacodylic acid |
| 1573 | **151** | Calcium arsenate |
| 1574 | **151** | Calcium arsenate and Calcium arsenite mixture, solid |
| 1574 | **151** | Calcium arsenite and Calcium arsenate mixture, solid |
| 1575 | **157** | Calcium cyanide |
| 1577 | **153** | Chlorodinitrobenzenes, liquid |
| 1577 | **153** | Chlorodinitrobenzenes, solid |
| 1577 | **153** | Dinitrochlorobenzenes |
| 1578 | **152** | Chloronitrobenzenes |
| 1578 | **152** | Chloronitrobenzenes, solid |
| 1579 | **153** | 4-Chloro-o-toluidine hydrochloride |
| 1579 | **153** | 4-Chloro-o-toluidine hydrochloride, solid |
| 1580 | **154** | Chloropicrin |
| 1581 | **123** | Chloropicrin and Methyl bromide mixture |
| 1581 | **123** | Methyl bromide and Chloropicrin mixture |
| 1582 | **119** | Chloropicrin and Methyl chloride mixture |
| 1582 | **119** | Methyl chloride and Chloropicrin mixture |
| 1583 | **154** | Chloropicrin mixture, n.o.s. |
| 1585 | **151** | Copper acetoarsenite |
| 1586 | **151** | Copper arsenite |
| 1587 | **151** | Copper cyanide |
| 1588 | **157** | Cyanides, inorganic, solid, n.o.s. |
| 1589 | **125** | CK |
| 1589 | **125** | Cyanogen chloride, stabilized |
| 1590 | **153** | Dichloroanilines, liquid |
| 1590 | **153** | Dichloroanilines, solid |
| 1591 | **152** | o-Dichlorobenzene |
| 1593 | **160** | Dichloromethane |

| ID No. | Guide No. | Name of Material |
|---|---|---|
| 1593 | **160** | Methylene chloride |
| 1594 | **152** | Diethyl sulfate |
| 1594 | **152** | Diethyl sulphate |
| 1595 | **156** | Dimethyl sulfate |
| 1595 | **156** | Dimethyl sulphate |
| 1596 | **153** | Dinitroanilines |
| 1597 | **152** | Dinitrobenzenes, liquid |
| 1597 | **152** | Dinitrobenzenes, solid |
| 1598 | **153** | Dinitro-o-cresol |
| 1599 | **153** | Dinitrophenol, solution |
| 1600 | **152** | Dinitrotoluenes, molten |
| 1601 | **151** | Disinfectant, solid, poisonous, n.o.s. |
| 1601 | **151** | Disinfectant, solid, toxic, n.o.s. |
| 1602 | **151** | Dye, liquid, poisonous, n.o.s. |
| 1602 | **151** | Dye, liquid, toxic, n.o.s. |
| 1602 | **151** | Dye intermediate, liquid, poisonous, n.o.s. |
| 1602 | **151** | Dye intermediate, liquid, toxic, n.o.s. |
| 1603 | **155** | Ethyl bromoacetate |
| 1604 | **132** | Ethylenediamine |
| 1605 | **154** | Ethylene dibromide |
| 1606 | **151** | Ferric arsenate |
| 1607 | **151** | Ferric arsenite |
| 1608 | **151** | Ferrous arsenate |
| 1611 | **151** | Hexaethyl tetraphosphate |
| 1612 | **123** | Compressed gas and hexaethyl tetraphosphate mixture |
| 1612 | **123** | Hexaethyl tetraphosphate and compressed gas mixture |
| 1613 | **154** | Hydrocyanic acid, aqueous solution, with less than 5% Hydrogen cyanide |
| 1613 | **154** | Hydrocyanic acid, aqueous solution, with not more than 20% Hydrogen cyanide |
| 1613 | **154** | Hydrogen cyanide, aqueous solution, with not more than 20% Hydrogen cyanide |
| 1614 | **152** | Hydrogen cyanide, stabilized (absorbed) |
| 1616 | **151** | Lead acetate |
| 1617 | **151** | Lead arsenates |
| 1618 | **151** | Lead arsenites |
| 1620 | **151** | Lead cyanide |
| 1621 | **151** | London purple |
| 1622 | **151** | Magnesium arsenate |
| 1623 | **151** | Mercuric arsenate |
| 1624 | **154** | Mercuric chloride |
| 1625 | **141** | Mercuric nitrate |
| 1626 | **157** | Mercuric potassium cyanide |
| 1627 | **141** | Mercurous nitrate |
| 1629 | **151** | Mercury acetate |
| 1630 | **151** | Mercury ammonium chloride |
| 1631 | **154** | Mercury benzoate |
| 1634 | **154** | Mercuric bromide |
| 1634 | **154** | Mercurous bromide |
| 1634 | **154** | Mercury bromides |
| 1636 | **154** | Mercuric cyanide |
| 1636 | **154** | Mercury cyanide |
| 1637 | **151** | Mercury gluconate |
| 1638 | **151** | Mercury iodide |
| 1639 | **151** | Mercury nucleate |
| 1640 | **151** | Mercury oleate |
| 1641 | **151** | Mercury oxide |
| 1642 | **151** | Mercuric oxycyanide |

| ID No. | Guide No. | Name of Material |
|---|---|---|
| 1642 | **151** | Mercury oxycyanide, desensitized |
| 1643 | **151** | Mercury potassium iodide |
| 1644 | **151** | Mercury salicylate |
| 1645 | **151** | Mercuric sulfate |
| 1645 | **151** | Mercuric sulphate |
| 1645 | **151** | Mercury sulfate |
| 1645 | **151** | Mercury sulphate |
| 1646 | **151** | Mercury thiocyanate |
| 1647 | **151** | Ethylene dibromide and Methyl bromide mixture, liquid |
| 1647 | **151** | Methyl bromide and Ethylene dibromide mixture, liquid |
| 1648 | **127** | Acetonitrile |
| 1649 | **131** | Motor fuel anti-knock mixture |
| 1650 | **153** | beta-Naphthylamine |
| 1650 | **153** | beta-Naphthylamine, solid |
| 1650 | **153** | Naphthylamine (beta) |
| 1650 | **153** | Naphthylamine (beta), solid |
| 1651 | **153** | Naphthylthiourea |
| 1652 | **153** | Naphthylurea |
| 1653 | **151** | Nickel cyanide |
| 1654 | **151** | Nicotine |
| 1655 | **151** | Nicotine compound, solid, n.o.s. |
| 1655 | **151** | Nicotine preparation, solid, n.o.s. |
| 1656 | **151** | Nicotine hydrochloride |
| 1656 | **151** | Nicotine hydrochloride, liquid |
| 1656 | **151** | Nicotine hydrochloride, solution |
| 1657 | **151** | Nicotine salicylate |
| 1658 | **151** | Nicotine sulfate, solid |
| 1658 | **151** | Nicotine sulfate, solution |
| 1658 | **151** | Nicotine sulphate, solid |
| 1658 | **151** | Nicotine sulphate, solution |
| 1659 | **151** | Nicotine tartrate |
| 1660 | **124** | Nitric oxide |
| 1660 | **124** | Nitric oxide, compressed |
| 1661 | **153** | Nitroanilines |
| 1662 | **152** | Nitrobenzene |
| 1663 | **153** | Nitrophenols |
| 1664 | **152** | Nitrotoluenes, liquid |
| 1664 | **152** | Nitrotoluenes, solid |
| 1665 | **152** | Nitroxylenes, liquid |
| 1665 | **152** | Nitroxylenes, solid |
| 1669 | **151** | Pentachloroethane |
| 1670 | **157** | Perchloromethyl mercaptan |
| 1671 | **153** | Phenol, solid |
| 1672 | **151** | Phenylcarbylamine chloride |
| 1673 | **153** | Phenylenediamines |
| 1674 | **151** | Phenylmercuric acetate |
| 1677 | **151** | Potassium arsenate |
| 1678 | **154** | Potassium arsenite |
| 1679 | **157** | Potassium cuprocyanide |
| 1680 | **157** | Potassium cyanide |
| 1680 | **157** | Potassium cyanide, solid |
| 1683 | **151** | Silver arsenite |
| 1684 | **151** | Silver cyanide |
| 1685 | **151** | Sodium arsenate |
| 1686 | **154** | Sodium arsenite, aqueous solution |
| 1687 | **153** | Sodium azide |
| 1688 | **152** | Sodium cacodylate |
| 1689 | **157** | Sodium cyanide |

| ID No. | Guide No. | Name of Material |
|---|---|---|
| 1689 | **157** | Sodium cyanide, solid |
| 1690 | **154** | Sodium fluoride |
| 1690 | **154** | Sodium fluoride, solid |
| 1691 | **151** | Strontium arsenite |
| 1692 | **151** | Strychnine |
| 1692 | **151** | Strychnine salts |
| 1693 | **159** | Tear gas devices |
| 1693 | **159** | Tear gas substance, liquid, n.o.s. |
| 1693 | **159** | Tear gas substance, solid, n.o.s. |
| 1694 | **159** | Bromobenzyl cyanides, liquid |
| 1694 | **159** | Bromobenzyl cyanides, solid |
| 1694 | **159** | CA |
| 1695 | **131** | Chloroacetone, stabilized |
| 1697 | **153** | Chloroacetophenone |
| 1697 | **153** | Chloroacetophenone, solid |
| 1697 | **153** | CN |
| 1698 | **154** | Adamsite |
| 1698 | **154** | Diphenylamine chloroarsine |
| 1698 | **154** | DM |
| 1699 | **151** | DA |
| 1699 | **151** | Diphenylchloroarsine, liquid |
| 1699 | **151** | Diphenylchloroarsine, solid |
| 1700 | **159** | Tear gas candles |
| 1700 | **159** | Tear gas grenades |
| 1701 | **152** | Xylyl bromide |
| 1701 | **152** | Xylyl bromide, liquid |
| 1702 | **151** | 1,1,2,2-Tetrachloroethane |
| 1702 | **151** | Tetrachloroethane |
| 1704 | **153** | Tetraethyl dithiopyrophosphate |
| 1707 | **151** | Thallium compound, n.o.s. |
| 1708 | **153** | Toluidines, liquid |
| 1708 | **153** | Toluidines, solid |
| 1709 | **151** | 2,4-Toluenediamine, solid |
| 1709 | **151** | 2,4-Toluylenediamine |
| 1709 | **151** | 2,4-Toluylenediamine, solid |
| 1710 | **160** | Trichloroethylene |
| 1711 | **153** | Xylidines, liquid |
| 1711 | **153** | Xylidines, solid |
| 1712 | **151** | Zinc arsenate |
| 1712 | **151** | Zinc arsenate and Zinc arsenite mixture |
| 1712 | **151** | Zinc arsenite |
| 1712 | **151** | Zinc arsenite and Zinc arsenate mixture |
| 1713 | **151** | Zinc cyanide |
| 1714 | **139** | Zinc phosphide |
| 1715 | **137** | Acetic anhydride |
| 1716 | **156** | Acetyl bromide |
| 1717 | **155** | Acetyl chloride |
| 1718 | **153** | Acid butyl phosphate |
| 1718 | **153** | Butyl acid phosphate |
| 1719 | **154** | Caustic alkali liquid, n.o.s. |
| 1722 | **155** | Allyl chlorocarbonate |
| 1722 | **155** | Allyl chloroformate |
| 1723 | **132** | Allyl iodide |
| 1724 | **155** | Allyltrichlorosilane, stabilized |
| 1725 | **137** | Aluminum bromide, anhydrous |
| 1726 | **137** | Aluminum chloride, anhydrous |
| 1727 | **154** | Ammonium bifluoride, solid |
| 1727 | **154** | Ammonium hydrogendifluoride, solid |
| 1728 | **155** | Amyltrichlorosilane |

| ID No. | Guide No. | Name of Material |
|---|---|---|
| 1729 | **156** | Anisoyl chloride |
| 1730 | **157** | Antimony pentachloride, liquid |
| 1731 | **157** | Antimony pentachloride, solution |
| 1732 | **157** | Antimony pentafluoride |
| 1733 | **157** | Antimony trichloride |
| 1733 | **157** | Antimony trichloride, liquid |
| 1733 | **157** | Antimony trichloride, solid |
| 1736 | **137** | Benzoyl chloride |
| 1737 | **156** | Benzyl bromide |
| 1738 | **156** | Benzyl chloride |
| 1739 | **137** | Benzyl chloroformate |
| 1740 | **154** | Hydrogendifluorides, n.o.s. |
| 1740 | **154** | Hydrogendifluorides, solid, n.o.s. |
| 1741 | **125** | Boron trichloride |
| 1742 | **157** | Boron trifluoride acetic acid complex |
| 1742 | **157** | Boron trifluoride acetic acid complex, liquid |
| 1743 | **157** | Boron trifluoride propionic acid complex |
| 1743 | **157** | Boron trifluoride propionic acid complex, liquid |
| 1744 | **154** | Bromine |
| 1744 | **154** | Bromine, solution |
| 1744 | **154** | Bromine, solution (Inhalation Hazard Zone A) |
| 1744 | **154** | Bromine, solution (Inhalation Hazard Zone B) |
| 1745 | **144** | Bromine pentafluoride |
| 1746 | **144** | Bromine trifluoride |
| 1747 | **155** | Butyltrichlorosilane |
| 1748 | **140** | Calcium hypochlorite, dry |
| 1748 | **140** | Calcium hypochlorite mixture, dry, with more than 39% available Chlorine (8.8% available Oxygen) |
| 1749 | **124** | Chlorine trifluoride |
| 1750 | **153** | Chloroacetic acid, solution |
| 1751 | **153** | Chloroacetic acid, solid |
| 1752 | **156** | Chloroacetyl chloride |
| 1753 | **156** | Chlorophenyltrichlorosilane |
| 1754 | **137** | Chlorosulfonic acid (with or without sulfur trioxide mixture) |
| 1754 | **137** | Chlorosulphonic acid (with or without sulphur trioxide mixture) |
| 1755 | **154** | Chromic acid, solution |
| 1756 | **154** | Chromic fluoride, solid |
| 1757 | **154** | Chromic fluoride, solution |
| 1758 | **137** | Chromium oxychloride |
| 1759 | **154** | Corrosive solid, n.o.s. |
| 1759 | **154** | Ferrous chloride, solid |
| 1760 | **154** | Chemical kit |
| 1760 | **154** | Compounds, cleaning liquid (corrosive) |
| 1760 | **154** | Compounds, tree or weed killing, liquid (corrosive) |
| 1760 | **154** | Corrosive liquid, n.o.s. |
| 1760 | **154** | Ferrous chloride, solution |
| 1761 | **154** | Cupriethylenediamine, solution |
| 1762 | **156** | Cyclohexenyltrichlorosilane |
| 1763 | **156** | Cyclohexyltrichlorosilane |
| 1764 | **153** | Dichloroacetic acid |
| 1765 | **156** | Dichloroacetyl chloride |
| 1766 | **156** | Dichlorophenyltrichlorosilane |
| 1767 | **155** | Diethyldichlorosilane |

| ID No. | Guide No. | Name of Material |
|---|---|---|
| 1768 | **154** | Difluorophosphoric acid, anhydrous |
| 1769 | **156** | Diphenyldichlorosilane |
| 1770 | **153** | Diphenylmethyl bromide |
| 1771 | **156** | Dodecyltrichlorosilane |
| 1773 | **157** | Ferric chloride, anhydrous |
| 1774 | **154** | Fire extinguisher charges, corrosive liquid |
| 1775 | **154** | Fluoroboric acid |
| 1776 | **154** | Fluorophosphoric acid, anhydrous |
| 1777 | **137** | Fluorosulfonic acid |
| 1777 | **137** | Fluorosulphonic acid |
| 1778 | **154** | Fluorosilicic acid |
| 1778 | **154** | Hydrofluorosilicic acid |
| 1779 | **153** | Formic acid |
| 1779 | **153** | Formic acid, with more than 85% acid |
| 1780 | **156** | Fumaryl chloride |
| 1781 | **156** | Hexadecyltrichlorosilane |
| 1782 | **154** | Hexafluorophosphoric acid |
| 1783 | **153** | Hexamethylenediamine, solution |
| 1784 | **156** | Hexyltrichlorosilane |
| 1786 | **157** | Hydrofluoric acid and Sulfuric acid mixture |
| 1786 | **157** | Hydrofluoric acid and Sulphuric acid mixture |
| 1786 | **157** | Sulfuric acid and Hydrofluoric acid mixture |
| 1786 | **157** | Sulphuric acid and Hydrofluoric acid mixture |
| 1787 | **154** | Hydriodic acid |
| 1788 | **154** | Hydrobromic acid |
| 1789 | **157** | Hydrochloric acid |
| 1789 | **157** | Muriatic acid |
| 1790 | **157** | Hydrofluoric acid |
| 1791 | **154** | Hypochlorite solution |
| 1791 | **154** | Sodium hypochlorite |
| 1792 | **157** | Iodine monochloride, solid |
| 1793 | **153** | Isopropyl acid phosphate |
| 1794 | **154** | Lead sulfate, with more than 3% free acid |
| 1794 | **154** | Lead sulphate, with more than 3% free acid |
| 1796 | **157** | Nitrating acid mixture with more than 50% nitric acid |
| 1796 | **157** | Nitrating acid mixture with not more than 50% nitric acid |
| 1798 | **157** | Aqua regia |
| 1798 | **157** | Nitrohydrochloric acid |
| 1799 | **156** | Nonyltrichlorosilane |
| 1800 | **156** | Octadecyltrichlorosilane |
| 1801 | **156** | Octyltrichlorosilane |
| 1802 | **140** | Perchloric acid, with not more than 50% acid |
| 1803 | **153** | Phenolsulfonic acid, liquid |
| 1803 | **153** | Phenolsulphonic acid, liquid |
| 1804 | **156** | Phenyltrichlorosilane |
| 1805 | **154** | Phosphoric acid, liquid |
| 1805 | **154** | Phosphoric acid, solid |
| 1805 | **154** | Phosphoric acid, solution |
| 1806 | **137** | Phosphorus pentachloride |
| 1807 | **137** | Phosphorus pentoxide |
| 1808 | **137** | Phosphorus tribromide |
| 1809 | **137** | Phosphorus trichloride |
| 1810 | **137** | Phosphorus oxychloride |
| 1811 | **154** | Potassium hydrogendifluoride |

| ID No. | Guide No. | Name of Material |
|---|---|---|
| 1811 | **154** | Potassium hydrogen difluoride, solid |
| 1812 | **154** | Potassium fluoride |
| 1812 | **154** | Potassium fluoride, solid |
| 1813 | **154** | Caustic potash, solid |
| 1813 | **154** | Potassium hydroxide, solid |
| 1814 | **154** | Caustic potash, solution |
| 1814 | **154** | Potassium hydroxide, solution |
| 1815 | **132** | Propionyl chloride |
| 1816 | **155** | Propyltrichlorosilane |
| 1817 | **137** | Pyrosulfuryl chloride |
| 1817 | **137** | Pyrosulphuryl chloride |
| 1818 | **157** | Silicon tetrachloride |
| 1819 | **154** | Sodium aluminate, solution |
| 1823 | **154** | Caustic soda, solid |
| 1823 | **154** | Sodium hydroxide, solid |
| 1824 | **154** | Caustic soda, solution |
| 1824 | **154** | Sodium hydroxide, solution |
| 1825 | **157** | Sodium monoxide |
| 1826 | **157** | Nitrating acid mixture, spent, with more than 50% nitric acid |
| 1826 | **157** | Nitrating acid mixture, spent, with not more than 50% nitric acid |
| 1827 | **137** | Stannic chloride, anhydrous |
| 1827 | **137** | Tin tetrachloride |
| 1828 | **137** | Sulfur chlorides |
| 1828 | **137** | Sulphur chlorides |
| 1829 | **137** | Sulfur trioxide, stabilized |
| 1829 | **137** | Sulphur trioxide, stabilized |
| 1830 | **137** | Sulfuric acid |
| 1830 | **137** | Sulfuric acid, with more than 51% acid |
| 1830 | **137** | Sulphuric acid |
| 1830 | **137** | Sulphuric acid, with more than 51% acid |
| 1831 | **137** | Sulfuric acid, fuming |
| 1831 | **137** | Sulfuric acid, fuming, with less than 30% free Sulfur trioxide |
| 1831 | **137** | Sulfuric acid, fuming, with not less than 30% free Sulfur trioxide |
| 1831 | **137** | Sulphuric acid, fuming |
| 1831 | **137** | Sulphuric acid, fuming, with less than 30% free Sulphur trioxide |
| 1831 | **137** | Sulphuric acid, fuming, with not less than 30% free Sulphur trioxide |
| 1832 | **137** | Sulfuric acid, spent |
| 1832 | **137** | Sulphuric acid, spent |
| 1833 | **154** | Sulfurous acid |
| 1833 | **154** | Sulphurous acid |
| 1834 | **137** | Sulfuryl chloride |
| 1834 | **137** | Sulphuryl chloride |
| 1835 | **153** | Tetramethylammonium hydroxide |
| 1835 | **153** | Tetramethylammonium hydroxide, solution |
| 1836 | **137** | Thionyl chloride |
| 1837 | **157** | Thiophosphoryl chloride |
| 1838 | **137** | Titanium tetrachloride |
| 1839 | **153** | Trichloroacetic acid |
| 1840 | **154** | Zinc chloride, solution |
| 1841 | **171** | Acetaldehyde ammonia |
| 1843 | **141** | Ammonium dinitro-o-cresolate |
| 1843 | **141** | Ammonium dinitro-o-cresolate, solid |
| 1845 | **120** | Carbon dioxide, solid |
| 1845 | **120** | Dry ice |

| ID No. | Guide No. | Name of Material |
|---|---|---|
| 1846 | **151** | Carbon tetrachloride |
| 1847 | **153** | Potassium sulfide, hydrated, with not less than 30% water of crystallization |
| 1847 | **153** | Potassium sulphide, hydrated, with not less than 30% water of crystallization |
| 1848 | **132** | Propionic acid |
| 1848 | **132** | Propionic acid, with not less than 10% and less than 90% acid |
| 1849 | **153** | Sodium sulfide, hydrated, with not less than 30% water |
| 1849 | **153** | Sodium sulphide, hydrated, with not less than 30% water |
| 1851 | **151** | Medicine, liquid, poisonous, n.o.s. |
| 1851 | **151** | Medicine, liquid, toxic, n.o.s. |
| 1854 | **135** | Barium alloys, pyrophoric |
| 1855 | **135** | Calcium, pyrophoric |
| 1855 | **135** | Calcium alloys, pyrophoric |
| 1856 | **133** | Rags, oily |
| 1857 | **133** | Textile waste, wet |
| 1858 | **126** | Hexafluoropropylene |
| 1858 | **126** | Hexafluoropropylene, compressed |
| 1858 | **126** | Refrigerant gas R-1216 |
| 1859 | **125** | Silicon tetrafluoride |
| 1859 | **125** | Silicon tetrafluoride, compressed |
| 1860 | **116P** | Vinyl fluoride, stabilized |
| 1862 | **130** | Ethyl crotonate |
| 1863 | **128** | Fuel, aviation, turbine engine |
| 1865 | **131** | n-Propyl nitrate |
| 1866 | **127** | Resin solution |
| 1868 | **134** | Decaborane |
| 1869 | **138** | Magnesium |
| 1869 | **138** | Magnesium, in pellets, turnings or ribbons |
| 1869 | **138** | Magnesium alloys, with more than 50% Magnesium, in pellets, turnings or ribbons |
| 1870 | **138** | Potassium borohydride |
| 1871 | **170** | Titanium hydride |
| 1872 | **141** | Lead dioxide |
| 1873 | **143** | Perchloric acid, with more than 50% but not more than 72% acid |
| 1884 | **157** | Barium oxide |
| 1885 | **153** | Benzidine |
| 1886 | **156** | Benzylidene chloride |
| 1887 | **160** | Bromochloromethane |
| 1888 | **151** | Chloroform |
| 1889 | **157** | Cyanogen bromide |
| 1891 | **131** | Ethyl bromide |
| 1892 | **151** | ED |
| 1892 | **151** | Ethyldichloroarsine |
| 1894 | **151** | Phenylmercuric hydroxide |
| 1895 | **151** | Phenylmercuric nitrate |
| 1897 | **160** | Perchloroethylene |
| 1897 | **160** | Tetrachloroethylene |
| 1898 | **156** | Acetyl iodide |
| 1902 | **153** | Diisooctyl acid phosphate |
| 1903 | **153** | Disinfectant, liquid, corrosive, n.o.s. |
| 1905 | **154** | Selenic acid |
| 1906 | **153** | Acid, sludge |
| 1906 | **153** | Sludge acid |
| 1907 | **154** | Soda lime, with more than 4% Sodium hydroxide |

| ID No. | Guide No. | Name of Material |
|---|---|---|
| 1908 | **154** | Chlorite solution |
| 1910 | **157** | Calcium oxide |
| 1911 | **119** | Diborane |
| 1911 | **119** | Diborane, compressed |
| 1911 | **119** | Diborane mixtures |
| 1912 | **115** | Methyl chloride and Methylene chloride mixture |
| 1912 | **115** | Methylene chloride and Methyl chloride mixture |
| 1913 | **120** | Neon, refrigerated liquid (cryogenic liquid) |
| 1914 | **130** | Butyl propionates |
| 1915 | **127** | Cyclohexanone |
| 1916 | **152** | 2,2'-Dichlorodiethyl ether |
| 1916 | **152** | Dichloroethyl ether |
| 1917 | **129P** | Ethyl acrylate, stabilized |
| 1918 | **130** | Cumene |
| 1918 | **130** | Isopropylbenzene |
| 1919 | **129P** | Methyl acrylate, stabilized |
| 1920 | **128** | Nonanes |
| 1921 | **131P** | Propyleneimine, stabilized |
| 1922 | **132** | Pyrrolidine |
| 1923 | **135** | Calcium dithionite |
| 1923 | **135** | Calcium hydrosulfite |
| 1923 | **135** | Calcium hydrosulphite |
| 1928 | **135** | Methyl magnesium bromide in Ethyl ether |
| 1929 | **135** | Potassium dithionite |
| 1929 | **135** | Potassium hydrosulfite |
| 1929 | **135** | Potassium hydrosulphite |
| 1931 | **171** | Zinc dithionite |
| 1931 | **171** | Zinc hydrosulfite |
| 1931 | **171** | Zinc hydrosulphite |
| 1932 | **135** | Zirconium scrap |
| 1935 | **157** | Cyanide solution, n.o.s. |
| 1938 | **156** | Bromoacetic acid |
| 1938 | **156** | Bromoacetic acid, solution |
| 1939 | **137** | Phosphorus oxybromide |
| 1939 | **137** | Phosphorus oxybromide, solid |
| 1940 | **153** | Thioglycolic acid |
| 1941 | **171** | Dibromodifluoromethane |
| 1941 | **171** | Refrigerant gas R-12B2 |
| 1942 | **140** | Ammonium nitrate, with not more than 0.2% combustible substances |
| 1944 | **133** | Matches, safety |
| 1945 | **133** | Matches, wax "vesta" |
| 1950 | **126** | Aerosols |
| 1951 | **120** | Argon, refrigerated liquid (cryogenic liquid) |
| 1952 | **126** | Carbon dioxide and Ethylene oxide mixtures, with not more than 9% Ethylene oxide |
| 1952 | **126** | Ethylene oxide and Carbon dioxide mixtures, with not more than 9% Ethylene oxide |
| 1953 | **119** | Compressed gas, poisonous, flammable, n.o.s. |
| 1953 | **119** | Compressed gas, poisonous, flammable, n.o.s. (Inhalation Hazard Zone A) |
| 1953 | **119** | Compressed gas, poisonous, flammable, n.o.s. (Inhalation Hazard Zone B) |
| 1953 | **119** | Compressed gas, poisonous, flammable, n.o.s. (Inhalation Hazard Zone C) |
| 1953 | **119** | Compressed gas, poisonous, flammable, n.o.s. (Inhalation Hazard Zone D) |

| ID No. | Guide No. | Name of Material |
|---|---|---|
| 1953 | **119** | Compressed gas, toxic, flammable, n.o.s. |
| 1953 | **119** | Compressed gas, toxic, flammable, n.o.s. (Inhalation Hazard Zone A) |
| 1953 | **119** | Compressed gas, toxic, flammable, n.o.s. (Inhalation Hazard Zone B) |
| 1953 | **119** | Compressed gas, toxic, flammable, n.o.s. (Inhalation Hazard Zone C) |
| 1953 | **119** | Compressed gas, toxic, flammable, n.o.s. (Inhalation Hazard Zone D) |
| 1954 | **115** | Compressed gas, flammable, n.o.s. |
| 1954 | **115** | Dispersant gases, n.o.s. (flammable) |
| 1954 | **115** | Refrigerant gases, n.o.s. (flammable) |
| 1955 | **123** | Compressed gas, poisonous, n.o.s. |
| 1955 | **123** | Compressed gas, poisonous, n.o.s. (Inhalation Hazard Zone A) |
| 1955 | **123** | Compressed gas, poisonous, n.o.s. (Inhalation Hazard Zone B) |
| 1955 | **123** | Compressed gas, poisonous, n.o.s. (Inhalation Hazard Zone C) |
| 1955 | **123** | Compressed gas, poisonous, n.o.s. (Inhalation Hazard Zone D) |
| 1955 | **123** | Compressed gas, toxic, n.o.s. |
| 1955 | **123** | Compressed gas, toxic, n.o.s. (Inhalation Hazard Zone A) |
| 1955 | **123** | Compressed gas, toxic, n.o.s. (Inhalation Hazard Zone B) |
| 1955 | **123** | Compressed gas, toxic, n.o.s. (Inhalation Hazard Zone C) |
| 1955 | **123** | Compressed gas, toxic, n.o.s. (Inhalation Hazard Zone D) |
| 1955 | **123** | Organic phosphate compound mixed with compressed gas |
| 1955 | **123** | Organic phosphate mixed with compressed gas |
| 1955 | **123** | Organic phosphorus compound mixed with compressed gas |
| 1956 | **126** | Compressed gas, n.o.s. |
| 1957 | **115** | Deuterium |
| 1957 | **115** | Deuterium, compressed |
| 1958 | **126** | 1,2-Dichloro-1,1,2,2-tetrafluoroethane |
| 1958 | **126** | Refrigerant gas R-114 |
| 1959 | **116P** | 1,1-Difluoroethylene |
| 1959 | **116P** | Refrigerant gas R-1132a |
| 1961 | **115** | Ethane, refrigerated liquid |
| 1961 | **115** | Ethane-Propane mixture, refrigerated liquid |
| 1961 | **115** | Propane-Ethane mixture, refrigerated liquid |
| 1962 | **116P** | Ethylene |
| 1962 | **116P** | Ethylene, compressed |
| 1963 | **120** | Helium, refrigerated liquid (cryogenic liquid) |
| 1964 | **115** | Hydrocarbon gas mixture, compressed, n.o.s. |
| 1965 | **115** | Hydrocarbon gas mixture, liquefied, n.o.s. |
| 1966 | **115** | Hydrogen, refrigerated liquid (cryogenic liquid) |
| 1967 | **123** | Insecticide gas, poisonous, n.o.s. |
| 1967 | **123** | Insecticide gas, toxic, n.o.s. |
| 1967 | **123** | Parathion and compressed gas mixture |

| ID No. | Guide No. | Name of Material |
|---|---|---|
| 1968 | **126** | Insecticide gas, n.o.s. |
| 1969 | **115** | Isobutane |
| 1970 | **120** | Krypton, refrigerated liquid (cryogenic liquid) |
| 1971 | **115** | Methane |
| 1971 | **115** | Methane, compressed |
| 1971 | **115** | Natural gas, compressed |
| 1972 | **115** | Liquefied natural gas (cryogenic liquid) |
| 1972 | **115** | LNG (cryogenic liquid) |
| 1972 | **115** | Methane, refrigerated liquid (cryogenic liquid) |
| 1972 | **115** | Natural gas, refrigerated liquid (cryogenic liquid) |
| 1973 | **126** | Chlorodifluoromethane and Chloropentafluoroethane mixture |
| 1973 | **126** | Chloropentafluoroethane and Chlorodifluoromethane mixture |
| 1973 | **126** | Refrigerant gas R-502 |
| 1974 | **126** | Chlorodifluorobromomethane |
| 1974 | **126** | Refrigerant gas R-12B1 |
| 1975 | **124** | Dinitrogen tetroxide and Nitric oxide mixture |
| 1975 | **124** | Nitric oxide and Dinitrogen tetroxide mixture |
| 1975 | **124** | Nitric oxide and Nitrogen dioxide mixture |
| 1975 | **124** | Nitric oxide and Nitrogen tetroxide mixture |
| 1975 | **124** | Nitrogen dioxide and Nitric oxide mixture |
| 1975 | **124** | Nitrogen tetroxide and Nitric oxide mixture |
| 1976 | **126** | Octafluorocyclobutane |
| 1976 | **126** | Refrigerant gas RC-318 |
| 1977 | **120** | Nitrogen, refrigerated liquid (cryogenic liquid) |
| 1978 | **115** | Propane |
| 1979 | **121** | Rare gases mixture, compressed |
| 1980 | **121** | Oxygen and Rare gases mixture, compressed |
| 1980 | **121** | Rare gases and Oxygen mixture, compressed |
| 1981 | **121** | Nitrogen and Rare gases mixture, compressed |
| 1981 | **121** | Rare gases and Nitrogen mixture, compressed |
| 1982 | **126** | Refrigerant gas R-14 |
| 1982 | **126** | Refrigerant gas R-14, compressed |
| 1982 | **126** | Tetrafluoromethane |
| 1982 | **126** | Tetrafluoromethane, compressed |
| 1983 | **126** | 1-Chloro-2,2,2-trifluoroethane |
| 1983 | **126** | Refrigerant gas R-133a |
| 1984 | **126** | Refrigerant gas R-23 |
| 1984 | **126** | Trifluoromethane |
| 1986 | **131** | Alcohols, flammable, poisonous, n.o.s. |
| 1986 | **131** | Alcohols, flammable, toxic, n.o.s. |
| 1987 | **127** | Alcohols, n.o.s. |
| 1987 | **127** | Denatured alcohol |
| 1988 | **131** | Aldehydes, flammable, poisonous, n.o.s. |
| 1988 | **131** | Aldehydes, flammable, toxic, n.o.s. |
| 1989 | **129** | Aldehydes, n.o.s. |
| 1990 | **129** | Benzaldehyde |
| 1991 | **131P** | Chloroprene, stabilized |

| ID No. | Guide No. | Name of Material |
|---|---|---|
| 1992 | **131** | Flammable liquid, poisonous, n.o.s. |
| 1992 | **131** | Flammable liquid, toxic, n.o.s. |
| 1993 | **128** | Combustible liquid, n.o.s. |
| 1993 | **128** | Compounds, cleaning liquid (flammable) |
| 1993 | **128** | Compounds, tree or weed killing, liquid (flammable) |
| 1993 | **128** | Diesel fuel |
| 1993 | **128** | Flammable liquid, n.o.s. |
| 1993 | **128** | Fuel oil |
| 1994 | **131** | Iron pentacarbonyl |
| 1999 | **130** | Asphalt |
| 1999 | **130** | Asphalt, cut back |
| 1999 | **130** | Tars, liquid |
| 2000 | **133** | Celluloid, in blocks, rods, rolls, sheets, tubes, etc., except scrap |
| 2001 | **133** | Cobalt naphthenates, powder |
| 2002 | **135** | Celluloid, scrap |
| 2003 | **135** | Metal alkyls, water-reactive, n.o.s. |
| 2003 | **135** | Metal aryls, water-reactive, n.o.s. |
| 2004 | **135** | Magnesium diamide |
| 2005 | **135** | Magnesium diphenyl |
| 2006 | **135** | Plastics, nitrocellulose-based, self-heating, n.o.s. |
| 2008 | **135** | Zirconium powder, dry |
| 2009 | **135** | Zirconium, dry, finished sheets, strips or coiled wire |
| 2010 | **138** | Magnesium hydride |
| 2011 | **139** | Magnesium phosphide |
| 2012 | **139** | Potassium phosphide |
| 2013 | **139** | Strontium phosphide |
| 2014 | **140** | Hydrogen peroxide, aqueous solution, with not less than 20% but not more than 60% Hydrogen peroxide (stabilized as necessary) |
| 2015 | **143** | Hydrogen peroxide, aqueous solution, stabilized, with more than 60% Hydrogen peroxide |
| 2015 | **143** | Hydrogen peroxide, stabilized |
| 2016 | **151** | Ammunition, poisonous, non-explosive |
| 2016 | **151** | Ammunition, toxic, non-explosive |
| 2017 | **159** | Ammunition, tear-producing, non-explosive |
| 2018 | **152** | Chloroanilines, solid |
| 2019 | **152** | Chloroanilines, liquid |
| 2020 | **153** | Chlorophenols, solid |
| 2021 | **153** | Chlorophenols, liquid |
| 2022 | **153** | Cresylic acid |
| 2023 | **131P** | 1-Chloro-2,3-epoxypropane |
| 2023 | **131P** | Epichlorohydrin |
| 2024 | **151** | Mercury compound, liquid, n.o.s. |
| 2025 | **151** | Mercury compound, solid, n.o.s. |
| 2026 | **151** | Phenylmercuric compound, n.o.s. |
| 2027 | **151** | Sodium arsenite, solid |
| 2028 | **153** | Bombs, smoke, non-explosive, with corrosive liquid, without initiating device |
| 2029 | **132** | Hydrazine, anhydrous |
| 2030 | **153** | Hydrazine, aqueous solution, with more than 37% Hydrazine |

| ID No. | Guide No. | Name of Material |
|---|---|---|
| 2030 | **153** | Hydrazine, aqueous solution, with not less than 37% but not more than 64% Hydrazine |
| 2030 | **153** | Hydrazine hydrate |
| 2031 | **157** | Nitric acid, other than red fuming, with more than 70% nitric acid |
| 2031 | **157** | Nitric acid, other than red fuming, with not more than 70% nitric acid |
| 2032 | **157** | Nitric acid, red fuming |
| 2033 | **154** | Potassium monoxide |
| 2034 | **115** | Hydrogen and Methane mixture, compressed |
| 2034 | **115** | Methane and Hydrogen mixture, compressed |
| 2035 | **115** | Refrigerant gas R-143a |
| 2035 | **115** | 1,1,1-Trifluoroethane |
| 2036 | **121** | Xenon |
| 2036 | **121** | Xenon, compressed |
| 2037 | **115** | Gas cartridges |
| 2037 | **115** | Receptacles, small, containing gas |
| 2038 | **152** | Dinitrotoluenes |
| 2038 | **152** | Dinitrotoluenes, liquid |
| 2038 | **152** | Dinitrotoluenes, solid |
| 2044 | **115** | 2,2-Dimethylpropane |
| 2045 | **130** | Isobutyl aldehyde |
| 2045 | **130** | Isobutyraldehyde |
| 2046 | **130** | Cymenes |
| 2047 | **129** | Dichloropropenes |
| 2048 | **130** | Dicyclopentadiene |
| 2049 | **130** | Diethylbenzene |
| 2050 | **128** | Diisobutylene, isomeric compounds |
| 2051 | **132** | 2-Dimethylaminoethanol |
| 2052 | **128** | Dipentene |
| 2053 | **129** | Methylamyl alcohol |
| 2053 | **129** | Methyl isobutyl carbinol |
| 2053 | **129** | M.I.B.C. |
| 2054 | **132** | Morpholine |
| 2055 | **128P** | Styrene monomer, stabilized |
| 2056 | **127** | Tetrahydrofuran |
| 2057 | **128** | Tripropylene |
| 2058 | **129** | Valeraldehyde |
| 2059 | **127** | Nitrocellulose, solution, flammable |
| 2067 | **140** | Ammonium nitrate based fertilizer |
| 2068 | **140** | Ammonium nitrate fertilizers, with Calcium carbonate |
| 2069 | **140** | Ammonium nitrate fertilizers, with Ammonium sulfate |
| 2069 | **140** | Ammonium nitrate fertilizers, with Ammonium sulphate |
| 2070 | **143** | Ammonium nitrate fertilizers, with Phosphate or Potash |
| 2071 | **140** | Ammonium nitrate based fertilizer |
| 2072 | **140** | Ammonium nitrate fertilizer, n.o.s. |
| 2073 | **125** | Ammonia, solution, with more than 35% but not more than 50% Ammonia |
| 2074 | **153P** | Acrylamide |
| 2074 | **153P** | Acrylamide, solid |
| 2075 | **153** | Chloral, anhydrous, stabilized |
| 2076 | **153** | Cresols, liquid |
| 2076 | **153** | Cresols, solid |
| 2077 | **153** | alpha-Naphthylamine |
| 2077 | **153** | Naphthylamine (alpha) |

| ID No. | Guide No. | Name of Material |
|---|---|---|
| 2078 | **156** | Toluene diisocyanate |
| 2079 | **154** | Diethylenetriamine |
| 2186 | **125** | Hydrogen chloride, refrigerated liquid |
| 2187 | **120** | Carbon dioxide, refrigerated liquid |
| 2188 | **119** | Arsine |
| 2188 | **119** | SA |
| 2189 | **119** | Dichlorosilane |
| 2190 | **124** | Oxygen difluoride |
| 2190 | **124** | Oxygen difluoride, compressed |
| 2191 | **123** | Sulfuryl fluoride |
| 2191 | **123** | Sulphuryl fluoride |
| 2192 | **119** | Germane |
| 2193 | **126** | Hexafluoroethane |
| 2193 | **126** | Hexafluoroethane, compressed |
| 2193 | **126** | Refrigerant gas R-116 |
| 2193 | **126** | Refrigerant gas R-116, compressed |
| 2194 | **125** | Selenium hexafluoride |
| 2195 | **125** | Tellurium hexafluoride |
| 2196 | **125** | Tungsten hexafluoride |
| 2197 | **125** | Hydrogen iodide, anhydrous |
| 2198 | **125** | Phosphorus pentafluoride |
| 2198 | **125** | Phosphorus pentafluoride, compressed |
| 2199 | **119** | Phosphine |
| 2200 | **116P** | Propadiene, stabilized |
| 2201 | **122** | Nitrous oxide, refrigerated liquid |
| 2202 | **117** | Hydrogen selenide, anhydrous |
| 2203 | **116** | Silane |
| 2203 | **116** | Silane, compressed |

| ID No. | Guide No. | Name of Material |
|---|---|---|
| 2204 | **119** | Carbonyl sulfide |
| 2204 | **119** | Carbonyl sulphide |
| 2205 | **153** | Adiponitrile |
| 2206 | **155** | Isocyanate solution, poisonous, n.o.s. |
| 2206 | **155** | Isocyanate solution, toxic, n.o.s. |
| 2206 | **155** | Isocyanates, poisonous, n.o.s. |
| 2206 | **155** | Isocyanates, toxic, n.o.s. |
| 2208 | **140** | Bleaching powder |
| 2208 | **140** | Calcium hypochlorite mixture, dry, with more than 10% but not more than 39% available Chlorine |
| 2209 | **132** | Formaldehyde, solution (corrosive) |
| 2209 | **132** | Formalin (corrosive) |
| 2210 | **135** | Maneb |
| 2210 | **135** | Maneb preparation, with not less than 60% Maneb |
| 2211 | **133** | Polymeric beads, expandable |
| 2211 | **133** | Polystyrene beads, expandable |
| 2212 | **171** | Asbestos |
| 2212 | **171** | Asbestos, amphibole |
| 2212 | **171** | Asbestos, blue |
| 2212 | **171** | Asbestos, brown |
| 2212 | **171** | Blue asbestos |
| 2212 | **171** | Brown asbestos |
| 2213 | **133** | Paraformaldehyde |
| 2214 | **156** | Phthalic anhydride |
| 2215 | **156** | Maleic anhydride |
| 2215 | **156** | Maleic anhydride, molten |
| 2216 | **171** | Fish meal, stabilized |
| 2216 | **171** | Fish scrap, stabilized |

| ID No. | Guide No. | Name of Material |
|---|---|---|
| 2217 | **135** | Seed cake, with not more than 1.5% oil and not more than 11% moisture |
| 2218 | **132P** | Acrylic acid, stabilized |
| 2219 | **129** | Allyl glycidyl ether |
| 2222 | **128** | Anisole |
| 2224 | **152** | Benzonitrile |
| 2225 | **156** | Benzenesulfonyl chloride |
| 2225 | **156** | Benzenesulphonyl chloride |
| 2226 | **156** | Benzotrichloride |
| 2227 | **130P** | n-Butyl methacrylate, stabilized |
| 2232 | **153** | Chloroacetaldehyde |
| 2232 | **153** | 2-Chloroethanal |
| 2233 | **152** | Chloroanisidines |
| 2234 | **130** | Chlorobenzotrifluorides |
| 2235 | **153** | Chlorobenzyl chlorides |
| 2235 | **153** | Chlorobenzyl chlorides, liquid |
| 2236 | **156** | 3-Chloro-4-methylphenyl isocyanate |
| 2236 | **156** | 3-Chloro-4-methylphenyl isocyanate, liquid |
| 2237 | **153** | Chloronitroanilines |
| 2238 | **129** | Chlorotoluenes |
| 2239 | **153** | Chlorotoluidines |
| 2239 | **153** | Chlorotoluidines, solid |
| 2240 | **154** | Chromosulfuric acid |
| 2240 | **154** | Chromosulphuric acid |
| 2241 | **128** | Cycloheptane |
| 2242 | **128** | Cycloheptene |
| 2243 | **130** | Cyclohexyl acetate |
| 2244 | **129** | Cyclopentanol |
| 2245 | **128** | Cyclopentanone |
| 2246 | **128** | Cyclopentene |
| 2247 | **128** | n-Decane |
| 2248 | **132** | Di-n-butylamine |
| 2249 | **131** | Dichlorodimethyl ether, symmetrical |
| 2250 | **156** | Dichlorophenyl isocyanates |
| 2251 | **128P** | Bicyclo[2.2.1]hepta-2,5-diene, stabilized |
| 2251 | **128P** | 2,5-Norbornadiene, stabilized |
| 2252 | **127** | 1,2-Dimethoxyethane |
| 2253 | **153** | N,N-Dimethylaniline |
| 2254 | **133** | Matches, fusee |
| 2256 | **130** | Cyclohexene |
| 2257 | **138** | Potassium |
| 2257 | **138** | Potassium, metal |
| 2258 | **132** | 1,2-Propylenediamine |
| 2259 | **153** | Triethylenetetramine |
| 2260 | **132** | Tripropylamine |
| 2261 | **153** | Xylenols |
| 2261 | **153** | Xylenols, solid |
| 2262 | **156** | Dimethylcarbamoyl chloride |
| 2263 | **128** | Dimethylcyclohexanes |
| 2264 | **132** | N,N-Dimethylcyclohexylamine |
| 2264 | **132** | Dimethylcyclohexylamine |
| 2265 | **129** | N,N-Dimethylformamide |
| 2266 | **132** | Dimethyl-N-propylamine |
| 2267 | **156** | Dimethyl thiophosphoryl chloride |
| 2269 | **153** | 3,3'-Iminodipropylamine |
| 2270 | **132** | Ethylamine, aqueous solution, with not less than 50% but not more than 70% Ethylamine |
| 2271 | **128** | Ethyl amyl ketone |
| 2272 | **153** | N-Ethylaniline |

| ID No. | Guide No. | Name of Material |
|---|---|---|
| 2273 | **153** | 2-Ethylaniline |
| 2274 | **153** | N-Ethyl-N-benzylaniline |
| 2275 | **129** | 2-Ethylbutanol |
| 2276 | **132** | 2-Ethylhexylamine |
| 2277 | **130P** | Ethyl methacrylate |
| 2277 | **130P** | Ethyl methacrylate, stabilized |
| 2278 | **128** | n-Heptene |
| 2279 | **151** | Hexachlorobutadiene |
| 2280 | **153** | Hexamethylenediamine, solid |
| 2281 | **156** | Hexamethylene diisocyanate |
| 2282 | **129** | Hexanols |
| 2283 | **130P** | Isobutyl methacrylate, stabilized |
| 2284 | **131** | Isobutyronitrile |
| 2285 | **156** | Isocyanatobenzotrifluorides |
| 2286 | **128** | Pentamethylheptane |
| 2287 | **128** | Isoheptenes |
| 2288 | **128** | Isohexenes |
| 2289 | **153** | Isophoronediamine |
| 2290 | **156** | IPDI |
| 2290 | **156** | Isophorone diisocyanate |
| 2291 | **151** | Lead compound, soluble, n.o.s. |
| 2293 | **128** | 4-Methoxy-4-methylpentan-2-one |
| 2294 | **153** | N-Methylaniline |
| 2295 | **155** | Methyl chloroacetate |
| 2296 | **128** | Methylcyclohexane |
| 2297 | **128** | Methylcyclohexanone |
| 2298 | **128** | Methylcyclopentane |
| 2299 | **155** | Methyl dichloroacetate |
| 2300 | **153** | 2-Methyl-5-ethylpyridine |
| 2301 | **128** | 2-Methylfuran |
| 2302 | **127** | 5-Methylhexan-2-one |
| 2303 | **128** | Isopropenylbenzene |
| 2304 | **133** | Naphthalene, molten |
| 2305 | **153** | Nitrobenzenesulfonic acid |
| 2305 | **153** | Nitrobenzenesulphonic acid |
| 2306 | **152** | Nitrobenzotrifluorides |
| 2306 | **152** | Nitrobenzotrifluorides, liquid |
| 2307 | **152** | 3-Nitro-4-chlorobenzotrifluoride |
| 2308 | **157** | Nitrosylsulfuric acid, liquid |
| 2308 | **157** | Nitrosylsulfuric acid, solid |
| 2308 | **157** | Nitrosylsulphuric acid, liquid |
| 2308 | **157** | Nitrosylsulphuric acid, solid |
| 2309 | **128P** | Octadiene |
| 2310 | **131** | Pentane-2,4-dione |
| 2311 | **153** | Phenetidines |
| 2312 | **153** | Phenol, molten |
| 2313 | **129** | Picolines |
| 2315 | **171** | Articles containing Polychlorinated biphenyls (PCB) |
| 2315 | **171** | PCB |
| 2315 | **171** | Polychlorinated biphenyls |
| 2315 | **171** | Polychlorinated biphenyls, liquid |
| 2316 | **157** | Sodium cuprocyanide, solid |
| 2317 | **157** | Sodium cuprocyanide, solution |
| 2318 | **135** | Sodium hydrosulfide, with less than 25% water of crystallization |
| 2318 | **135** | Sodium hydrosulphide, with less than 25% water of crystallization |
| 2319 | **128** | Terpene hydrocarbons, n.o.s. |
| 2320 | **153** | Tetraethylenepentamine |

| ID No. | Guide No. | Name of Material |
|---|---|---|
| 2321 | **153** | Trichlorobenzenes, liquid |
| 2322 | **152** | Trichlorobutene |
| 2323 | **130** | Triethyl phosphite |
| 2324 | **128** | Triisobutylene |
| 2325 | **129** | 1,3,5-Trimethylbenzene |
| 2326 | **153** | Trimethylcyclohexylamine |
| 2327 | **153** | Trimethylhexamethylenediamines |
| 2328 | **156** | Trimethylhexamethylene diisocyanate |
| 2329 | **130** | Trimethyl phosphite |
| 2330 | **128** | Undecane |
| 2331 | **154** | Zinc chloride, anhydrous |
| 2332 | **129** | Acetaldehyde oxime |
| 2333 | **131** | Allyl acetate |
| 2334 | **131** | Allylamine |
| 2335 | **131** | Allyl ethyl ether |
| 2336 | **131** | Allyl formate |
| 2337 | **131** | Phenyl mercaptan |
| 2338 | **127** | Benzotrifluoride |
| 2339 | **130** | 2-Bromobutane |
| 2340 | **130** | 2-Bromoethyl ethyl ether |
| 2341 | **130** | 1-Bromo-3-methylbutane |
| 2342 | **130** | Bromomethylpropanes |
| 2343 | **130** | 2-Bromopentane |
| 2344 | **129** | Bromopropanes |
| 2345 | **130** | 3-Bromopropyne |
| 2346 | **127** | Butanedione |
| 2346 | **127** | Diacetyl |
| 2347 | **130** | Butyl mercaptan |
| 2348 | **129P** | Butyl acrylates, stabilized |
| 2350 | **127** | Butyl methyl ether |
| 2351 | **129** | Butyl nitrites |
| 2352 | **127P** | Butyl vinyl ether, stabilized |
| 2353 | **132** | Butyryl chloride |
| 2354 | **131** | Chloromethyl ethyl ether |
| 2356 | **129** | 2-Chloropropane |
| 2357 | **132** | Cyclohexylamine |
| 2358 | **128P** | Cyclooctatetraene |
| 2359 | **132** | Diallylamine |
| 2360 | **131P** | Diallyl ether |
| 2361 | **132** | Diisobutylamine |
| 2362 | **130** | 1,1-Dichloroethane |
| 2363 | **129** | Ethyl mercaptan |
| 2364 | **128** | n-Propyl benzene |
| 2366 | **128** | Diethyl carbonate |
| 2367 | **130** | alpha-Methylvaleraldehyde |
| 2367 | **130** | Methyl valeraldehyde (alpha) |
| 2368 | **128** | alpha-Pinene |
| 2368 | **128** | Pinene (alpha) |
| 2370 | **128** | 1-Hexene |
| 2371 | **128** | Isopentenes |
| 2372 | **129** | 1,2-Di-(dimethylamino)ethane |
| 2373 | **127** | Diethoxymethane |
| 2374 | **127** | 3,3-Diethoxypropene |
| 2375 | **129** | Diethyl sulfide |
| 2375 | **129** | Diethyl sulphide |
| 2376 | **127** | 2,3-Dihydropyran |
| 2377 | **127** | 1,1-Dimethoxyethane |
| 2378 | **131** | 2-Dimethylaminoacetonitrile |
| 2379 | **132** | 1,3-Dimethylbutylamine |
| 2380 | **127** | Dimethyldiethoxysilane |
| 2381 | **130** | Dimethyl disulfide |

| ID No. | Guide No. | Name of Material |
|---|---|---|
| 2381 | **130** | Dimethyl disulphide |
| 2382 | **131** | Dimethylhydrazine, symmetrical |
| 2383 | **132** | Dipropylamine |
| 2384 | **127** | Di-n-propyl ether |
| 2385 | **129** | Ethyl isobutyrate |
| 2386 | **132** | 1-Ethylpiperidine |
| 2387 | **130** | Fluorobenzene |
| 2388 | **130** | Fluorotoluenes |
| 2389 | **128** | Furan |
| 2390 | **129** | 2-Iodobutane |
| 2391 | **129** | Iodomethylpropanes |
| 2392 | **129** | Iodopropanes |
| 2393 | **129** | Isobutyl formate |
| 2394 | **129** | Isobutyl propionate |
| 2395 | **132** | Isobutyryl chloride |
| 2396 | **131P** | Methacrylaldehyde, stabilized |
| 2397 | **127** | 3-Methylbutan-2-one |
| 2398 | **127** | Methyl tert-butyl ether |
| 2399 | **132** | 1-Methylpiperidine |
| 2400 | **130** | Methyl isovalerate |
| 2401 | **132** | Piperidine |
| 2402 | **130** | Propanethiols |
| 2403 | **129P** | Isopropenyl acetate |
| 2404 | **131** | Propionitrile |
| 2405 | **129** | Isopropyl butyrate |
| 2406 | **127** | Isopropyl isobutyrate |
| 2407 | **155** | Isopropyl chloroformate |
| 2409 | **129** | Isopropyl propionate |
| 2410 | **129** | 1,2,3,6-Tetrahydropyridine |
| 2411 | **131** | Butyronitrile |
| 2412 | **130** | Tetrahydrothiophene |
| 2413 | **128** | Tetrapropyl orthotitanate |
| 2414 | **130** | Thiophene |
| 2416 | **129** | Trimethyl borate |
| 2417 | **125** | Carbonyl fluoride |
| 2417 | **125** | Carbonyl fluoride, compressed |
| 2418 | **125** | Sulfur tetrafluoride |
| 2418 | **125** | Sulphur tetrafluoride |
| 2419 | **116** | Bromotrifluoroethylene |
| 2420 | **125** | Hexafluoroacetone |
| 2421 | **124** | Nitrogen trioxide |
| 2422 | **126** | Octafluorobut-2-ene |
| 2422 | **126** | Refrigerant gas R-1318 |
| 2424 | **126** | Octafluoropropane |
| 2424 | **126** | Refrigerant gas R-218 |
| 2426 | **140** | Ammonium nitrate, liquid (hot concentrated solution) |
| 2427 | **140** | Potassium chlorate, aqueous solution |
| 2428 | **140** | Sodium chlorate, aqueous solution |
| 2429 | **140** | Calcium chlorate, aqueous solution |
| 2430 | **153** | Alkylphenols, solid, n.o.s. (including C2-C12 homologues) |
| 2431 | **153** | Anisidines |
| 2431 | **153** | Anisidines, liquid |
| 2431 | **153** | Anisidines, solid |
| 2432 | **153** | N,N-Diethylaniline |
| 2433 | **152** | Chloronitrotoluenes, liquid |
| 2433 | **152** | Chloronitrotoluenes, solid |
| 2434 | **156** | Dibenzyldichlorosilane |
| 2435 | **156** | Ethylphenyldichlorosilane |
| 2436 | **129** | Thioacetic acid |

| ID No. | Guide No. | Name of Material |
|---|---|---|
| 2437 | **156** | Methylphenyldichlorosilane |
| 2438 | **132** | Trimethylacetyl chloride |
| 2439 | **154** | Sodium hydrogendifluoride |
| 2440 | **154** | Stannic chloride, pentahydrate |
| 2441 | **135** | Titanium trichloride, pyrophoric |
| 2441 | **135** | Titanium trichloride mixture, pyrophoric |
| 2442 | **156** | Trichloroacetyl chloride |
| 2443 | **137** | Vanadium oxytrichloride |
| 2444 | **137** | Vanadium tetrachloride |
| 2445 | **135** | Lithium alkyls |
| 2445 | **135** | Lithium alkyls, liquid |
| 2446 | **153** | Nitrocresols |
| 2446 | **153** | Nitrocresols, solid |
| 2447 | **136** | Phosphorus, white, molten |
| 2447 | **136** | White phosphorus, molten |
| 2448 | **133** | Molten sulfur |
| 2448 | **133** | Molten sulphur |
| 2448 | **133** | Sulfur, molten |
| 2448 | **133** | Sulphur, molten |
| 2451 | **122** | Nitrogen trifluoride |
| 2451 | **122** | Nitrogen trifluoride, compressed |
| 2452 | **116P** | Ethylacetylene, stabilized |
| 2453 | **115** | Ethyl fluoride |
| 2453 | **115** | Refrigerant gas R-161 |
| 2454 | **115** | Methyl fluoride |
| 2454 | **115** | Refrigerant gas R-41 |
| 2455 | **116** | Methyl nitrite |
| 2456 | **130P** | 2-Chloropropene |
| 2457 | **128** | 2,3-Dimethylbutane |
| 2458 | **130** | Hexadiene |
| 2459 | **128** | 2-Methyl-1-butene |
| 2460 | **128** | 2-Methyl-2-butene |
| 2461 | **128** | Methylpentadiene |
| 2463 | **138** | Aluminum hydride |
| 2464 | **141** | Beryllium nitrate |
| 2465 | **140** | Dichloroisocyanuric acid, dry |
| 2465 | **140** | Dichloroisocyanuric acid salts |
| 2465 | **140** | Sodium dichloroisocyanurate |
| 2465 | **140** | Sodium dichloro-s-triazinetrione |
| 2466 | **143** | Potassium superoxide |
| 2468 | **140** | Trichloroisocyanuric acid, dry |
| 2469 | **140** | Zinc bromate |
| 2470 | **152** | Phenylacetonitrile, liquid |
| 2471 | **154** | Osmium tetroxide |
| 2473 | **154** | Sodium arsanilate |
| 2474 | **157** | Thiophosgene |
| 2475 | **157** | Vanadium trichloride |
| 2477 | **131** | Methyl isothiocyanate |
| 2478 | **155** | Isocyanate solution, flammable, poisonous, n.o.s. |
| 2478 | **155** | Isocyanate solution, flammable, toxic, n.o.s. |
| 2478 | **155** | Isocyanates, flammable, poisonous, n.o.s. |
| 2478 | **155** | Isocyanates, flammable, toxic, n.o.s. |
| 2480 | **155** | Methyl isocyanate |
| 2481 | **155** | Ethyl isocyanate |
| 2482 | **155** | n-Propyl isocyanate |
| 2483 | **155** | Isopropyl isocyanate |
| 2484 | **155** | tert-Butyl isocyanate |
| 2485 | **155** | n-Butyl isocyanate |

| ID No. | Guide No. | Name of Material |
|---|---|---|
| 2486 | **155** | Isobutyl isocyanate |
| 2487 | **155** | Phenyl isocyanate |
| 2488 | **155** | Cyclohexyl isocyanate |
| 2490 | **153** | Dichloroisopropyl ether |
| 2491 | **153** | Ethanolamine |
| 2491 | **153** | Ethanolamine, solution |
| 2491 | **153** | Monoethanolamine |
| 2493 | **132** | Hexamethyleneimine |
| 2495 | **144** | Iodine pentafluoride |
| 2496 | **156** | Propionic anhydride |
| 2498 | **129** | 1,2,3,6-Tetrahydrobenzaldehyde |
| 2501 | **152** | Tris-(1-aziridinyl)phosphine oxide, solution |
| 2502 | **132** | Valeryl chloride |
| 2503 | **137** | Zirconium tetrachloride |
| 2504 | **159** | Acetylene tetrabromide |
| 2504 | **159** | Tetrabromoethane |
| 2505 | **154** | Ammonium fluoride |
| 2506 | **154** | Ammonium hydrogen sulfate |
| 2506 | **154** | Ammonium hydrogen sulphate |
| 2507 | **154** | Chloroplatinic acid, solid |
| 2508 | **156** | Molybdenum pentachloride |
| 2509 | **154** | Potassium hydrogen sulfate |
| 2509 | **154** | Potassium hydrogen sulphate |
| 2511 | **153** | 2-Chloropropionic acid |
| 2511 | **153** | 2-Chloropropionic acid, solid |
| 2511 | **153** | 2-Chloropropionic acid, solution |
| 2512 | **152** | Aminophenols |
| 2513 | **156** | Bromoacetyl bromide |
| 2514 | **130** | Bromobenzene |
| 2515 | **159** | Bromoform |
| 2516 | **151** | Carbon tetrabromide |
| 2517 | **115** | 1-Chloro-1,1-difluoroethane |
| 2517 | **115** | Difluorochloroethanes |
| 2517 | **115** | Refrigerant gas R-142b |
| 2518 | **153** | 1,5,9-Cyclododecatriene |
| 2520 | **130P** | Cyclooctadienes |
| 2521 | **131P** | Diketene, stabilized |
| 2522 | **153P** | 2-Dimethylaminoethyl methacrylate |
| 2524 | **129** | Ethyl orthoformate |
| 2525 | **156** | Ethyl oxalate |
| 2526 | **132** | Furfurylamine |
| 2527 | **129P** | Isobutyl acrylate, stabilized |
| 2528 | **130** | Isobutyl isobutyrate |
| 2529 | **132** | Isobutyric acid |
| 2531 | **153P** | Methacrylic acid, stabilized |
| 2533 | **156** | Methyl trichloroacetate |
| 2534 | **119** | Methylchlorosilane |
| 2535 | **132** | 4-Methylmorpholine |
| 2535 | **132** | N-Methylmorpholine |
| 2536 | **127** | Methyltetrahydrofuran |
| 2538 | **133** | Nitronaphthalene |
| 2541 | **128** | Terpinolene |
| 2542 | **153** | Tributylamine |
| 2545 | **135** | Hafnium powder, dry |
| 2546 | **135** | Titanium powder, dry |
| 2547 | **143** | Sodium superoxide |
| 2548 | **124** | Chlorine pentafluoride |
| 2552 | **151** | Hexafluoroacetone hydrate |
| 2552 | **151** | Hexafluoroacetone hydrate, liquid |
| 2554 | **130P** | Methylallyl chloride |

| ID No. | Guide No. | Name of Material |
|---|---|---|
| 2555 | **113** | Nitrocellulose with water, not less than 25% water |
| 2556 | **113** | Nitrocellulose with alcohol |
| 2556 | **113** | Nitrocellulose with not less than 25% alcohol |
| 2557 | **133** | Nitrocellulose mixture, without pigment |
| 2557 | **133** | Nitrocellulose mixture, without plasticizer |
| 2557 | **133** | Nitrocellulose mixture, with pigment |
| 2557 | **133** | Nitrocellulose mixture, with plasticizer |
| 2558 | **131** | Epibromohydrin |
| 2560 | **129** | 2-Methylpentan-2-ol |
| 2561 | **128** | 3-Methyl-1-butene |
| 2564 | **153** | Trichloroacetic acid, solution |
| 2565 | **153** | Dicyclohexylamine |
| 2567 | **154** | Sodium pentachlorophenate |
| 2570 | **154** | Cadmium compound |
| 2571 | **156** | Alkylsulfuric acids |
| 2571 | **156** | Alkylsulphuric acids |
| 2572 | **153** | Phenylhydrazine |
| 2573 | **141** | Thallium chlorate |
| 2574 | **151** | Tricresyl phosphate |
| 2576 | **137** | Phosphorus oxybromide, molten |
| 2577 | **156** | Phenylacetyl chloride |
| 2578 | **157** | Phosphorus trioxide |
| 2579 | **153** | Piperazine |
| 2580 | **154** | Aluminum bromide, solution |
| 2581 | **154** | Aluminum chloride, solution |
| 2582 | **154** | Ferric chloride, solution |
| 2583 | **153** | Alkyl sulfonic acids, solid, with more than 5% free Sulfuric acid |
| 2583 | **153** | Alkyl sulphonic acids, solid, with more than 5% free Sulphuric acid |
| 2583 | **153** | Aryl sulfonic acids, solid, with more than 5% free Sulfuric acid |
| 2583 | **153** | Aryl sulphonic acids, solid, with more than 5% free Sulphuric acid |
| 2584 | **153** | Alkyl sulfonic acids, liquid, with more than 5% free Sulfuric acid |
| 2584 | **153** | Alkyl sulphonic acids, liquid, with more than 5% free Sulphuric acid |
| 2584 | **153** | Aryl sulfonic acids, liquid, with more than 5% free Sulfuric acid |
| 2584 | **153** | Aryl sulphonic acids, liquid, with more than 5% free Sulphuric acid |
| 2585 | **153** | Alkyl sulfonic acids, solid, with not more than 5% free Sulfuric acid |
| 2585 | **153** | Alkyl sulphonic acids, solid, with not more than 5% free Sulphuric acid |
| 2585 | **153** | Aryl sulfonic acids, solid, with not more than 5% free Sulfuric acid |
| 2585 | **153** | Aryl sulphonic acids, solid, with not more than 5% free Sulphuric acid |
| 2586 | **153** | Alkyl sulfonic acids, liquid, with not more than 5% free Sulfuric acid |
| 2586 | **153** | Alkyl sulphonic acids, liquid, with not more than 5% free Sulphuric acid |

| ID No. | Guide No. | Name of Material |
|---|---|---|
| 2586 | **153** | Aryl sulfonic acids, liquid, with not more than 5% free Sulfuric acid |
| 2586 | **153** | Aryl sulphonic acids, liquid, with not more than 5% free Sulphuric acid |
| 2587 | **153** | Benzoquinone |
| 2588 | **151** | Pesticide, solid, poisonous, n.o.s. |
| 2588 | **151** | Pesticide, solid, toxic, n.o.s. |
| 2589 | **155** | Vinyl chloroacetate |
| 2590 | **171** | Asbestos, chrysolite |
| 2590 | **171** | Asbestos, white |
| 2590 | **171** | White asbestos |
| 2591 | **120** | Xenon, refrigerated liquid (cryogenic liquid) |
| 2599 | **126** | Chlorotrifluoromethane and Trifluoromethane azeotropic mixture with approximately 60% Chlorotrifluoromethane |
| 2599 | **126** | Refrigerant gas R-503 |
| 2599 | **126** | Trifluoromethane and Chlorotrifluoromethane azeotropic mixture with approximately 60% Chlorotrifluoromethane |
| 2600 | **119** | Carbon monoxide and Hydrogen mixture, compressed |
| 2600 | **119** | Hydrogen and Carbon monoxide mixture, compressed |
| 2601 | **115** | Cyclobutane |
| 2602 | **126** | Dichlorodifluoromethane and Difluoroethane azeotropic mixture with approximately 74% Dichlorodifluoromethane |
| 2602 | **126** | Difluoroethane and Dichlorodifluoromethane azeotropic mixture with approximately 74% Dichlorodifluoromethane |
| 2602 | **126** | Refrigerant gas R-500 |
| 2603 | **131** | Cycloheptatriene |
| 2604 | **132** | Boron trifluoride diethyl etherate |
| 2605 | **155** | Methoxymethyl isocyanate |
| 2606 | **155** | Methyl orthosilicate |
| 2607 | **129P** | Acrolein dimer, stabilized |
| 2608 | **129** | Nitropropanes |
| 2609 | **156** | Triallyl borate |
| 2610 | **132** | Triallylamine |
| 2611 | **131** | Propylene chlorohydrin |
| 2612 | **127** | Methyl propyl ether |
| 2614 | **129** | Methallyl alcohol |
| 2615 | **127** | Ethyl propyl ether |
| 2616 | **129** | Triisopropyl borate |
| 2617 | **129** | Methylcyclohexanols |
| 2618 | **130P** | Vinyltoluenes, stabilized |
| 2619 | **132** | Benzyldimethylamine |
| 2620 | **130** | Amyl butyrates |
| 2621 | **127** | Acetyl methyl carbinol |
| 2622 | **131P** | Glycidaldehyde |
| 2623 | **133** | Firelighters, solid, with flammable liquid |
| 2624 | **138** | Magnesium silicide |
| 2626 | **140** | Chloric acid, aqueous solution, with not more than 10% Chloric acid |
| 2627 | **140** | Nitrites, inorganic, n.o.s. |
| 2628 | **151** | Potassium fluoroacetate |
| 2629 | **151** | Sodium fluoroacetate |
| 2630 | **151** | Selenates |
| 2630 | **151** | Selenites |
| 2642 | **154** | Fluoroacetic acid |

| ID No. | Guide No. | Name of Material |
|---|---|---|
| 2643 | **155** | Methyl bromoacetate |
| 2644 | **151** | Methyl iodide |
| 2645 | **153** | Phenacyl bromide |
| 2646 | **151** | Hexachlorocyclopentadiene |
| 2647 | **153** | Malononitrile |
| 2648 | **154** | 1,2-Dibromobutan-3-one |
| 2649 | **153** | 1,3-Dichloroacetone |
| 2650 | **153** | 1,1-Dichloro-1-nitroethane |
| 2651 | **153** | 4,4'-Diaminodiphenylmethane |
| 2653 | **156** | Benzyl iodide |
| 2655 | **151** | Potassium fluorosilicate |
| 2655 | **151** | Potassium silicofluoride |
| 2656 | **154** | Quinoline |
| 2657 | **153** | Selenium disulfide |
| 2657 | **153** | Selenium disulphide |
| 2659 | **151** | Sodium chloroacetate |
| 2660 | **153** | Mononitrotoluidines |
| 2660 | **153** | Nitrotoluidines (mono) |
| 2661 | **153** | Hexachloroacetone |
| 2662 | **153** | Hydroquinone |
| 2664 | **160** | Dibromomethane |
| 2667 | **152** | Butyltoluenes |
| 2668 | **131** | Chloroacetonitrile |
| 2669 | **152** | Chlorocresols |
| 2669 | **152** | Chlorocresols, solution |
| 2670 | **157** | Cyanuric chloride |
| 2671 | **153** | Aminopyridines |
| 2672 | **154** | Ammonia, solution, with more than 10% but not more than 35% Ammonia |
| 2672 | **154** | Ammonium hydroxide |
| 2672 | **154** | Ammonium hydroxide, with more than 10% but not more than 35% Ammonia |
| 2673 | **151** | 2-Amino-4-chlorophenol |
| 2674 | **154** | Sodium fluorosilicate |
| 2674 | **154** | Sodium silicofluoride |
| 2676 | **119** | Stibine |
| 2677 | **154** | Rubidium hydroxide, solution |
| 2678 | **154** | Rubidium hydroxide |
| 2678 | **154** | Rubidium hydroxide, solid |
| 2679 | **154** | Lithium hydroxide, solution |
| 2680 | **154** | Lithium hydroxide |
| 2680 | **154** | Lithium hydroxide, monohydrate |
| 2681 | **154** | Caesium hydroxide, solution |
| 2681 | **154** | Cesium hydroxide, solution |
| 2682 | **157** | Caesium hydroxide |
| 2682 | **157** | Cesium hydroxide |
| 2683 | **132** | Ammonium sulfide, solution |
| 2683 | **132** | Ammonium sulphide, solution |
| 2684 | **132** | 3-Diethylaminopropylamine |
| 2684 | **132** | Diethylaminopropylamine |
| 2685 | **132** | N,N-Diethylethylenediamine |
| 2686 | **132** | 2-Diethylaminoethanol |
| 2687 | **133** | Dicyclohexylammonium nitrite |
| 2688 | **159** | 1-Bromo-3-chloropropane |
| 2689 | **153** | Glycerol alpha-monochlorohydrin |
| 2690 | **152** | N,n-Butylimidazole |
| 2691 | **137** | Phosphorus pentabromide |
| 2692 | **157** | Boron tribromide |
| 2693 | **154** | Bisulfites, aqueous solution, n.o.s. |

| ID No. | Guide No. | Name of Material |
|---|---|---|
| 2693 | **154** | Bisulphites, aqueous solution, n.o.s. |
| 2698 | **156** | Tetrahydrophthalic anhydrides |
| 2699 | **154** | Trifluoroacetic acid |
| 2705 | **153P** | 1-Pentol |
| 2707 | **127** | Dimethyldioxanes |
| 2709 | **128** | Butylbenzenes |
| 2710 | **128** | Dipropyl ketone |
| 2713 | **153** | Acridine |
| 2714 | **133** | Zinc resinate |
| 2715 | **133** | Aluminum resinate |
| 2716 | **153** | 1,4-Butynediol |
| 2717 | **133** | Camphor |
| 2717 | **133** | Camphor, synthetic |
| 2719 | **141** | Barium bromate |
| 2720 | **141** | Chromium nitrate |
| 2721 | **141** | Copper chlorate |
| 2722 | **140** | Lithium nitrate |
| 2723 | **140** | Magnesium chlorate |
| 2724 | **140** | Manganese nitrate |
| 2725 | **140** | Nickel nitrate |
| 2726 | **140** | Nickel nitrite |
| 2727 | **141** | Thallium nitrate |
| 2728 | **140** | Zirconium nitrate |
| 2729 | **152** | Hexachlorobenzene |
| 2730 | **152** | Nitroanisoles, liquid |
| 2730 | **152** | Nitroanisoles, solid |
| 2732 | **152** | Nitrobromobenzenes, liquid |
| 2732 | **152** | Nitrobromobenzenes, solid |
| 2733 | **132** | Amines, flammable, corrosive, n.o.s. |
| 2733 | **132** | Polyalkylamines, n.o.s. |
| 2733 | **132** | Polyamines, flammable, corrosive, n.o.s. |
| 2734 | **132** | Amines, liquid, corrosive, flammable, n.o.s. |
| 2734 | **132** | Polyalkylamines, n.o.s. |
| 2734 | **132** | Polyamines, liquid, corrosive, flammable, n.o.s. |
| 2735 | **153** | Amines, liquid, corrosive, n.o.s. |
| 2735 | **153** | Polyalkylamines, n.o.s. |
| 2735 | **153** | Polyamines, liquid, corrosive, n.o.s. |
| 2738 | **153** | N-Butylaniline |
| 2739 | **156** | Butyric anhydride |
| 2740 | **155** | n-Propyl chloroformate |
| 2741 | **141** | Barium hypochlorite, with more than 22% available Chlorine |
| 2742 | **155** | sec-Butyl chloroformate |
| 2742 | **155** | Chloroformates, poisonous, corrosive, flammable, n.o.s. |
| 2742 | **155** | Chloroformates, toxic, corrosive, flammable, n.o.s. |
| 2742 | **155** | Isobutyl chloroformate |
| 2743 | **155** | n-Butyl chloroformate |
| 2744 | **155** | Cyclobutyl chloroformate |
| 2745 | **157** | Chloromethyl chloroformate |
| 2746 | **156** | Phenyl chloroformate |
| 2747 | **156** | tert-Butylcyclohexyl chloroformate |
| 2748 | **156** | 2-Ethylhexyl chloroformate |
| 2749 | **130** | Tetramethylsilane |
| 2750 | **153** | 1,3-Dichloropropanol-2 |
| 2751 | **155** | Diethylthiophosphoryl chloride |
| 2752 | **127** | 1,2-Epoxy-3-ethoxypropane |
| 2753 | **153** | N-Ethylbenzyltoluidines, liquid |

| ID No. | Guide No. | Name of Material |
| --- | --- | --- |
| 2753 | **153** | N-Ethylbenzyltoluidines, solid |
| 2754 | **153** | N-Ethyltoluidines |
| 2757 | **151** | Carbamate pesticide, solid, poisonous |
| 2757 | **151** | Carbamate pesticide, solid, toxic |
| 2758 | **131** | Carbamate pesticide, liquid, flammable, poisonous |
| 2758 | **131** | Carbamate pesticide, liquid, flammable, toxic |
| 2759 | **151** | Arsenical pesticide, solid, poisonous |
| 2759 | **151** | Arsenical pesticide, solid, toxic |
| 2760 | **131** | Arsenical pesticide, liquid, flammable, poisonous |
| 2760 | **131** | Arsenical pesticide, liquid, flammable, toxic |
| 2761 | **151** | Organochlorine pesticide, solid, poisonous |
| 2761 | **151** | Organochlorine pesticide, solid, toxic |
| 2762 | **131** | Organochlorine pesticide, liquid, flammable, poisonous |
| 2762 | **131** | Organochlorine pesticide, liquid, flammable, toxic |
| 2763 | **151** | Triazine pesticide, solid, poisonous |
| 2763 | **151** | Triazine pesticide, solid, toxic |
| 2764 | **131** | Triazine pesticide, liquid, flammable, poisonous |
| 2764 | **131** | Triazine pesticide, liquid, flammable, toxic |
| 2771 | **151** | Thiocarbamate pesticide, solid, poisonous |
| 2771 | **151** | Thiocarbamate pesticide, solid, toxic |
| 2772 | **131** | Thiocarbamate pesticide, liquid, flammable, poisonous |

| ID No. | Guide No. | Name of Material |
| --- | --- | --- |
| 2772 | **131** | Thiocarbamate pesticide, liquid, flammable, toxic |
| 2775 | **151** | Copper based pesticide, solid, poisonous |
| 2775 | **151** | Copper based pesticide, solid, toxic |
| 2776 | **131** | Copper based pesticide, liquid, flammable, poisonous |
| 2776 | **131** | Copper based pesticide, liquid, flammable, toxic |
| 2777 | **151** | Mercury based pesticide, solid, poisonous |
| 2777 | **151** | Mercury based pesticide, solid, toxic |
| 2778 | **131** | Mercury based pesticide, liquid, flammable, poisonous |
| 2778 | **131** | Mercury based pesticide, liquid, flammable, toxic |
| 2779 | **153** | Substituted nitrophenol pesticide, solid, poisonous |
| 2779 | **153** | Substituted nitrophenol pesticide, solid, toxic |
| 2780 | **131** | Substituted nitrophenol pesticide, liquid, flammable, poisonous |
| 2780 | **131** | Substituted nitrophenol pesticide, liquid, flammable, toxic |
| 2781 | **151** | Bipyridilium pesticide, solid, poisonous |
| 2781 | **151** | Bipyridilium pesticide, solid, toxic |
| 2782 | **131** | Bipyridilium pesticide, liquid, flammable, poisonous |
| 2782 | **131** | Bipyridilium pesticide, liquid, flammable, toxic |
| 2783 | **152** | Organophosphorus pesticide, solid, poisonous |
| 2783 | **152** | Organophosphorus pesticide, solid, toxic |

| ID No. | Guide No. | Name of Material |
|---|---|---|
| 2784 | **131** | Organophosphorus pesticide, liquid, flammable, poisonous |
| 2784 | **131** | Organophosphorus pesticide, liquid, flammable, toxic |
| 2785 | **152** | 4-Thiapentanal |
| 2786 | **153** | Organotin pesticide, solid, poisonous |
| 2786 | **153** | Organotin pesticide, solid, toxic |
| 2787 | **131** | Organotin pesticide, liquid, flammable, poisonous |
| 2787 | **131** | Organotin pesticide, liquid, flammable, toxic |
| 2788 | **153** | Organotin compound, liquid, n.o.s. |
| 2789 | **132** | Acetic acid, glacial |
| 2789 | **132** | Acetic acid, solution, more than 80% acid |
| 2790 | **153** | Acetic acid, solution, more than 10% but not more than 80% acid |
| 2793 | **170** | Ferrous metal borings, shavings, turnings or cuttings |
| 2794 | **154** | Batteries, wet, filled with acid |
| 2795 | **154** | Batteries, wet, filled with alkali |
| 2796 | **157** | Battery fluid, acid |
| 2796 | **157** | Sulfuric acid, with not more than 51% acid |
| 2796 | **157** | Sulphuric acid, with not more than 51% acid |
| 2797 | **154** | Battery fluid, alkali |
| 2798 | **137** | Benzene phosphorus dichloride |
| 2798 | **137** | Phenylphosphorus dichloride |
| 2799 | **137** | Benzene phosphorus thiodichloride |
| 2799 | **137** | Phenylphosphorus thiodichloride |
| 2800 | **154** | Batteries, wet, non-spillable |

| ID No. | Guide No. | Name of Material |
|---|---|---|
| 2801 | **154** | Dye, liquid, corrosive, n.o.s. |
| 2801 | **154** | Dye intermediate, liquid, corrosive, n.o.s. |
| 2802 | **154** | Copper chloride |
| 2803 | **172** | Gallium |
| 2805 | **138** | Lithium hydride, fused solid |
| 2806 | **138** | Lithium nitride |
| 2807 | **171** | Magnetized material |
| 2809 | **172** | Mercury |
| 2809 | **172** | Mercury metal |
| 2810 | **153** | Buzz |
| 2810 | **153** | BZ |
| 2810 | **153** | Compounds, tree or weed killing, liquid (toxic) |
| 2810 | **153** | CS |
| 2810 | **153** | DC |
| 2810 | **153** | GA |
| 2810 | **153** | GB |
| 2810 | **153** | GD |
| 2810 | **153** | GF |
| 2810 | **153** | H |
| 2810 | **153** | HD |
| 2810 | **153** | HL |
| 2810 | **153** | HN-1 |
| 2810 | **153** | HN-2 |
| 2810 | **153** | HN-3 |
| 2810 | **153** | L (Lewisite) |
| 2810 | **153** | Lewisite |
| 2810 | **153** | Mustard |
| 2810 | **153** | Mustard Lewisite |
| 2810 | **153** | Poisonous liquid, organic, n.o.s. |

| ID No. | Guide No. | Name of Material |
|---|---|---|
| 2810 | **153** | Sarin |
| 2810 | **153** | Soman |
| 2810 | **153** | Tabun |
| 2810 | **153** | Thickened GD |
| 2810 | **153** | Toxic liquid, organic, n.o.s. |
| 2810 | **153** | VX |
| 2811 | **154** | CX |
| 2811 | **154** | Poisonous solid, organic, n.o.s. |
| 2811 | **154** | Toxic solid, organic, n.o.s. |
| 2812 | **154** | Sodium aluminate, solid |
| 2813 | **138** | Water-reactive solid, n.o.s. |
| 2814 | **158** | Infectious substance, affecting humans |
| 2815 | **153** | N-Aminoethylpiperazine |
| 2817 | **154** | Ammonium bifluoride, solution |
| 2817 | **154** | Ammonium hydrogendifluoride, solution |
| 2818 | **154** | Ammonium polysulfide, solution |
| 2818 | **154** | Ammonium polysulphide, solution |
| 2819 | **153** | Amyl acid phosphate |
| 2820 | **153** | Butyric acid |
| 2821 | **153** | Phenol solution |
| 2822 | **153** | 2-Chloropyridine |
| 2823 | **153** | Crotonic acid |
| 2823 | **153** | Crotonic acid, liquid |
| 2823 | **153** | Crotonic acid, solid |
| 2826 | **155** | Ethyl chlorothioformate |
| 2829 | **153** | Caproic acid |
| 2829 | **153** | Hexanoic acid |
| 2830 | **139** | Lithium ferrosilicon |
| 2831 | **160** | 1,1,1-Trichloroethane |
| 2834 | **154** | Phosphorous acid |
| 2835 | **138** | Sodium aluminum hydride |
| 2837 | **154** | Bisulfates, aqueous solution |
| 2837 | **154** | Bisulphates, aqueous solution |
| 2837 | **154** | Sodium bisulfate, solution |
| 2837 | **154** | Sodium bisulphate, solution |
| 2838 | **129P** | Vinyl butyrate, stabilized |
| 2839 | **153** | Aldol |
| 2840 | **129** | Butyraldoxime |
| 2841 | **131** | Di-n-amylamine |
| 2842 | **129** | Nitroethane |
| 2844 | **138** | Calcium manganese silicon |
| 2845 | **135** | Ethyl phosphonous dichloride, anhydrous |
| 2845 | **135** | Methyl phosphonous dichloride |
| 2845 | **135** | Pyrophoric liquid, organic, n.o.s. |
| 2846 | **135** | Pyrophoric solid, organic, n.o.s. |
| 2849 | **153** | 3-Chloropropanol-1 |
| 2850 | **128** | Propylene tetramer |
| 2851 | **157** | Boron trifluoride, dihydrate |
| 2852 | **113** | Dipicryl sulfide, wetted with not less than 10% water |
| 2852 | **113** | Dipicryl sulphide, wetted with not less than 10% water |
| 2853 | **151** | Magnesium fluorosilicate |
| 2853 | **151** | Magnesium silicofluoride |
| 2854 | **151** | Ammonium fluorosilicate |
| 2854 | **151** | Ammonium silicofluoride |
| 2855 | **151** | Zinc fluorosilicate |
| 2855 | **151** | Zinc silicofluoride |
| 2856 | **151** | Fluorosilicates, n.o.s. |
| 2856 | **151** | Silicofluorides, n.o.s. |

| ID No. | Guide No. | Name of Material |
|---|---|---|
| 2857 | **126** | Refrigerating machines, containing Ammonia solutions (UN2672) |
| 2857 | **126** | Refrigerating machines, containing non-flammable, non-poisonous gases |
| 2857 | **126** | Refrigerating machines, containing non-flammable, non-toxic gases |
| 2858 | **170** | Zirconium, dry, coiled wire, finished metal sheets or strip |
| 2859 | **154** | Ammonium metavanadate |
| 2861 | **151** | Ammonium polyvanadate |
| 2862 | **151** | Vanadium pentoxide |
| 2863 | **154** | Sodium ammonium vanadate |
| 2864 | **151** | Potassium metavanadate |
| 2865 | **154** | Hydroxylamine sulfate |
| 2865 | **154** | Hydroxylamine sulphate |
| 2869 | **157** | Titanium trichloride mixture |
| 2870 | **135** | Aluminum borohydride |
| 2870 | **135** | Aluminum borohydride in devices |
| 2871 | **170** | Antimony powder |
| 2872 | **159** | Dibromochloropropanes |
| 2873 | **153** | Dibutylaminoethanol |
| 2874 | **153** | Furfuryl alcohol |
| 2875 | **151** | Hexachlorophene |
| 2876 | **153** | Resorcinol |
| 2878 | **170** | Titanium sponge granules |
| 2878 | **170** | Titanium sponge powders |
| 2879 | **157** | Selenium oxychloride |
| 2880 | **140** | Calcium hypochlorite, hydrated, with not less than 5.5% but not more than 16% water |
| 2880 | **140** | Calcium hypochlorite, hydrated mixture, with not less than 5.5% but not more than 16% water |
| 2881 | **135** | Metal catalyst, dry |
| 2881 | **135** | Nickel catalyst, dry |
| 2900 | **158** | Infectious substance, affecting animals only |
| 2901 | **124** | Bromine chloride |
| 2902 | **151** | Pesticide, liquid, poisonous, n.o.s. |
| 2902 | **151** | Pesticide, liquid, toxic, n.o.s. |
| 2903 | **131** | Pesticide, liquid, poisonous, flammable, n.o.s. |
| 2903 | **131** | Pesticide, liquid, toxic, flammable, n.o.s. |
| 2904 | **154** | Chlorophenolates, liquid |
| 2904 | **154** | Phenolates, liquid |
| 2905 | **154** | Chlorophenolates, solid |
| 2905 | **154** | Phenolates, solid |
| 2907 | **133** | Isosorbide dinitrate mixture |
| 2908 | **161** | Radioactive material, excepted package, empty packaging |
| 2909 | **161** | Radioactive material, excepted package, articles manufactured from depleted Uranium |
| 2909 | **161** | Radioactive material, excepted package, articles manufactured from natural Thorium |
| 2909 | **161** | Radioactive material, excepted package, articles manufactured from natural Uranium |
| 2910 | **161** | Radioactive material, excepted package, limited quantity of material |

| ID No. | Guide No. | Name of Material |
|---|---|---|
| 2911 | **161** | Radioactive material, excepted package, instruments or articles |
| 2912 | **162** | Radioactive material, low specific activity (LSA-I), non fissile or fissile-excepted |
| 2913 | **162** | Radioactive material, surface contaminated objects (SCO-I), non fissile or fissile-excepted |
| 2913 | **162** | Radioactive material, surface contaminated objects (SCO-II), non fissile or fissile-excepted |
| 2915 | **163** | Radioactive material, Type A package, non-special form, non fissile or fissile-excepted |
| 2916 | **163** | Radioactive material, Type B(U) package, non fissile or fissile-excepted |
| 2917 | **163** | Radioactive material, Type B(M) package, non fissile or fissile-excepted |
| 2919 | **163** | Radioactive material, transported under special arrangement, non fissile or fissile-excepted |
| 2920 | **132** | Corrosive liquid, flammable, n.o.s. |
| 2921 | **134** | Corrosive solid, flammable, n.o.s. |
| 2922 | **154** | Corrosive liquid, poisonous, n.o.s. |
| 2922 | **154** | Corrosive liquid, toxic, n.o.s. |
| 2923 | **154** | Corrosive solid, poisonous, n.o.s. |
| 2923 | **154** | Corrosive solid, toxic, n.o.s. |
| 2924 | **132** | Flammable liquid, corrosive, n.o.s |
| 2925 | **134** | Flammable solid, corrosive, organic, n.o.s. |
| 2926 | **134** | Flammable solid, poisonous, organic, n.o.s. |
| 2926 | **134** | Flammable solid, toxic, organic, n.o.s. |
| 2927 | **154** | Ethyl phosphonothioic dichloride, anhydrous |
| 2927 | **154** | Ethyl phosphorodichloridate |
| 2927 | **154** | Poisonous liquid, corrosive, organic, n.o.s. |
| 2927 | **154** | Toxic liquid, corrosive, organic, n.o.s. |
| 2928 | **154** | Poisonous solid, corrosive, organic, n.o.s. |
| 2928 | **154** | Toxic solid, corrosive, organic, n.o.s. |
| 2929 | **131** | Poisonous liquid, flammable, organic, n.o.s. |
| 2929 | **131** | Toxic liquid, flammable, organic, n.o.s. |
| 2930 | **134** | Poisonous solid, flammable, organic, n.o.s. |
| 2930 | **134** | Toxic solid, flammable, organic, n.o.s. |
| 2931 | **151** | Vanadyl sulfate |
| 2931 | **151** | Vanadyl sulphate |
| 2933 | **129** | Methyl 2-chloropropionate |
| 2934 | **129** | Isopropyl 2-chloropropionate |
| 2935 | **129** | Ethyl 2-chloropropionate |
| 2936 | **153** | Thiolactic acid |
| 2937 | **153** | alpha-Methylbenzyl alcohol |
| 2937 | **153** | alpha-Methylbenzyl alcohol, liquid |
| 2937 | **153** | Methylbenzyl alcohol (alpha) |
| 2940 | **135** | Cyclooctadiene phosphines |
| 2940 | **135** | 9-Phosphabicyclononanes |
| 2941 | **153** | Fluoroanilines |

| ID No. | Guide No. | Name of Material |
|---|---|---|
| 2942 | **153** | 2-Trifluoromethylaniline |
| 2943 | **129** | Tetrahydrofurfurylamine |
| 2945 | **132** | N-Methylbutylamine |
| 2946 | **153** | 2-Amino-5-diethylaminopentane |
| 2947 | **155** | Isopropyl chloroacetate |
| 2948 | **153** | 3-Trifluoromethylaniline |
| 2949 | **154** | Sodium hydrosulfide, hydrated, with not less than 25% water of crystallization |
| 2949 | **154** | Sodium hydrosulfide, with not less than 25% water of crystallization |
| 2949 | **154** | Sodium hydrosulphide, hydrated, with not less than 25% water of crystallization |
| 2949 | **154** | Sodium hydrosulphide, with not less than 25% water of crystallization |
| 2950 | **138** | Magnesium granules, coated |
| 2956 | **149** | 5-tert-Butyl-2,4,6-trinitro-m-xylene |
| 2956 | **149** | Musk xylene |
| 2965 | **139** | Boron trifluoride dimethyl etherate |
| 2966 | **153** | Thioglycol |
| 2967 | **154** | Sulfamic acid |
| 2967 | **154** | Sulphamic acid |
| 2968 | **135** | Maneb, stabilized |
| 2968 | **135** | Maneb preparation, stabilized |
| 2969 | **171** | Castor beans, meal, pomace or flake |
| 2977 | **166** | Radioactive material, Uranium hexafluoride, fissile |
| 2977 | **166** | Uranium hexafluoride, radioactive material, fissile |
| 2978 | **166** | Radioactive material, Uranium hexafluoride, non fissile or fissile-excepted |
| 2978 | **166** | Uranium hexafluoride, radioactive material, non fissile or fissile-excepted |
| 2983 | **129P** | Ethylene oxide and Propylene oxide mixture, with not more than 30% Ethylene oxide |
| 2983 | **129P** | Propylene oxide and Ethylene oxide mixture, with not more than 30% Ethylene oxide |
| 2984 | **140** | Hydrogen peroxide, aqueous solution, with not less than 8% but less than 20% Hydrogen peroxide |
| 2985 | **155** | Chlorosilanes, flammable, corrosive, n.o.s. |
| 2986 | **155** | Chlorosilanes, corrosive, flammable, n.o.s. |
| 2987 | **156** | Chlorosilanes, corrosive, n.o.s. |
| 2988 | **139** | Chlorosilanes, water-reactive, flammable, corrosive, n.o.s. |
| 2989 | **133** | Lead phosphite, dibasic |
| 2990 | **171** | Life-saving appliances, self-inflating |
| 2991 | **131** | Carbamate pesticide, liquid, poisonous, flammable |
| 2991 | **131** | Carbamate pesticide, liquid, toxic, flammable |
| 2992 | **151** | Carbamate pesticide, liquid, poisonous |
| 2992 | **151** | Carbamate pesticide, liquid, toxic |
| 2993 | **131** | Arsenical pesticide, liquid, poisonous, flammable |
| 2993 | **131** | Arsenical pesticide, liquid, toxic, flammable |
| 2994 | **151** | Arsenical pesticide, liquid, poisonous |

| ID No. | Guide No. | Name of Material |
|---|---|---|
| 2994 | **151** | Arsenical pesticide, liquid, toxic |
| 2995 | **131** | Organochlorine pesticide, liquid, poisonous, flammable |
| 2995 | **131** | Organochlorine pesticide, liquid, toxic, flammable |
| 2996 | **151** | Organochlorine pesticide, liquid, poisonous |
| 2996 | **151** | Organochlorine pesticide, liquid, toxic |
| 2997 | **131** | Triazine pesticide, liquid, poisonous, flammable |
| 2997 | **131** | Triazine pesticide, liquid, toxic, flammable |
| 2998 | **151** | Triazine pesticide, liquid, poisonous |
| 2998 | **151** | Triazine pesticide, liquid, toxic |
| 3002 | **151** | Phenyl urea pesticide, liquid, poisonous |
| 3002 | **151** | Phenyl urea pesticide, liquid, toxic |
| 3005 | **131** | Thiocarbamate pesticide, liquid, poisonous, flammable |
| 3005 | **131** | Thiocarbamate pesticide, liquid, toxic, flammable |
| 3006 | **151** | Thiocarbamate pesticide, liquid, poisonous |
| 3006 | **151** | Thiocarbamate pesticide, liquid, toxic |
| 3009 | **131** | Copper based pesticide, liquid, poisonous, flammable |
| 3009 | **131** | Copper based pesticide, liquid, toxic, flammable |
| 3010 | **151** | Copper based pesticide, liquid, poisonous |
| 3010 | **151** | Copper based pesticide, liquid, toxic |
| 3011 | **131** | Mercury based pesticide, liquid, poisonous, flammable |
| 3011 | **131** | Mercury based pesticide, liquid, toxic, flammable |
| 3012 | **151** | Mercury based pesticide, liquid, poisonous |
| 3012 | **151** | Mercury based pesticide, liquid, toxic |
| 3013 | **131** | Substituted nitrophenol pesticide, liquid, poisonous, flammable |
| 3013 | **131** | Substituted nitrophenol pesticide, liquid, toxic, flammable |
| 3014 | **153** | Substituted nitrophenol pesticide, liquid, poisonous |
| 3014 | **153** | Substituted nitrophenol pesticide, liquid, toxic |
| 3015 | **131** | Bipyridilium pesticide, liquid, poisonous, flammable |
| 3015 | **131** | Bipyridilium pesticide, liquid, toxic, flammable |
| 3016 | **151** | Bipyridilium pesticide, liquid, poisonous |
| 3016 | **151** | Bipyridilium pesticide, liquid, toxic |
| 3017 | **131** | Organophosphorus pesticide, liquid, poisonous, flammable |
| 3017 | **131** | Organophosphorus pesticide, liquid, toxic, flammable |
| 3018 | **152** | Organophosphorus pesticide, liquid, poisonous |
| 3018 | **152** | Organophosphorus pesticide, liquid, toxic |
| 3019 | **131** | Organotin pesticide, liquid, poisonous, flammable |
| 3019 | **131** | Organotin pesticide, liquid, toxic, flammable |
| 3020 | **153** | Organotin pesticide, liquid, poisonous |
| 3020 | **153** | Organotin pesticide, liquid, toxic |

| ID No. | Guide No. | Name of Material |
|---|---|---|
| 3021 | **131** | Pesticide, liquid, flammable, poisonous, n.o.s. |
| 3021 | **131** | Pesticide, liquid, flammable, toxic, n.o.s. |
| 3022 | **127P** | 1,2-Butylene oxide, stabilized |
| 3023 | **131** | 2-Methyl-2-heptanethiol |
| 3024 | **131** | Coumarin derivative pesticide, liquid, flammable, poisonous |
| 3024 | **131** | Coumarin derivative pesticide, liquid, flammable, toxic |
| 3025 | **131** | Coumarin derivative pesticide, liquid, poisonous, flammable |
| 3025 | **131** | Coumarin derivative pesticide, liquid, toxic, flammable |
| 3026 | **151** | Coumarin derivative pesticide, liquid, poisonous |
| 3026 | **151** | Coumarin derivative pesticide, liquid, toxic |
| 3027 | **151** | Coumarin derivative pesticide, solid, poisonous |
| 3027 | **151** | Coumarin derivative pesticide, solid, toxic |
| 3028 | **154** | Batteries, dry, containing Potassium hydroxide solid |
| 3048 | **157** | Aluminum phosphide pesticide |
| 3049 | **138** | Metal alkyl halides, water-reactive, n.o.s. |
| 3049 | **138** | Metal aryl halides, water-reactive, n.o.s. |
| 3050 | **138** | Metal alkyl hydrides, water-reactive, n.o.s. |
| 3050 | **138** | Metal aryl hydrides, water-reactive, n.o.s. |
| 3051 | **135** | Aluminum alkyls |
| 3052 | **135** | Aluminum alkyl halides, liquid |
| 3052 | **135** | Aluminum alkyl halides, solid |
| 3053 | **135** | Magnesium alkyls |
| 3054 | **129** | Cyclohexanethiol |
| 3054 | **129** | Cyclohexyl mercaptan |
| 3055 | **154** | 2-(2-Aminoethoxy)ethanol |
| 3056 | **129** | n-Heptaldehyde |
| 3057 | **125** | Trifluoroacetyl chloride |
| 3064 | **127** | Nitroglycerin, solution in alcohol, with more than 1% but not more than 5% Nitroglycerin |
| 3065 | **127** | Alcoholic beverages |
| 3066 | **153** | Paint (corrosive) |
| 3066 | **153** | Paint related material (corrosive) |
| 3070 | **126** | Dichlorodifluoromethane and Ethylene oxide mixture, with not more than 12.5% Ethylene oxide |
| 3070 | **126** | Ethylene oxide and Dichlorodifluoromethane mixture, with not more than 12.5% Ethylene oxide |
| 3071 | **131** | Mercaptan mixture, liquid, poisonous, flammable, n.o.s. |
| 3071 | **131** | Mercaptan mixture, liquid, toxic, flammable, n.o.s. |
| 3071 | **131** | Mercaptans, liquid, poisonous, flammable, n.o.s. |
| 3071 | **131** | Mercaptans, liquid, toxic, flammable, n.o.s. |
| 3072 | **171** | Life-saving appliances, not self-inflating |
| 3073 | **131P** | Vinylpyridines, stabilized |
| 3076 | **138** | Aluminum alkyl hydrides |
| 3077 | **171** | Environmentally hazardous substance, solid, n.o.s. |
| 3077 | **171** | Hazardous waste, solid, n.o.s. |
| 3077 | **171** | Other regulated substances, solid, n.o.s. |

| ID No. | Guide No. | Name of Material |
|---|---|---|
| 3078 | **138** | Cerium, turnings or gritty powder |
| 3079 | **131P** | Methacrylonitrile, stabilized |
| 3080 | **155** | Isocyanate solution, poisonous, flammable, n.o.s. |
| 3080 | **155** | Isocyanate solution, toxic, flammable, n.o.s. |
| 3080 | **155** | Isocyanates, poisonous, flammable, n.o.s. |
| 3080 | **155** | Isocyanates, toxic, flammable, n.o.s. |
| 3082 | **171** | Environmentally hazardous substance, liquid, n.o.s. |
| 3082 | **171** | Hazardous waste, liquid, n.o.s. |
| 3082 | **171** | Other regulated substances, liquid, n.o.s. |
| 3083 | **124** | Perchloryl fluoride |
| 3084 | **140** | Corrosive solid, oxidizing, n.o.s. |
| 3085 | **140** | Oxidizing solid, corrosive, n.o.s. |
| 3086 | **141** | Poisonous solid, oxidizing, n.o.s. |
| 3086 | **141** | Toxic solid, oxidizing, n.o.s. |
| 3087 | **141** | Oxidizing solid, poisonous, n.o.s. |
| 3087 | **141** | Oxidizing solid, toxic, n.o.s. |
| 3088 | **135** | Self-heating solid, organic, n.o.s. |
| 3089 | **170** | Metal powder, flammable, n.o.s. |
| 3090 | **138** | Lithium batteries |
| 3090 | **138** | Lithium metal batteries (including lithium alloy batteries) |
| 3091 | **138** | Lithium batteries contained in equipment |
| 3091 | **138** | Lithium batteries packed with equipment |
| 3091 | **138** | Lithium metal batteries contained in equipment (including lithium alloy batteries) |
| 3091 | **138** | Lithium metal batteries packed with equipment (including lithium alloy batteries) |
| 3092 | **129** | 1-Methoxy-2-propanol |
| 3093 | **140** | Corrosive liquid, oxidizing, n.o.s. |
| 3094 | **138** | Corrosive liquid, water-reactive, n.o.s. |
| 3095 | **136** | Corrosive solid, self-heating, n.o.s. |
| 3096 | **138** | Corrosive solid, water-reactive, n.o.s. |
| 3097 | **140** | Flammable solid, oxidizing, n.o.s. |
| 3098 | **140** | Oxidizing liquid, corrosive, n.o.s. |
| 3099 | **142** | Oxidizing liquid, poisonous, n.o.s. |
| 3099 | **142** | Oxidizing liquid, toxic, n.o.s. |
| 3100 | **135** | Oxidizing solid, self-heating, n.o.s. |
| 3101 | **146** | Organic peroxide type B, liquid |
| 3102 | **146** | Organic peroxide type B, solid |
| 3103 | **146** | Organic peroxide type C, liquid |
| 3104 | **146** | Organic peroxide type C, solid |
| 3105 | **145** | Organic peroxide type D, liquid |
| 3106 | **145** | Organic peroxide type D, solid |
| 3107 | **145** | Organic peroxide type E, liquid |
| 3108 | **145** | Organic peroxide type E, solid |
| 3109 | **145** | Organic peroxide type F, liquid |
| 3110 | **145** | Organic peroxide type F, solid |
| 3111 | **148** | Organic peroxide type B, liquid, temperature controlled |

| ID No. | Guide No. | Name of Material |
|---|---|---|
| 3112 | **148** | Organic peroxide type B, solid, temperature controlled |
| 3113 | **148** | Organic peroxide type C, liquid, temperature controlled |
| 3114 | **148** | Organic peroxide type C, solid, temperature controlled |
| 3115 | **148** | Organic peroxide type D, liquid, temperature controlled |
| 3116 | **148** | Organic peroxide type D, solid, temperature controlled |
| 3117 | **148** | Organic peroxide type E, liquid, temperature controlled |
| 3118 | **148** | Organic peroxide type E, solid, temperature controlled |
| 3119 | **148** | Organic peroxide type F, liquid, temperature controlled |
| 3120 | **148** | Organic peroxide type F, solid, temperature controlled |
| 3121 | **144** | Oxidizing solid, water-reactive, n.o.s. |
| 3122 | **142** | Poisonous liquid, oxidizing, n.o.s. |
| 3122 | **142** | Toxic liquid, oxidizing, n.o.s. |
| 3123 | **139** | Poisonous liquid, water-reactive, n.o.s. |
| 3123 | **139** | Toxic liquid, water-reactive, n.o.s. |
| 3124 | **136** | Poisonous solid, self-heating, n.o.s. |
| 3124 | **136** | Toxic solid, self-heating, n.o.s. |
| 3125 | **139** | Poisonous solid, water-reactive, n.o.s. |
| 3125 | **139** | Toxic solid, water-reactive, n.o.s. |
| 3126 | **136** | Self-heating solid, corrosive, organic, n.o.s. |
| 3127 | **135** | Self-heating solid, oxidizing, n.o.s. |
| 3128 | **136** | Self-heating solid, poisonous, organic, n.o.s. |
| 3128 | **136** | Self-heating solid, toxic, organic, n.o.s. |
| 3129 | **138** | Water-reactive liquid, corrosive, n.o.s. |
| 3130 | **139** | Water-reactive liquid, poisonous, n.o.s. |
| 3130 | **139** | Water-reactive liquid, toxic, n.o.s. |
| 3131 | **138** | Water-reactive solid, corrosive, n.o.s. |
| 3132 | **138** | Water-reactive solid, flammable, n.o.s. |
| 3133 | **138** | Water-reactive solid, oxidizing, n.o.s. |
| 3134 | **139** | Water-reactive solid, poisonous, n.o.s. |
| 3134 | **139** | Water-reactive solid, toxic, n.o.s. |
| 3135 | **138** | Water-reactive solid, self-heating, n.o.s. |
| 3136 | **120** | Trifluoromethane, refrigerated liquid |
| 3137 | **140** | Oxidizing solid, flammable, n.o.s. |
| 3138 | **115** | Acetylene, Ethylene and Propylene in mixture, refrigerated liquid containing at least 71.5% Ethylene with not more than 22.5% Acetylene and not more than 6% Propylene |
| 3138 | **115** | Ethylene, Acetylene and Propylene in mixture, refrigerated liquid containing at least 71.5% Ethylene with not more than 22.5% Acetylene and not more than 6% Propylene |

| ID No. | Guide No. | Name of Material |
|---|---|---|
| 3138 | **115** | Propylene, Ethylene and Acetylene in mixture, refrigerated liquid containing at least 71.5% Ethylene with not more than 22.5% Acetylene and not more than 6% Propylene |
| 3139 | **140** | Oxidizing liquid, n.o.s. |
| 3140 | **151** | Alkaloids, liquid, n.o.s. (poisonous) |
| 3140 | **151** | Alkaloid salts, liquid, n.o.s. (poisonous) |
| 3141 | **157** | Antimony compound, inorganic, liquid, n.o.s. |
| 3142 | **151** | Disinfectant, liquid, poisonous, n.o.s. |
| 3142 | **151** | Disinfectant, liquid, toxic, n.o.s. |
| 3143 | **151** | Dye, solid, poisonous, n.o.s. |
| 3143 | **151** | Dye, solid, toxic, n.o.s. |
| 3143 | **151** | Dye intermediate, solid, poisonous, n.o.s. |
| 3143 | **151** | Dye intermediate, solid, toxic, n.o.s. |
| 3144 | **151** | Nicotine compound, liquid, n.o.s. |
| 3144 | **151** | Nicotine preparation, liquid, n.o.s. |
| 3145 | **153** | Alkylphenols, liquid, n.o.s. (including C2-C12 homologues) |
| 3146 | **153** | Organotin compound, solid, n.o.s. |
| 3147 | **154** | Dye, solid, corrosive, n.o.s. |
| 3147 | **154** | Dye intermediate, solid, corrosive, n.o.s. |
| 3148 | **138** | Water-reactive liquid, n.o.s. |
| 3149 | **140** | Hydrogen peroxide and Peroxyacetic acid mixture, with acid(s), water and not more than 5% Peroxyacetic acid, stabilized |
| 3149 | **140** | Peroxyacetic acid and hydrogen peroxide mixture, with acid(s), water and not more than 5% Peroxyacetic acid, stabilized |
| 3150 | **115** | Devices, small, hydrocarbon gas powered, with release device |
| 3150 | **115** | Hydrocarbon gas refills for small devices, with release device |
| 3151 | **171** | Halogenated monomethyldiphenylmethanes, liquid |
| 3151 | **171** | Polyhalogenated biphenyls, liquid |
| 3151 | **171** | Polyhalogenated terphenyls, liquid |
| 3152 | **171** | Halogenated monomethyldiphenylmethanes, solid |
| 3152 | **171** | Polyhalogenated biphenyls, solid |
| 3152 | **171** | Polyhalogenated terphenyls, solid |
| 3153 | **115** | Perfluoro(methyl vinyl ether) |
| 3154 | **115** | Perfluoro(ethyl vinyl ether) |
| 3155 | **154** | Pentachlorophenol |
| 3156 | **122** | Compressed gas, oxidizing, n.o.s. |
| 3157 | **122** | Liquefied gas, oxidizing, n.o.s. |
| 3158 | **120** | Gas, refrigerated liquid, n.o.s. |
| 3159 | **126** | Refrigerant gas R-134a |
| 3159 | **126** | 1,1,1,2-Tetrafluoroethane |

| ID No. | Guide No. | Name of Material |
|---|---|---|
| 3160 | **119** | Liquefied gas, poisonous, flammable, n.o.s. |
| 3160 | **119** | Liquefied gas, poisonous, flammable, n.o.s. (Inhalation Hazard Zone A) |
| 3160 | **119** | Liquefied gas, poisonous, flammable, n.o.s. (Inhalation Hazard Zone B) |
| 3160 | **119** | Liquefied gas, poisonous, flammable, n.o.s. (Inhalation Hazard Zone C) |
| 3160 | **119** | Liquefied gas, poisonous, flammable, n.o.s. (Inhalation Hazard Zone D) |
| 3160 | **119** | Liquefied gas, toxic, flammable, n.o.s. |
| 3160 | **119** | Liquefied gas, toxic, flammable, n.o.s. (Inhalation Hazard Zone A) |
| 3160 | **119** | Liquefied gas, toxic, flammable, n.o.s. (Inhalation Hazard Zone B) |
| 3160 | **119** | Liquefied gas, toxic, flammable, n.o.s. (Inhalation Hazard Zone C) |
| 3160 | **119** | Liquefied gas, toxic, flammable, n.o.s. (Inhalation Hazard Zone D) |
| 3161 | **115** | Liquefied gas, flammable, n.o.s. |
| 3162 | **123** | Liquefied gas, poisonous, n.o.s. |
| 3162 | **123** | Liquefied gas, poisonous, n.o.s. (Inhalation Hazard Zone A) |
| 3162 | **123** | Liquefied gas, poisonous, n.o.s. (Inhalation Hazard Zone B) |
| 3162 | **123** | Liquefied gas, poisonous, n.o.s. (Inhalation Hazard Zone C) |
| 3162 | **123** | Liquefied gas, poisonous, n.o.s. (Inhalation Hazard Zone D) |
| 3162 | **123** | Liquefied gas, toxic, n.o.s. |
| 3162 | **123** | Liquefied gas, toxic, n.o.s. (Inhalation Hazard Zone A) |
| 3162 | **123** | Liquefied gas, toxic, n.o.s. (Inhalation Hazard Zone B) |
| 3162 | **123** | Liquefied gas, toxic, n.o.s. (Inhalation Hazard Zone C) |
| 3162 | **123** | Liquefied gas, toxic, n.o.s. (Inhalation Hazard Zone D) |
| 3163 | **126** | Liquefied gas, n.o.s. |
| 3164 | **126** | Articles, pressurized, hydraulic (containing non-flammable gas) |
| 3164 | **126** | Articles, pressurized, pneumatic (containing non-flammable gas) |
| 3165 | **131** | Aircraft hydraulic power unit fuel tank |
| 3166 | **115** | Engine, fuel cell, flammable gas powered |
| 3166 | **128** | Engine, fuel cell, flammable liquid powered |
| 3166 | **128** | Engine, internal combustion |
| 3166 | **115** | Engines, internal combustion, flammable gas powered |
| 3166 | **128** | Engines, internal combustion, flammable liquid powered |
| 3166 | **115** | Vehicle, flammable gas powered |
| 3166 | **128** | Vehicle, flammable liquid powered |
| 3166 | **115** | Vehicle, fuel cell, flammable gas powered |
| 3166 | **128** | Vehicle, fuel cell, flammable liquid powered |
| 3167 | **115** | Gas sample, non-pressurized, flammable, n.o.s., not refrigerated liquid |
| 3168 | **119** | Gas sample, non-pressurized, poisonous, flammable, n.o.s., not refrigerated liquid |

| ID No. | Guide No. | Name of Material |
|---|---|---|
| 3168 | **119** | Gas sample, non-pressurized, toxic, flammable, n.o.s., not refrigerated liquid |
| 3169 | **123** | Gas sample, non-pressurized, poisonous, n.o.s., not refrigerated liquid |
| 3169 | **123** | Gas sample, non-pressurized, toxic, n.o.s., not refrigerated liquid |
| 3170 | **138** | Aluminum dross |
| 3170 | **138** | Aluminum remelting by-products |
| 3170 | **138** | Aluminum smelting by-products |
| 3171 | **154** | Battery-powered equipment (wet battery) |
| 3171 | **147** | Battery-powered equipment (with lithium ion batteries) |
| 3171 | **138** | Battery-powered equipment (with lithium metal batteries) |
| 3171 | **138** | Battery-powered equipment (with sodium batteries) |
| 3171 | **154** | Battery-powered vehicle (wet battery) |
| 3171 | **147** | Battery-powered vehicle (with lithium ion batteries) |
| 3171 | **138** | Battery-powered vehicle (with sodium batteries) |
| 3171 | **154** | Wheelchair, electric, with batteries |
| 3172 | **153** | Toxins, extracted from living sources, liquid, n.o.s. |
| 3172 | **153** | Toxins, extracted from living sources, solid, n.o.s. |
| 3174 | **135** | Titanium disulfide |
| 3174 | **135** | Titanium disulphide |
| 3175 | **133** | Solids containing flammable liquid, n.o.s. |
| 3176 | **133** | Flammable solid, organic, molten, n.o.s. |
| 3178 | **133** | Flammable solid, inorganic, n.o.s. |
| 3178 | **133** | Smokeless powder for small arms |
| 3179 | **134** | Flammable solid, poisonous, inorganic, n.o.s. |
| 3179 | **134** | Flammable solid, toxic, inorganic, n.o.s. |
| 3180 | **134** | Flammable solid, corrosive, inorganic, n.o.s. |
| 3181 | **133** | Metal salts of organic compounds, flammable, n.o.s. |
| 3182 | **170** | Metal hydrides, flammable, n.o.s. |
| 3183 | **135** | Self-heating liquid, organic, n.o.s. |
| 3184 | **136** | Self-heating liquid, poisonous, organic, n.o.s. |
| 3184 | **136** | Self-heating liquid, toxic, organic, n.o.s. |
| 3185 | **136** | Self-heating liquid, corrosive, organic, n.o.s. |
| 3186 | **135** | Self-heating liquid, inorganic, n.o.s. |
| 3187 | **136** | Self-heating liquid, poisonous, inorganic, n.o.s. |
| 3187 | **136** | Self-heating liquid, toxic, inorganic, n.o.s. |
| 3188 | **136** | Self-heating liquid, corrosive, inorganic, n.o.s. |
| 3189 | **135** | Metal powder, self-heating, n.o.s. |
| 3190 | **135** | Self-heating solid, inorganic, n.o.s. |
| 3191 | **136** | Self-heating solid, poisonous, inorganic, n.o.s. |
| 3191 | **136** | Self-heating solid, toxic, inorganic, n.o.s. |

| ID No. | Guide No. | Name of Material |
|---|---|---|
| 3192 | **136** | Self-heating solid, corrosive, inorganic, n.o.s. |
| 3194 | **135** | Pyrophoric liquid, inorganic, n.o.s. |
| 3200 | **135** | Pyrophoric solid, inorganic, n.o.s. |
| 3203 | **135** | Pyrophoric organometallic compound, water-reactive, n.o.s. |
| 3205 | **135** | Alkaline earth metal alcoholates, n.o.s. |
| 3206 | **136** | Alkali metal alcoholates, self-heating, corrosive, n.o.s. |
| 3207 | **138** | Organometallic compound, water-reactive, flammable, n.o.s. |
| 3207 | **138** | Organometallic compound dispersion, water-reactive, flammable, n.o.s. |
| 3207 | **138** | Organometallic compound solution, water-reactive, flammable, n.o.s. |
| 3208 | **138** | Metallic substance, water-reactive, n.o.s. |
| 3209 | **138** | Metallic substance, water-reactive, self-heating, n.o.s. |
| 3210 | **140** | Chlorates, inorganic, aqueous solution, n.o.s. |
| 3211 | **140** | Perchlorates, inorganic, aqueous solution, n.o.s. |
| 3212 | **140** | Hypochlorites, inorganic, n.o.s. |
| 3213 | **140** | Bromates, inorganic, aqueous solution, n.o.s. |
| 3214 | **140** | Permanganates, inorganic, aqueous solution, n.o.s. |
| 3215 | **140** | Persulfates, inorganic, n.o.s. |
| 3215 | **140** | Persulphates, inorganic, n.o.s. |
| 3216 | **140** | Persulfates, inorganic, aqueous solution, n.o.s. |
| 3216 | **140** | Persulphates, inorganic, aqueous solution, n.o.s. |
| 3218 | **140** | Nitrates, inorganic, aqueous solution, n.o.s. |
| 3219 | **140** | Nitrites, inorganic, aqueous solution, n.o.s. |
| 3220 | **126** | Pentafluoroethane |
| 3220 | **126** | Refrigerant gas R-125 |
| 3221 | **149** | Self-reactive liquid type B |
| 3222 | **149** | Self-reactive solid type B |
| 3223 | **149** | Self-reactive liquid type C |
| 3224 | **149** | Self-reactive solid type C |
| 3225 | **149** | Self-reactive liquid type D |
| 3226 | **149** | Self-reactive solid type D |
| 3227 | **149** | Self-reactive liquid type E |
| 3228 | **149** | Self-reactive solid type E |
| 3229 | **149** | Self-reactive liquid type F |
| 3230 | **149** | Self-reactive solid type F |
| 3231 | **150** | Self-reactive liquid type B, temperature controlled |
| 3232 | **150** | Self-reactive solid type B, temperature controlled |
| 3233 | **150** | Self-reactive liquid type C, temperature controlled |
| 3234 | **150** | Self-reactive solid type C, temperature controlled |
| 3235 | **150** | Self-reactive liquid type D, temperature controlled |
| 3236 | **150** | Self-reactive solid type D, temperature controlled |
| 3237 | **150** | Self-reactive liquid type E, temperature controlled |
| 3238 | **150** | Self-reactive solid type E, temperature controlled |
| 3239 | **150** | Self-reactive liquid type F, temperature controlled |

| ID No. | Guide No. | Name of Material |
|---|---|---|
| 3240 | **150** | Self-reactive solid type F, temperature controlled |
| 3241 | **133** | 2-Bromo-2-nitropropane-1, 3-diol |
| 3242 | **149** | Azodicarbonamide |
| 3243 | **151** | Solids containing poisonous liquid, n.o.s. |
| 3243 | **151** | Solids containing toxic liquid, n.o.s. |
| 3244 | **154** | Solids containing corrosive liquid, n.o.s. |
| 3245 | **171** | Genetically modified micro-organisms |
| 3245 | **171** | Genetically modified organisms |
| 3246 | **156** | Methanesulfonyl chloride |
| 3246 | **156** | Methanesulphonyl chloride |
| 3247 | **140** | Sodium peroxoborate, anhydrous |
| 3248 | **131** | Medicine, liquid, flammable, poisonous, n.o.s. |
| 3248 | **131** | Medicine, liquid, flammable, toxic, n.o.s. |
| 3249 | **151** | Medicine, solid, poisonous, n.o.s. |
| 3249 | **151** | Medicine, solid, toxic, n.o.s. |
| 3250 | **153** | Chloroacetic acid, molten |
| 3251 | **133** | Isosorbide-5-mononitrate |
| 3252 | **115** | Difluoromethane |
| 3252 | **115** | Refrigerant gas R-32 |
| 3253 | **154** | Disodium trioxosilicate |
| 3254 | **135** | Tributylphosphane |
| 3255 | **135** | tert-Butyl hypochlorite |
| 3256 | **128** | Elevated temperature liquid, flammable, n.o.s., with flash point above 37.8°C (100°F), at or above its flash point |
| 3256 | **128** | Elevated temperature liquid, flammable, n.o.s., with flash point above 60°C (140°F), at or above its flash point |
| 3257 | **128** | Elevated temperature liquid, n.o.s., at or above 100°C (212°F), and below its flash point |
| 3258 | **171** | Elevated temperature solid, n.o.s., at or above 240°C (464°F) |
| 3259 | **154** | Amines, solid, corrosive, n.o.s. |
| 3259 | **154** | Polyamines, solid, corrosive, n.o.s. |
| 3260 | **154** | Corrosive solid, acidic, inorganic, n.o.s. |
| 3261 | **154** | Corrosive solid, acidic, organic, n.o.s. |
| 3262 | **154** | Corrosive solid, basic, inorganic, n.o.s. |
| 3263 | **154** | Corrosive solid, basic, organic, n.o.s. |
| 3264 | **154** | Corrosive liquid, acidic, inorganic, n.o.s. |
| 3265 | **153** | Corrosive liquid, acidic, organic, n.o.s. |
| 3266 | **154** | Corrosive liquid, basic, inorganic, n.o.s. |
| 3267 | **153** | Corrosive liquid, basic, organic, n.o.s. |
| 3268 | **171** | Air bag inflators |
| 3268 | **171** | Air bag modules |
| 3268 | **171** | Safety devices |
| 3268 | **171** | Seat-belt pre-tensioners |
| 3269 | **128** | Polyester resin kit |
| 3269 | **128** | Polyester resin kit, liquid base material |
| 3270 | **133** | Nitrocellulose membrane filters |

| ID No. | Guide No. | Name of Material |
|---|---|---|
| 3271 | **127** | Ethers, n.o.s. |
| 3272 | **127** | Esters, n.o.s. |
| 3273 | **131** | Nitriles, flammable, poisonous, n.o.s. |
| 3273 | **131** | Nitriles, flammable, toxic, n.o.s. |
| 3274 | **132** | Alcoholates solution, n.o.s., in alcohol |
| 3275 | **131** | Nitriles, poisonous, flammable, n.o.s. |
| 3275 | **131** | Nitriles, toxic, flammable, n.o.s. |
| 3276 | **151** | Nitriles, liquid, poisonous, n.o.s. |
| 3276 | **151** | Nitriles, liquid, toxic, n.o.s. |
| 3276 | **151** | Nitriles, poisonous, liquid, n.o.s. |
| 3276 | **151** | Nitriles, poisonous, n.o.s. |
| 3276 | **151** | Nitriles, toxic, liquid, n.o.s. |
| 3276 | **151** | Nitriles, toxic, n.o.s. |
| 3277 | **154** | Chloroformates, poisonous, corrosive, n.o.s. |
| 3277 | **154** | Chloroformates, toxic, corrosive, n.o.s. |
| 3278 | **151** | Organophosphorus compound, liquid, poisonous, n.o.s. |
| 3278 | **151** | Organophosphorus compound, liquid, toxic, n.o.s. |
| 3278 | **151** | Organophosphorus compound, poisonous, liquid, n.o.s. |
| 3278 | **151** | Organophosphorus compound, poisonous, n.o.s. |
| 3278 | **151** | Organophosphorus compound, toxic, liquid, n.o.s. |
| 3278 | **151** | Organophosphorus compound, toxic, n.o.s. |
| 3279 | **131** | Organophosphorus compound, poisonous, flammable, n.o.s. |
| 3279 | **131** | Organophosphorus compound, toxic, flammable, n.o.s. |
| 3280 | **151** | Organoarsenic compound, liquid, n.o.s. |
| 3280 | **151** | Organoarsenic compound, n.o.s. |
| 3281 | **151** | Metal carbonyls, liquid, n.o.s. |
| 3281 | **151** | Metal carbonyls, n.o.s. |
| 3282 | **151** | Organometallic compound, liquid, poisonous, n.o.s. |
| 3282 | **151** | Organometallic compound, liquid, toxic, n.o.s. |
| 3282 | **151** | Organometallic compound, poisonous, liquid, n.o.s. |
| 3282 | **151** | Organometallic compound, poisonous, n.o.s. |
| 3282 | **151** | Organometallic compound, toxic, liquid, n.o.s. |
| 3282 | **151** | Organometallic compound, toxic, n.o.s. |
| 3283 | **151** | Selenium compound, n.o.s. |
| 3283 | **151** | Selenium compound, solid, n.o.s. |
| 3284 | **151** | Tellurium compound, n.o.s. |
| 3285 | **151** | Vanadium compound, n.o.s. |
| 3286 | **131** | Flammable liquid, poisonous, corrosive, n.o.s. |
| 3286 | **131** | Flammable liquid, toxic, corrosive, n.o.s. |
| 3287 | **151** | Poisonous liquid, inorganic, n.o.s. |
| 3287 | **151** | Toxic liquid, inorganic, n.o.s. |
| 3288 | **151** | Poisonous solid, inorganic, n.o.s. |
| 3288 | **151** | Toxic solid, inorganic, n.o.s. |
| 3289 | **154** | Poisonous liquid, corrosive, inorganic, n.o.s. |
| 3289 | **154** | Toxic liquid, corrosive, inorganic, n.o.s. |

| ID No. | Guide No. | Name of Material |
|---|---|---|
| 3290 | **154** | Poisonous solid, corrosive, inorganic, n.o.s. |
| 3290 | **154** | Toxic solid, corrosive, inorganic, n.o.s. |
| 3291 | **158** | (Bio)Medical waste, n.o.s. |
| 3291 | **158** | Clinical waste, unspecified, n.o.s. |
| 3291 | **158** | Medical waste, n.o.s. |
| 3291 | **158** | Regulated medical waste, n.o.s. |
| 3292 | **138** | Batteries, containing Sodium |
| 3292 | **138** | Cells, containing Sodium |
| 3292 | **138** | Sodium, batteries containing |
| 3293 | **152** | Hydrazine, aqueous solution, with not more than 37% Hydrazine |
| 3294 | **131** | Hydrogen cyanide, solution in alcohol, with not more than 45% Hydrogen cyanide |
| 3295 | **128** | Hydrocarbons, liquid, n.o.s. |
| 3296 | **126** | Heptafluoropropane |
| 3296 | **126** | Refrigerant gas R-227 |
| 3297 | **126** | Chlorotetrafluoroethane and Ethylene oxide mixture, with not more than 8.8% Ethylene oxide |
| 3297 | **126** | Ethylene oxide and Chlorotetrafluoroethane mixture, with not more than 8.8% Ethylene oxide |
| 3298 | **126** | Ethylene oxide and Pentafluoroethane mixture, with not more than 7.9% Ethylene oxide |
| 3298 | **126** | Pentafluoroethane and Ethylene oxide mixture, with not more than 7.9% Ethylene oxide |
| 3299 | **126** | Ethylene oxide and Tetrafluoroethane mixture, with not more than 5.6% Ethylene oxide |
| 3299 | **126** | Tetrafluoroethane and Ethylene oxide mixture, with not more than 5.6% Ethylene oxide |
| 3300 | **119P** | Carbon dioxide and Ethylene oxide mixture, with more than 87% Ethylene oxide |
| 3300 | **119P** | Ethylene oxide and Carbon dioxide mixture, with more than 87% Ethylene oxide |
| 3301 | **136** | Corrosive liquid, self-heating, n.o.s. |
| 3302 | **152** | 2-Dimethylaminoethyl acrylate |
| 3303 | **124** | Compressed gas, poisonous, oxidizing, n.o.s. |
| 3303 | **124** | Compressed gas, poisonous, oxidizing, n.o.s. (Inhalation Hazard Zone A) |
| 3303 | **124** | Compressed gas, poisonous, oxidizing, n.o.s. (Inhalation Hazard Zone B) |
| 3303 | **124** | Compressed gas, poisonous, oxidizing, n.o.s. (Inhalation Hazard Zone C) |
| 3303 | **124** | Compressed gas, poisonous, oxidizing, n.o.s. (Inhalation Hazard Zone D) |
| 3303 | **124** | Compressed gas, toxic, oxidizing, n.o.s. |
| 3303 | **124** | Compressed gas, toxic, oxidizing, n.o.s. (Inhalation Hazard Zone A) |
| 3303 | **124** | Compressed gas, toxic, oxidizing, n.o.s. (Inhalation Hazard Zone B) |
| 3303 | **124** | Compressed gas, toxic, oxidizing, n.o.s. (Inhalation Hazard Zone C) |

| ID No. | Guide No. | Name of Material |
|---|---|---|
| 3303 | **124** | Compressed gas, toxic, oxidizing, n.o.s. (Inhalation Hazard Zone D) |
| 3304 | **123** | Compressed gas, poisonous, corrosive, n.o.s. |
| 3304 | **123** | Compressed gas, poisonous, corrosive, n.o.s. (Inhalation Hazard Zone A) |
| 3304 | **123** | Compressed gas, poisonous, corrosive, n.o.s. (Inhalation Hazard Zone B) |
| 3304 | **123** | Compressed gas, poisonous, corrosive, n.o.s. (Inhalation Hazard Zone C) |
| 3304 | **123** | Compressed gas, poisonous, corrosive, n.o.s. (Inhalation Hazard Zone D) |
| 3304 | **123** | Compressed gas, toxic, corrosive, n.o.s. |
| 3304 | **123** | Compressed gas, toxic, corrosive, n.o.s. (Inhalation Hazard Zone A) |
| 3304 | **123** | Compressed gas, toxic, corrosive, n.o.s. (Inhalation Hazard Zone B) |
| 3304 | **123** | Compressed gas, toxic, corrosive, n.o.s. (Inhalation Hazard Zone C) |
| 3304 | **123** | Compressed gas, toxic, corrosive, n.o.s. (Inhalation Hazard Zone D) |
| 3305 | **119** | Compressed gas, poisonous, flammable, corrosive, n.o.s. |
| 3305 | **119** | Compressed gas, poisonous, flammable, corrosive, n.o.s. (Inhalation Hazard Zone A) |
| 3305 | **119** | Compressed gas, poisonous, flammable, corrosive, n.o.s. (Inhalation Hazard Zone B) |
| 3305 | **119** | Compressed gas, poisonous, flammable, corrosive, n.o.s. (Inhalation Hazard Zone C) |
| 3305 | **119** | Compressed gas, poisonous, flammable, corrosive, n.o.s. (Inhalation Hazard Zone D) |
| 3305 | **119** | Compressed gas, toxic, flammable, corrosive, n.o.s. |
| 3305 | **119** | Compressed gas, toxic, flammable, corrosive, n.o.s. (Inhalation Hazard Zone A) |
| 3305 | **119** | Compressed gas, toxic, flammable, corrosive, n.o.s. (Inhalation Hazard Zone B) |
| 3305 | **119** | Compressed gas, toxic, flammable, corrosive, n.o.s. (Inhalation Hazard Zone C) |
| 3305 | **119** | Compressed gas, toxic, flammable, corrosive, n.o.s. (Inhalation Hazard Zone D) |
| 3306 | **124** | Compressed gas, poisonous, oxidizing, corrosive, n.o.s. |
| 3306 | **124** | Compressed gas, poisonous, oxidizing, corrosive, n.o.s. (Inhalation Hazard Zone A) |
| 3306 | **124** | Compressed gas, poisonous, oxidizing, corrosive, n.o.s. (Inhalation Hazard Zone B) |
| 3306 | **124** | Compressed gas, poisonous, oxidizing, corrosive, n.o.s. (Inhalation Hazard Zone C) |
| 3306 | **124** | Compressed gas, poisonous, oxidizing, corrosive, n.o.s. (Inhalation Hazard Zone D) |
| 3306 | **124** | Compressed gas, toxic, oxidizing, corrosive, n.o.s. |
| 3306 | **124** | Compressed gas, toxic, oxidizing, corrosive, n.o.s. (Inhalation Hazard Zone A) |
| 3306 | **124** | Compressed gas, toxic, oxidizing, corrosive, n.o.s. (Inhalation Hazard Zone B) |
| 3306 | **124** | Compressed gas, toxic, oxidizing, corrosive, n.o.s. (Inhalation Hazard Zone C) |

| ID No. | Guide No. | Name of Material |
|---|---|---|
| 3306 | **124** | Compressed gas, toxic, oxidizing, corrosive, n.o.s. (Inhalation Hazard Zone D) |
| 3307 | **124** | Liquefied gas, poisonous, oxidizing, n.o.s. |
| 3307 | **124** | Liquefied gas, poisonous, oxidizing, n.o.s. (Inhalation Hazard Zone A) |
| 3307 | **124** | Liquefied gas, poisonous, oxidizing, n.o.s. (Inhalation Hazard Zone B) |
| 3307 | **124** | Liquefied gas, poisonous, oxidizing, n.o.s. (Inhalation Hazard Zone C) |
| 3307 | **124** | Liquefied gas, poisonous, oxidizing, n.o.s. (Inhalation Hazard Zone D) |
| 3307 | **124** | Liquefied gas, toxic, oxidizing, n.o.s. |
| 3307 | **124** | Liquefied gas, toxic, oxidizing, n.o.s. (Inhalation Hazard Zone A) |
| 3307 | **124** | Liquefied gas, toxic, oxidizing, n.o.s. (Inhalation Hazard Zone B) |
| 3307 | **124** | Liquefied gas, toxic, oxidizing, n.o.s. (Inhalation Hazard Zone C) |
| 3307 | **124** | Liquefied gas, toxic, oxidizing, n.o.s. (Inhalation Hazard Zone D) |
| 3308 | **123** | Liquefied gas, poisonous, corrosive, n.o.s. |
| 3308 | **123** | Liquefied gas, poisonous, corrosive, n.o.s. (Inhalation Hazard Zone A) |
| 3308 | **123** | Liquefied gas, poisonous, corrosive, n.o.s. (Inhalation Hazard Zone B) |
| 3308 | **123** | Liquefied gas, poisonous, corrosive, n.o.s. (Inhalation Hazard Zone C) |

| ID No. | Guide No. | Name of Material |
|---|---|---|
| 3308 | **123** | Liquefied gas, poisonous, corrosive, n.o.s. (Inhalation Hazard Zone D) |
| 3308 | **123** | Liquefied gas, toxic, corrosive, n.o.s. |
| 3308 | **123** | Liquefied gas, toxic, corrosive, n.o.s. (Inhalation Hazard Zone A) |
| 3308 | **123** | Liquefied gas, toxic, corrosive, n.o.s. (Inhalation Hazard Zone B) |
| 3308 | **123** | Liquefied gas, toxic, corrosive, n.o.s. (Inhalation Hazard Zone C) |
| 3308 | **123** | Liquefied gas, toxic, corrosive, n.o.s. (Inhalation Hazard Zone D) |
| 3309 | **119** | Liquefied gas, poisonous, flammable, corrosive, n.o.s. |
| 3309 | **119** | Liquefied gas, poisonous, flammable, corrosive, n.o.s. (Inhalation Hazard Zone A) |
| 3309 | **119** | Liquefied gas, poisonous, flammable, corrosive, n.o.s. (Inhalation Hazard Zone B) |
| 3309 | **119** | Liquefied gas, poisonous, flammable, corrosive, n.o.s. (Inhalation Hazard Zone C) |
| 3309 | **119** | Liquefied gas, poisonous, flammable, corrosive, n.o.s. (Inhalation Hazard Zone D) |
| 3309 | **119** | Liquefied gas, toxic, flammable, corrosive, n.o.s. |
| 3309 | **119** | Liquefied gas, toxic, flammable, corrosive, n.o.s. (Inhalation Hazard Zone A) |
| 3309 | **119** | Liquefied gas, toxic, flammable, corrosive, n.o.s. (Inhalation Hazard Zone B) |
| 3309 | **119** | Liquefied gas, toxic, flammable, corrosive, n.o.s. (Inhalation Hazard Zone C) |

| ID No. | Guide No. | Name of Material |
|---|---|---|
| 3309 | **119** | Liquefied gas, toxic, flammable, corrosive, n.o.s. (Inhalation Hazard Zone D) |
| 3310 | **124** | Liquefied gas, poisonous, oxidizing, corrosive, n.o.s. |
| 3310 | **124** | Liquefied gas, poisonous, oxidizing, corrosive, n.o.s. (Inhalation Hazard Zone A) |
| 3310 | **124** | Liquefied gas, poisonous, oxidizing, corrosive, n.o.s. (Inhalation Hazard Zone B) |
| 3310 | **124** | Liquefied gas, poisonous, oxidizing, corrosive, n.o.s. (Inhalation Hazard Zone C) |
| 3310 | **124** | Liquefied gas, poisonous, oxidizing, corrosive, n.o.s. (Inhalation Hazard Zone D) |
| 3310 | **124** | Liquefied gas, toxic, oxidizing, corrosive, n.o.s. |
| 3310 | **124** | Liquefied gas, toxic, oxidizing, corrosive, n.o.s. (Inhalation Hazard Zone A) |
| 3310 | **124** | Liquefied gas, toxic, oxidizing, corrosive, n.o.s. (Inhalation Hazard Zone B) |
| 3310 | **124** | Liquefied gas, toxic, oxidizing, corrosive, n.o.s. (Inhalation Hazard Zone C) |
| 3310 | **124** | Liquefied gas, toxic, oxidizing, corrosive, n.o.s. (Inhalation Hazard Zone D) |
| 3311 | **122** | Gas, refrigerated liquid, oxidizing, n.o.s. |
| 3312 | **115** | Gas, refrigerated liquid, flammable, n.o.s. |
| 3313 | **135** | Organic pigments, self-heating |
| 3314 | **171** | Plastic molding compound |
| 3314 | **171** | Plastics moulding compound |
| 3315 | **151** | Chemical sample, poisonous |
| 3315 | **151** | Chemical sample, toxic |
| 3316 | **171** | Chemical kit |
| 3316 | **171** | First aid kit |
| 3317 | **113** | 2-Amino-4,6-dinitrophenol, wetted with not less than 20% water |
| 3318 | **125** | Ammonia solution, with more than 50% Ammonia |
| 3319 | **113** | Nitroglycerin mixture, desensitized, solid, n.o.s., with more than 2% but not more than 10% Nitroglycerin |
| 3320 | **157** | Sodium borohydride and Sodium hydroxide solution, with not more than 12% Sodium borohydride and not more than 40% Sodium hydroxide |
| 3321 | **162** | Radioactive material, low specific activity (LSA-II), non fissile or fissile-excepted |
| 3322 | **162** | Radioactive material, low specific activity (LSA-III), non fissile or fissile-excepted |
| 3323 | **163** | Radioactive material, Type C package, non-fissile or fissile excepted |
| 3324 | **165** | Radioactive material, low specific activity (LSA-II), fissile |
| 3325 | **165** | Radioactive material, low specific activity (LSA-III), fissile |
| 3326 | **165** | Radioactive material, surface contaminated objects (SCO-I), fissile |
| 3326 | **165** | Radioactive material, surface contaminated objects (SCO-II), fissile |
| 3327 | **165** | Radioactive material, Type A package, fissile, non-special form |
| 3328 | **165** | Radioactive material, Type B(U) package, fissile |

| ID No. | Guide No. | Name of Material |
|---|---|---|
| 3329 | **165** | Radioactive material, Type B(M) package, fissile |
| 3330 | **165** | Radioactive material, Type C package, fissile |
| 3331 | **165** | Radioactive material, transported under special arrangement, fissile |
| 3332 | **164** | Radioactive material, Type A package, special form, non fissile or fissile-excepted |
| 3333 | **165** | Radioactive material, Type A package, special form, fissile |
| 3334 | **171** | Aviation regulated liquid, n.o.s. |
| 3334 | **171** | Self-defense spray, non-pressurized |
| 3335 | **171** | Aviation regulated solid, n.o.s. |
| 3336 | **130** | Mercaptan mixture, liquid, flammable, n.o.s. |
| 3336 | **130** | Mercaptans, liquid, flammable, n.o.s. |
| 3337 | **126** | Refrigerant gas R-404A |
| 3338 | **126** | Refrigerant gas R-407A |
| 3339 | **126** | Refrigerant gas R-407B |
| 3340 | **126** | Refrigerant gas R-407C |
| 3341 | **135** | Thiourea dioxide |
| 3342 | **135** | Xanthates |
| 3343 | **113** | Nitroglycerin mixture, desensitized, liquid, flammable, n.o.s., with not more than 30% Nitroglycerin |
| 3344 | **113** | Pentaerythrite tetranitrate mixture, desensitized, solid, n.o.s., with more than 10% but not more than 20% PETN |
| 3344 | **113** | Pentaerythritol tetranitrate mixture, desensitized, solid, n.o.s., with more than 10% but not more than 20% PETN |
| 3344 | **113** | PETN mixture, desensitized, solid, n.o.s., with more than 10% but not more than 20% PETN |
| 3345 | **153** | Phenoxyacetic acid derivative pesticide, solid, poisonous |
| 3345 | **153** | Phenoxyacetic acid derivative pesticide, solid, toxic |
| 3346 | **131** | Phenoxyacetic acid derivative pesticide, liquid, flammable, poisonous |
| 3346 | **131** | Phenoxyacetic acid derivative pesticide, liquid, flammable, toxic |
| 3347 | **131** | Phenoxyacetic acid derivative pesticide, liquid, poisonous, flammable |
| 3347 | **131** | Phenoxyacetic acid derivative pesticide, liquid, toxic, flammable |
| 3348 | **153** | Phenoxyacetic acid derivative pesticide, liquid, poisonous |
| 3348 | **153** | Phenoxyacetic acid derivative pesticide, liquid, toxic |
| 3349 | **151** | Pyrethroid pesticide, solid, poisonous |
| 3349 | **151** | Pyrethroid pesticide, solid, toxic |
| 3350 | **131** | Pyrethroid pesticide, liquid, flammable, poisonous |
| 3350 | **131** | Pyrethroid pesticide, liquid, flammable, toxic |
| 3351 | **131** | Pyrethroid pesticide, liquid, poisonous, flammable |
| 3351 | **131** | Pyrethroid pesticide, liquid, toxic, flammable |
| 3352 | **151** | Pyrethroid pesticide, liquid, poisonous |
| 3352 | **151** | Pyrethroid pesticide, liquid, toxic |

| ID No. | Guide No. | Name of Material |
|---|---|---|
| 3354 | **115** | Insecticide gas, flammable, n.o.s. |
| 3355 | **119** | Insecticide gas, poisonous, flammable, n.o.s. |
| 3355 | **119** | Insecticide gas, poisonous, flammable, n.o.s. (Inhalation Hazard Zone A) |
| 3355 | **119** | Insecticide gas, poisonous, flammable, n.o.s. (Inhalation Hazard Zone B) |
| 3355 | **119** | Insecticide gas, poisonous, flammable, n.o.s. (Inhalation Hazard Zone C) |
| 3355 | **119** | Insecticide gas, poisonous, flammable, n.o.s. (Inhalation Hazard Zone D) |
| 3355 | **119** | Insecticide gas, toxic, flammable, n.o.s. |
| 3355 | **119** | Insecticide gas, toxic, flammable, n.o.s. (Inhalation Hazard Zone A) |
| 3355 | **119** | Insecticide gas, toxic, flammable, n.o.s. (Inhalation Hazard Zone B) |
| 3355 | **119** | Insecticide gas, toxic, flammable, n.o.s. (Inhalation Hazard Zone C) |
| 3355 | **119** | Insecticide gas, toxic, flammable, n.o.s. (Inhalation Hazard Zone D) |
| 3356 | **140** | Oxygen generator, chemical |
| 3356 | **140** | Oxygen generator, chemical, spent |
| 3357 | **113** | Nitroglycerin mixture, desensitized, liquid, n.o.s., with not more than 30% Nitroglycerin |
| 3358 | **115** | Refrigerating machines, containing flammable, non-poisonous, liquefied gas |
| 3358 | **115** | Refrigerating machines, containing flammable, non-toxic, liquefied gas |
| 3359 | **171** | Fumigated cargo transport unit |
| 3359 | **171** | Fumigated unit |
| 3360 | **133** | Fibers, vegetable, dry |
| 3360 | **133** | Fibres, vegetable, dry |
| 3361 | **156** | Chlorosilanes, poisonous, corrosive, n.o.s. |
| 3361 | **156** | Chlorosilanes, toxic, corrosive, n.o.s. |
| 3362 | **155** | Chlorosilanes, poisonous, corrosive, flammable, n.o.s. |
| 3362 | **155** | Chlorosilanes, toxic, corrosive, flammable, n.o.s. |
| 3363 | **171** | Dangerous goods in apparatus |
| 3363 | **171** | Dangerous goods in machinery |
| 3364 | **113** | Picric acid, wetted with not less than 10% water |
| 3364 | **113** | Trinitrophenol, wetted with not less than 10% water |
| 3365 | **113** | Picryl chloride, wetted with not less than 10% water |
| 3365 | **113** | Trinitrochlorobenzene, wetted with not less than 10% water |
| 3366 | **113** | TNT, wetted with not less than 10% water |
| 3366 | **113** | Trinitrotoluene, wetted with not less than 10% water |
| 3367 | **113** | Trinitrobenzene, wetted with not less than 10% water |
| 3368 | **113** | Trinitrobenzoic acid, wetted with not less than 10% water |
| 3369 | **113** | Sodium dinitro-o-cresolate, wetted with not less than 10% water |
| 3370 | **113** | Urea nitrate, wetted with not less than 10% water |

| ID No. | Guide No. | Name of Material |
|---|---|---|
| 3371 | **129** | 2-Methylbutanal |
| 3373 | **158** | Biological substance, category B |
| 3374 | **116** | Acetylene, solvent free |
| 3375 | **140** | Ammonium nitrate emulsion |
| 3375 | **140** | Ammonium nitrate gel |
| 3375 | **140** | Ammonium nitrate suspension |
| 3376 | **113** | 4-Nitrophenylhydrazine, with not less than 30% water |
| 3377 | **140** | Sodium perborate monohydrate |
| 3378 | **140** | Sodium carbonate peroxyhydrate |
| 3379 | **128** | Desensitized explosive, liquid, n.o.s. |
| 3380 | **133** | Desensitized explosive, solid, n.o.s. |
| 3381 | **151** | Poisonous by inhalation liquid, n.o.s. (Inhalation Hazard Zone A) |
| 3381 | **151** | Toxic by inhalation liquid, n.o.s. (Inhalation Hazard Zone A) |
| 3382 | **151** | Poisonous by inhalation liquid, n.o.s. (Inhalation Hazard Zone B) |
| 3382 | **151** | Toxic by inhalation liquid, n.o.s. (Inhalation Hazard Zone B) |
| 3383 | **131** | Poisonous by inhalation liquid, flammable, n.o.s. (Inhalation Hazard Zone A) |
| 3383 | **131** | Toxic by inhalation liquid, flammable, n.o.s. (Inhalation Hazard Zone A) |
| 3384 | **131** | Poisonous by inhalation liquid, flammable, n.o.s. (Inhalation Hazard Zone B) |
| 3384 | **131** | Toxic by inhalation liquid, flammable, n.o.s. (Inhalation Hazard Zone B) |
| 3385 | **139** | Poisonous by inhalation liquid, water-reactive, n.o.s. (Inhalation Hazard Zone A) |
| 3385 | **139** | Toxic by inhalation liquid, water-reactive, n.o.s. (Inhalation Hazard Zone A) |
| 3386 | **139** | Poisonous by inhalation liquid, water-reactive, n.o.s. (Inhalation Hazard Zone B) |
| 3386 | **139** | Toxic by inhalation liquid, water-reactive, n.o.s. (Inhalation Hazard Zone B) |
| 3387 | **142** | Poisonous by inhalation liquid, oxidizing, n.o.s. (Inhalation Hazard Zone A) |
| 3387 | **142** | Toxic by inhalation liquid, oxidizing, n.o.s. (Inhalation Hazard Zone A) |
| 3388 | **142** | Poisonous by inhalation liquid, oxidizing, n.o.s. (Inhalation Hazard Zone B) |
| 3388 | **142** | Toxic by inhalation liquid, oxidizing, n.o.s. (Inhalation Hazard Zone B) |
| 3389 | **154** | Poisonous by inhalation liquid, corrosive, n.o.s. (Inhalation Hazard Zone A) |
| 3389 | **154** | Toxic by inhalation liquid, corrosive, n.o.s. (Inhalation Hazard Zone A) |
| 3390 | **154** | Poisonous by inhalation liquid, corrosive, n.o.s. (Inhalation Hazard Zone B) |
| 3390 | **154** | Toxic by inhalation liquid, corrosive, n.o.s. (Inhalation Hazard Zone B) |
| 3391 | **135** | Organometallic substance, solid, pyrophoric |
| 3392 | **135** | Organometallic substance, liquid, pyrophoric |
| 3393 | **135** | Organometallic substance, solid, pyrophoric, water-reactive |

| ID No. | Guide No. | Name of Material |
|---|---|---|
| 3394 | **135** | Organometallic substance, liquid, pyrophoric, water-reactive |
| 3395 | **135** | Organometallic substance, solid, water-reactive |
| 3396 | **138** | Organometallic substance, solid, water-reactive, flammable |
| 3397 | **138** | Organometallic substance, solid, water-reactive, self-heating |
| 3398 | **135** | Organometallic substance, liquid, water-reactive |
| 3399 | **138** | Organometallic substance, liquid, water-reactive, flammable |
| 3400 | **138** | Organometallic substance, solid, self-heating |
| 3401 | **138** | Alkali metal amalgam, solid |
| 3402 | **138** | Alkaline earth metal amalgam, solid |
| 3403 | **138** | Potassium, metal alloys, solid |
| 3404 | **138** | Potassium sodium alloys, solid |
| 3404 | **138** | Sodium potassium alloys, solid |
| 3405 | **141** | Barium chlorate, solution |
| 3406 | **141** | Barium perchlorate, solution |
| 3407 | **140** | Chlorate and Magnesium chloride mixture, solution |
| 3407 | **140** | Magnesium chloride and Chlorate mixture, solution |
| 3408 | **141** | Lead perchlorate, solution |
| 3409 | **152** | Chloronitrobenzenes, liquid |
| 3410 | **153** | 4-Chloro-o-toluidine hydrochloride, solution |
| 3411 | **153** | beta-Naphthylamine, solution |
| 3411 | **153** | Naphthylamine (beta), solution |
| 3412 | **153** | Formic acid, with not less than 5% but less than 10% acid |
| 3412 | **153** | Formic acid, with not less than 10% but not more than 85% acid |
| 3413 | **157** | Potassium cyanide, solution |
| 3414 | **157** | Sodium cyanide, solution |
| 3415 | **154** | Sodium fluoride, solution |
| 3416 | **153** | Chloroacetophenone, liquid |
| 3416 | **153** | CN |
| 3417 | **152** | Xylyl bromide, solid |
| 3418 | **151** | 2,4-Toluenediamine, solution |
| 3418 | **151** | 2,4-Toluylenediamine, solution |
| 3419 | **157** | Boron trifluoride acetic acid complex, solid |
| 3420 | **157** | Boron trifluoride propionic acid complex, solid |
| 3421 | **154** | Potassium hydrogen difluoride, solution |
| 3422 | **154** | Potassium fluoride, solution |
| 3423 | **153** | Tetramethylammonium hydroxide, solid |
| 3424 | **141** | Ammonium dinitro-o-cresolate, solution |
| 3425 | **156** | Bromoacetic acid, solid |
| 3426 | **153P** | Acrylamide, solution |
| 3427 | **153** | Chlorobenzyl chlorides, solid |
| 3428 | **156** | 3-Chloro-4-methylphenyl isocyanate, solid |
| 3429 | **153** | Chlorotoluidines, liquid |
| 3430 | **153** | Xylenols, liquid |
| 3431 | **152** | Nitrobenzotrifluorides, solid |
| 3432 | **171** | Polychlorinated biphenyls, solid |
| 3433 | **135** | Lithium alkyls, solid |
| 3434 | **153** | Nitrocresols, liquid |
| 3435 | **153** | Hydroquinone, solution |

| ID No. | Guide No. | Name of Material |
|---|---|---|
| 3436 | **151** | Hexafluoroacetone hydrate, solid |
| 3437 | **152** | Chlorocresols, solid |
| 3438 | **153** | alpha-Methylbenzyl alcohol, solid |
| 3439 | **151** | Nitriles, poisonous, solid, n.o.s. |
| 3439 | **151** | Nitriles, solid, poisonous, n.o.s. |
| 3439 | **151** | Nitriles, solid, toxic, n.o.s. |
| 3439 | **151** | Nitriles, toxic, solid, n.o.s. |
| 3440 | **151** | Selenium compound, liquid, n.o.s. |
| 3441 | **153** | Chlorodinitrobenzenes, solid |
| 3442 | **153** | Dichloroanilines, solid |
| 3443 | **152** | Dinitrobenzenes, solid |
| 3444 | **151** | Nicotine hydrochloride, solid |
| 3445 | **151** | Nicotine sulfate, solid |
| 3445 | **151** | Nicotine sulphate, solid |
| 3446 | **152** | Nitrotoluenes, solid |
| 3447 | **152** | Nitroxylenes, solid |
| 3448 | **159** | Tear gas substance, solid, n.o.s. |
| 3449 | **159** | Bromobenzyl cyanides, solid |
| 3450 | **151** | Diphenylchloroarsine, solid |
| 3451 | **153** | Toluidines, solid |
| 3452 | **153** | Xylidines, solid |
| 3453 | **154** | Phosphoric acid, solid |
| 3454 | **152** | Dinitrotoluenes, solid |
| 3455 | **153** | Cresols, solid |
| 3456 | **157** | Nitrosylsulfuric acid, solid |
| 3456 | **157** | Nitrosylsulphuric acid, solid |
| 3457 | **152** | Chloronitrotoluenes, solid |
| 3458 | **152** | Nitroanisoles, solid |
| 3459 | **152** | Nitrobromobenzenes, solid |
| 3460 | **153** | N-Ethylbenzyltoluidines, solid |
| 3461 | **135** | Aluminum alkyl halides, solid |
| 3462 | **153** | Toxins, extracted from living sources, solid, n.o.s. |
| 3463 | **132** | Propionic acid, with not less than 90% acid |
| 3464 | **151** | Organophosphorus compound, poisonous, solid, n.o.s. |
| 3464 | **151** | Organophosphorus compound, solid, poisonous, n.o.s. |
| 3464 | **151** | Organophosphorus compound, solid, toxic, n.o.s. |
| 3464 | **151** | Organophosphorus compound, toxic, solid, n.o.s. |
| 3465 | **151** | Organoarsenic compound, solid, n.o.s. |
| 3466 | **151** | Metal carbonyls, solid, n.o.s. |
| 3467 | **151** | Organometallic compound, poisonous, solid, n.o.s. |
| 3467 | **151** | Organometallic compound, solid, poisonous, n.o.s. |
| 3467 | **151** | Organometallic compound, solid, toxic, n.o.s. |
| 3467 | **151** | Organometallic compound, toxic, solid, n.o.s. |
| 3468 | **115** | Hydrogen in a metal hydride storage system |
| 3468 | **115** | Hydrogen in a metal hydride storage system contained in equipment |
| 3468 | **115** | Hydrogen in a metal hydride storage system packed with equipment |
| 3469 | **132** | Paint, flammable, corrosive |
| 3469 | **132** | Paint related material, flammable, corrosive |
| 3470 | **132** | Paint, corrosive, flammable |

| ID No. | Guide No. | Name of Material |
|---|---|---|
| 3470 | **132** | Paint related material, corrosive, flammable |
| 3471 | **154** | Hydrogendifluorides, solution, n.o.s. |
| 3472 | **153** | Crotonic acid, liquid |
| 3473 | **128** | Fuel cell cartridges, contained in equipment, containing flammable liquids |
| 3473 | **128** | Fuel cell cartridges containing flammable liquids |
| 3473 | **128** | Fuel cell cartridges packed with equipment, containing flammable liquids |
| 3474 | **113** | 1-Hydroxybenzotriazole, anhydrous, wetted with not less than 20% water |
| 3474 | **113** | 1-Hydroxybenzotriazole, monohydrate |
| 3475 | **127** | Ethanol and gasoline mixture, with more than 10% ethanol |
| 3475 | **127** | Ethanol and motor spirit mixture, with more than 10% ethanol |
| 3475 | **127** | Ethanol and petrol mixture, with more than 10% ethanol |
| 3475 | **127** | Gasoline and ethanol mixture, with more than 10% ethanol |
| 3475 | **127** | Motor spirit and ethanol mixture, with more than 10% ethanol |
| 3475 | **127** | Petrol and ethanol mixture, with more than 10% ethanol |
| 3476 | **138** | Fuel cell cartridges contained in equipment, containing water-reactive substances |
| 3476 | **138** | Fuel cell cartridges, containing water-reactive substances |
| 3476 | **138** | Fuel cell cartridges packed with equipment, containing water-reactive substances |
| 3477 | **153** | Fuel cell cartridges contained in equipment, containing corrosive substances |
| 3477 | **153** | Fuel cell cartridges, containing corrosive substances |
| 3477 | **153** | Fuel cell cartridges packed with equipment, containing corrosive substances |
| 3478 | **115** | Fuel cell cartridges contained in equipment, containing liquefied flammable gas |
| 3478 | **115** | Fuel cell cartridges, containing liquefied flammable gas |
| 3478 | **115** | Fuel cell cartridges packed with equipment, containing liquefied flammable gas |
| 3479 | **115** | Fuel cell cartridges contained in equipment, containing hydrogen in metal hydride |
| 3479 | **115** | Fuel cell cartridges, containing hydrogen in metal hydride |
| 3479 | **115** | Fuel cell cartridges packed with equipment, containing hydrogen in metal hydride |
| 3480 | **147** | Lithium ion batteries (including lithium ion polymer batteries) |
| 3481 | **147** | Lithium ion batteries contained in equipment (including lithium ion polymer batteries) |
| 3481 | **147** | Lithium ion batteries packed with equipment (including lithium ion polymer batteries) |
| 3482 | **138** | Alkali metal dispersion, flammable |
| 3482 | **138** | Alkaline earth metal dispersion, flammable |
| 3483 | **131** | Motor fuel anti-knock mixture, flammable |
| 3484 | **132** | Hydrazine aqueous solution, flammable, with more than 37% hydrazine, by mass |

| ID No. | Guide No. | Name of Material |
|---|---|---|
| 3485 | **140** | Calcium hypochlorite, dry, corrosive, with more than 39% available chlorine (8.8% available oxygen) |
| 3485 | **140** | Calcium hypochlorite mixture, dry, corrosive, with more than 39% available chlorine (8.8% available oxygen) |
| 3486 | **140** | Calcium hypochlorite mixture, dry, corrosive, with more than 10% but not more than 39% available chlorine |
| 3487 | **140** | Calcium hypochlorite, hydrated, corrosive, with not less than 5.5% but not more than 16% water |
| 3487 | **140** | Calcium hypochlorite, hydrated mixture, corrosive, with not less than 5.5% but not more than 16% water |
| 3488 | **131** | Poisonous by inhalation liquid, flammable, corrosive, n.o.s. (Inhalation Hazard Zone A) |
| 3488 | **131** | Toxic by inhalation liquid, flammable, corrosive, n.o.s. (Inhalation Hazard Zone A) |
| 3489 | **131** | Poisonous by inhalation liquid, flammable, corrosive, n.o.s. (Inhalation Hazard Zone B) |
| 3489 | **131** | Toxic by inhalation liquid, flammable, corrosive, n.o.s. (Inhalation Hazard Zone B) |
| 3490 | **155** | Poisonous by inhalation liquid, water-reactive, flammable, n.o.s. (Inhalation Hazard Zone A) |
| 3490 | **155** | Toxic by inhalation liquid, water-reactive, flammable, n.o.s. (Inhalation Hazard Zone A) |
| 3491 | **155** | Poisonous by inhalation liquid, water-reactive, flammable, n.o.s. (Inhalation Hazard Zone B) |
| 3491 | **155** | Toxic by inhalation liquid, water-reactive, flammable, n.o.s. (Inhalation Hazard Zone B) |
| 3492 | **131** | Poisonous by inhalation liquid, corrosive, flammable, n.o.s. (Inhalation Hazard Zone A) |
| 3492 | **131** | Toxic by inhalation liquid, corrosive, flammable, n.o.s. (Inhalation Hazard Zone A) |
| 3493 | **131** | Poisonous by inhalation liquid, corrosive, flammable, n.o.s. (Inhalation Hazard Zone B) |
| 3493 | **131** | Toxic by inhalation liquid, corrosive, flammable, n.o.s. (Inhalation Hazard Zone B) |
| 3494 | **131** | Petroleum sour crude oil, flammable, poisonous |
| 3494 | **131** | Petroleum sour crude oil, flammable, toxic |
| 3495 | **154** | Iodine |
| 3496 | **171** | Batteries, nickel-metal hydride |
| 3497 | **133** | Krill meal |
| 3498 | **157** | Iodine monochloride, liquid |
| 3499 | **171** | Capacitor, electric double layer |
| 3500 | **126** | Chemical under pressure, n.o.s. |
| 3501 | **115** | Chemical under pressure, flammable, n.o.s. |
| 3502 | **123** | Chemical under pressure, poisonous, n.o.s. |
| 3502 | **123** | Chemical under pressure, toxic, n.o.s. |
| 3503 | **125** | Chemical under pressure, corrosive, n.o.s. |
| 3504 | **119** | Chemical under pressure, flammable, poisonous, n.o.s. |
| 3504 | **119** | Chemical under pressure, flammable, toxic, n.o.s. |
| 3505 | **118** | Chemical under pressure, flammable, corrosive, n.o.s. |
| 3506 | **172** | Mercury contained in manufactured articles |

| ID No. | Guide No. | Name of Material |
|---|---|---|
| 3507 | **166** | Uranium hexafluoride, radioactive material, excepted package, less than 0.1 kg per package, non-fissile or fissile-excepted |
| 3508 | **171** | Capacitor, asymmetric |
| 3509 | **171** | Packaging discarded, empty, uncleaned |
| 3510 | **174** | Adsorbed gas, flammable, n.o.s. |
| 3511 | **174** | Adsorbed gas, n.o.s. |
| 3512 | **173** | Adsorbed gas, poisonous, n.o.s. |
| 3512 | **173** | Adsorbed gas, poisonous, n.o.s. (Inhalation hazard zone A) |
| 3512 | **173** | Adsorbed gas, poisonous, n.o.s. (Inhalation hazard zone B) |
| 3512 | **173** | Adsorbed gas, poisonous, n.o.s. (Inhalation hazard zone C) |
| 3512 | **173** | Adsorbed gas, poisonous, n.o.s. (Inhalation hazard zone D) |
| 3512 | **173** | Adsorbed gas, toxic, n.o.s. |
| 3512 | **173** | Adsorbed gas, toxic, n.o.s. (Inhalation hazard zone A) |
| 3512 | **173** | Adsorbed gas, toxic, n.o.s. (Inhalation hazard zone B) |
| 3512 | **173** | Adsorbed gas, toxic, n.o.s. (Inhalation hazard zone C) |
| 3512 | **173** | Adsorbed gas, toxic, n.o.s. (Inhalation hazard zone D) |
| 3513 | **174** | Adsorbed gas, oxidizing, n.o.s. |
| 3514 | **173** | Adsorbed gas, poisonous, flammable, n.o.s. |
| 3514 | **173** | Adsorbed gas, poisonous, flammable, n.o.s. (Inhalation hazard zone A) |
| 3514 | **173** | Adsorbed gas, poisonous, flammable, n.o.s. (Inhalation hazard zone B) |
| 3514 | **173** | Adsorbed gas, poisonous, flammable, n.o.s. (Inhalation hazard zone C) |
| 3514 | **173** | Adsorbed gas, poisonous, flammable, n.o.s. (Inhalation hazard zone D) |
| 3514 | **173** | Adsorbed gas, toxic, flammable, n.o.s. |
| 3514 | **173** | Adsorbed gas, toxic, flammable, n.o.s. (Inhalation hazard zone A) |
| 3514 | **173** | Adsorbed gas, toxic, flammable, n.o.s. (Inhalation hazard zone B) |
| 3514 | **173** | Adsorbed gas, toxic, flammable, n.o.s. (Inhalation hazard zone C) |
| 3514 | **173** | Adsorbed gas, toxic, flammable, n.o.s. (Inhalation hazard zone D) |
| 3515 | **173** | Adsorbed gas, poisonous, oxidizing, n.o.s. |
| 3515 | **173** | Adsorbed gas, poisonous, oxidizing, n.o.s. (Inhalation hazard zone A) |
| 3515 | **173** | Adsorbed gas, poisonous, oxidizing, n.o.s. (Inhalation hazard zone B) |
| 3515 | **173** | Adsorbed gas, poisonous, oxidizing, n.o.s. (Inhalation hazard zone C) |
| 3515 | **173** | Adsorbed gas, poisonous, oxidizing, n.o.s. (Inhalation hazard zone D) |
| 3515 | **173** | Adsorbed gas, toxic, oxidizing, n.o.s. |
| 3515 | **173** | Adsorbed gas, toxic, oxidizing, n.o.s. (Inhalation hazard zone A) |
| 3515 | **173** | Adsorbed gas, toxic, oxidizing, n.o.s. (Inhalation hazard zone B) |

| ID No. | Guide No. | Name of Material |
|---|---|---|
| 3515 | **173** | Adsorbed gas, toxic, oxidizing, n.o.s. (Inhalation hazard zone C) |
| 3515 | **173** | Adsorbed gas, toxic, oxidizing, n.o.s. (Inhalation hazard zone D) |
| 3516 | **173** | Adsorbed gas, poisonous, corrosive, n.o.s. |
| 3516 | **173** | Adsorbed gas, poisonous, corrosive, n.o.s. (Inhalation hazard zone A) |
| 3516 | **173** | Adsorbed gas, poisonous, corrosive, n.o.s. (Inhalation hazard zone B) |
| 3516 | **173** | Adsorbed gas, poisonous, corrosive, n.o.s. (Inhalation hazard zone C) |
| 3516 | **173** | Adsorbed gas, poisonous, corrosive, n.o.s. (Inhalation hazard zone D) |
| 3516 | **173** | Adsorbed gas, toxic, corrosive, n.o.s. |
| 3516 | **173** | Adsorbed gas, toxic, corrosive, n.o.s. (Inhalation hazard zone A) |
| 3516 | **173** | Adsorbed gas, toxic, corrosive, n.o.s. (Inhalation hazard zone B) |
| 3516 | **173** | Adsorbed gas, toxic, corrosive, n.o.s. (Inhalation hazard zone C) |
| 3516 | **173** | Adsorbed gas, toxic, corrosive, n.o.s. (Inhalation hazard zone D) |
| 3517 | **173** | Adsorbed gas, poisonous, flammable, corrosive, n.o.s. |
| 3517 | **173** | Adsorbed gas, poisonous, flammable, corrosive, n.o.s. (Inhalation hazard zone A) |
| 3517 | **173** | Adsorbed gas, poisonous, flammable, corrosive, n.o.s. (Inhalation hazard zone B) |

| ID No. | Guide No. | Name of Material |
|---|---|---|
| 3517 | **173** | Adsorbed gas, poisonous, flammable, corrosive, n.o.s. (Inhalation hazard zone C) |
| 3517 | **173** | Adsorbed gas, poisonous, flammable, corrosive, n.o.s. (Inhalation hazard zone D) |
| 3517 | **173** | Adsorbed gas, toxic, flammable, corrosive, n.o.s. |
| 3517 | **173** | Adsorbed gas, toxic, flammable, corrosive, n.o.s. (Inhalation hazard zone A) |
| 3517 | **173** | Adsorbed gas, toxic, flammable, corrosive, n.o.s. (Inhalation hazard zone B) |
| 3517 | **173** | Adsorbed gas, toxic, flammable, corrosive, n.o.s. (Inhalation hazard zone C) |
| 3517 | **173** | Adsorbed gas, toxic, flammable, corrosive, n.o.s. (Inhalation hazard zone D) |
| 3518 | **173** | Adsorbed gas, poisonous, oxidizing, corrosive, n.o.s. |
| 3518 | **173** | Adsorbed gas, poisonous, oxidizing, corrosive, n.o.s. (Inhalation hazard zone A) |
| 3518 | **173** | Adsorbed gas, poisonous, oxidizing, corrosive, n.o.s. (Inhalation hazard zone B) |
| 3518 | **173** | Adsorbed gas, poisonous, oxidizing, corrosive, n.o.s. (Inhalation hazard zone C) |
| 3518 | **173** | Adsorbed gas, poisonous, oxidizing, corrosive, n.o.s. (Inhalation hazard zone D) |
| 3518 | **173** | Adsorbed gas, toxic, oxidizing, corrosive, n.o.s. |
| 3518 | **173** | Adsorbed gas, toxic, oxidizing, corrosive, n.o.s. (Inhalation hazard zone A) |
| 3518 | **173** | Adsorbed gas, toxic, oxidizing, corrosive, n.o.s. (Inhalation hazard zone B) |

| ID No. | Guide No. | Name of Material |
|---|---|---|
| 3518 | **173** | Adsorbed gas, toxic, oxidizing, corrosive, n.o.s. (Inhalation hazard zone C) |
| 3518 | **173** | Adsorbed gas, toxic, oxidizing, corrosive, n.o.s. (Inhalation hazard zone D) |
| 3519 | **173** | Boron trifluoride, adsorbed |
| 3520 | **173** | Chlorine, adsorbed |
| 3521 | **173** | Silicon tetrafluoride, adsorbed |
| 3522 | **173** | Arsine, adsorbed |
| 3523 | **173** | Germane, adsorbed |
| 3524 | **173** | Phosphorus pentafluoride, adsorbed |
| 3525 | **173** | Phosphine, adsorbed |
| 3526 | **173** | Hydrogen selenide, adsorbed |
| 3527 | **128P** | Polyester resin kit, solid base material |
| 3528 | **128** | Engine, fuel cell, flammable liquid powered |
| 3528 | **128** | Engine, internal combustion flammable liquid powered |
| 3528 | **128** | Machinery, fuel cell, flammable liquid powered |
| 3528 | **128** | Machinery, internal combustion, flammable liquid powered |
| 3529 | **115** | Engine, fuel cell, flammable gas powered |
| 3529 | **115** | Engine, internal combustion flammable gas powered |
| 3529 | **115** | Machinery, fuel cell, flammable gas powered |
| 3529 | **115** | Machinery, internal combustion, flammable gas powered |
| 3530 | **171** | Engine, internal combustion |
| 3530 | **171** | Machinery, internal combustion |
| 3531 | **149P** | Polymerizing substance, solid, stabilized, n.o.s. |
| 3532 | **149P** | Polymerizing substance, liquid, stabilized, n.o.s. |
| 3533 | **150P** | Polymerizing substance, solid, temperature controlled, n.o.s. |
| 3534 | **150P** | Polymerizing substance, liquid, temperature controlled, n.o.s. |
| 8000 | **171** | Consumer commodity |
| 9035 | **123** | Gas identification set |
| 9191 | **143** | Chlorine dioxide, hydrate, frozen |
| 9202 | **168** | Carbon monoxide, refrigerated liquid (cryogenic liquid) |
| 9206 | **137** | Methyl phosphonic dichloride |
| 9260 | **169** | Aluminum, molten |
| 9263 | **156** | Chloropivaloyl chloride |
| 9264 | **151** | 3,5-Dichloro-2,4,6-trifluoropyridine |
| 9269 | **132** | Trimethoxysilane |
| 9279 | **115** | Hydrogen absorbed in metal hydride |

## GREEN HIGHLIGHTED ENTRIES IN BLUE PAGES

For entries highlighted in green follow these steps:

- **IF THERE IS NO FIRE**:
  - Go directly to **Table 1** (green-bordered pages)
  - Look up the ID number and name of material
  - Identify initial isolation and protective action distances

- **IF A FIRE IS INVOLVED**:
  - Also consult the assigned orange guide
  - If applicable, apply the evacuation information shown under PUBLIC SAFETY

**Note 1:** If the name in **Table 1** is shown with ***"(when spilled in water)"***, these materials produce large amounts of Toxic Inhalation Hazard (TIH) (PIH in the US) gases when spilled in water. Some Water Reactive materials are also TIH materials themselves (e.g., Bromine trifluoride (UN1746), Thionyl chloride (UN1836), etc.). In these instances, two entries are provided in **Table 1** for land-based and water-based spills. If the Water Reactive material **is NOT** a TIH and this material **is NOT** spilled in water, **Table 1** and **Table 2 do NOT** apply and safety distances will be found within the appropriate orange guide.

**Note 2:** **Explosives** are not individually listed by their name because in an emergency situation, the response will be based only on the division of the explosive, not on the individual explosive.

**For divisions 1.1, 1.2, 1.3 and 1.5, refer to GUIDE 112.**

**For divisions 1.4 and 1.6, refer to GUIDE 114.**

| Name of Material | Guide No. | ID No. |
|---|---|---|
| AC | **117** | 1051 |
| Acetal | **127** | 1088 |
| Acetaldehyde | **129P** | 1089 |
| Acetaldehyde ammonia | **171** | 1841 |
| Acetaldehyde oxime | **129** | 2332 |
| Acetic acid, glacial | **132** | 2789 |
| Acetic acid, solution, more than 10% but not more than 80% acid | **153** | 2790 |
| Acetic acid, solution, more than 80% acid | **132** | 2789 |
| Acetic anhydride | **137** | 1715 |
| Acetone | **127** | 1090 |
| Acetone cyanohydrin, stabilized | **155** | 1541 |
| Acetone oils | **127** | 1091 |
| Acetonitrile | **127** | 1648 |
| Acetyl bromide | **156** | 1716 |
| Acetyl chloride | **155** | 1717 |
| Acetylene, dissolved | **116** | 1001 |
| Acetylene, Ethylene and Propylene in mixture, refrigerated liquid containing at least 71.5% Ethylene with not more than 22.5% Acetylene and not more than 6% Propylene | **115** | 3138 |
| Acetylene, solvent free | **116** | 3374 |
| Acetylene tetrabromide | **159** | 2504 |
| Acetyl iodide | **156** | 1898 |
| Acetyl methyl carbinol | **127** | 2621 |
| Acid, sludge | **153** | 1906 |
| Acid butyl phosphate | **153** | 1718 |
| Acridine | **153** | 2713 |
| Acrolein, stabilized | **131P** | 1092 |
| Acrolein dimer, stabilized | **129P** | 2607 |
| Acrylamide | **153P** | 2074 |
| Acrylamide, solid | **153P** | 2074 |
| Acrylamide, solution | **153P** | 3426 |
| Acrylic acid, stabilized | **132P** | 2218 |
| Acrylonitrile, stabilized | **131P** | 1093 |
| Adamsite | **154** | 1698 |
| Adhesives (flammable) | **128** | 1133 |
| Adiponitrile | **153** | 2205 |
| Adsorbed gas, flammable, n.o.s. | **174** | 3510 |
| Adsorbed gas, n.o.s. | **174** | 3511 |
| Adsorbed gas, oxidizing, n.o.s. | **174** | 3513 |
| Adsorbed gas, poisonous, corrosive, n.o.s. | **173** | 3516 |
| Adsorbed gas, poisonous, corrosive, n.o.s. (Inhalation hazard zone A) | **173** | 3516 |
| Adsorbed gas, poisonous, corrosive, n.o.s. (Inhalation hazard zone B) | **173** | 3516 |
| Adsorbed gas, poisonous, corrosive, n.o.s. (Inhalation hazard zone C) | **173** | 3516 |
| Adsorbed gas, poisonous, corrosive, n.o.s. (Inhalation hazard zone D) | **173** | 3516 |
| Adsorbed gas, poisonous, flammable, corrosive, n.o.s. | **173** | 3517 |
| Adsorbed gas, poisonous, flammable, corrosive, n.o.s. (Inhalation hazard zone A) | **173** | 3517 |
| Adsorbed gas, poisonous, flammable, corrosive, n.o.s. (Inhalation hazard zone B) | **173** | 3517 |
| Adsorbed gas, poisonous, flammable, corrosive, n.o.s. (Inhalation hazard zone C) | **173** | 3517 |

| Name of Material | Guide No. | ID No. |
|---|---|---|
| Adsorbed gas, poisonous, flammable, corrosive, n.o.s. (Inhalation hazard zone D) | **173** | 3517 |
| Adsorbed gas, poisonous, flammable, n.o.s. | **173** | 3514 |
| Adsorbed gas, poisonous, flammable, n.o.s. (Inhalation hazard zone A) | **173** | 3514 |
| Adsorbed gas, poisonous, flammable, n.o.s. (Inhalation hazard zone B) | **173** | 3514 |
| Adsorbed gas, poisonous, flammable, n.o.s. (Inhalation hazard zone C) | **173** | 3514 |
| Adsorbed gas, poisonous, flammable, n.o.s. (Inhalation hazard zone D) | **173** | 3514 |
| Adsorbed gas, poisonous, n.o.s. | **173** | 3512 |
| Adsorbed gas, poisonous, n.o.s. (Inhalation hazard zone A) | **173** | 3512 |
| Adsorbed gas, poisonous, n.o.s. (Inhalation hazard zone B) | **173** | 3512 |
| Adsorbed gas, poisonous, n.o.s. (Inhalation hazard zone C) | **173** | 3512 |
| Adsorbed gas, poisonous, n.o.s. (Inhalation hazard zone D) | **173** | 3512 |
| Adsorbed gas, poisonous, oxidizing, corrosive, n.o.s. | **173** | 3518 |
| Adsorbed gas, poisonous, oxidizing, corrosive, n.o.s. (Inhalation hazard zone A) | **173** | 3518 |
| Adsorbed gas, poisonous, oxidizing, corrosive, n.o.s. (Inhalation hazard zone B) | **173** | 3518 |
| Adsorbed gas, poisonous, oxidizing, corrosive, n.o.s. (Inhalation hazard zone C) | **173** | 3518 |
| Adsorbed gas, poisonous, oxidizing, corrosive, n.o.s. (Inhalation hazard zone D) | **173** | 3518 |
| Adsorbed gas, poisonous, oxidizing, n.o.s. | **173** | 3515 |
| Adsorbed gas, poisonous, oxidizing, n.o.s. (Inhalation hazard zone A) | **173** | 3515 |
| Adsorbed gas, poisonous, oxidizing, n.o.s. (Inhalation hazard zone B) | **173** | 3515 |
| Adsorbed gas, poisonous, oxidizing, n.o.s. (Inhalation hazard zone C) | **173** | 3515 |
| Adsorbed gas, poisonous, oxidizing, n.o.s. (Inhalation hazard zone D) | **173** | 3515 |
| Adsorbed gas, toxic, corrosive, n.o.s. | **173** | 3516 |
| Adsorbed gas, toxic, corrosive, n.o.s. (Inhalation hazard zone A) | **173** | 3516 |
| Adsorbed gas, toxic, corrosive, n.o.s. (Inhalation hazard zone B) | **173** | 3516 |
| Adsorbed gas, toxic, corrosive, n.o.s. (Inhalation hazard zone C) | **173** | 3516 |
| Adsorbed gas, toxic, corrosive, n.o.s. (Inhalation hazard zone D) | **173** | 3516 |
| Adsorbed gas, toxic, flammable, corrosive, n.o.s. | **173** | 3517 |
| Adsorbed gas, toxic, flammable, corrosive, n.o.s. (Inhalation hazard zone A) | **173** | 3517 |
| Adsorbed gas, toxic, flammable, corrosive, n.o.s. (Inhalation hazard zone B) | **173** | 3517 |
| Adsorbed gas, toxic, flammable, corrosive, n.o.s. (Inhalation hazard zone C) | **173** | 3517 |

| Name of Material | Guide No. | ID No. |
|---|---|---|
| Adsorbed gas, toxic, flammable, corrosive, n.o.s. (Inhalation hazard zone D) | **173** | 3517 |
| Adsorbed gas, toxic, flammable, n.o.s. | **173** | 3514 |
| Adsorbed gas, toxic, flammable, n.o.s. (Inhalation hazard zone A) | **173** | 3514 |
| Adsorbed gas, toxic, flammable, n.o.s. (Inhalation hazard zone B) | **173** | 3514 |
| Adsorbed gas, toxic, flammable, n.o.s. (Inhalation hazard zone C) | **173** | 3514 |
| Adsorbed gas, toxic, flammable, n.o.s. (Inhalation hazard zone D) | **173** | 3514 |
| Adsorbed gas, toxic, n.o.s. | **173** | 3512 |
| Adsorbed gas, toxic, n.o.s. (Inhalation hazard zone A) | **173** | 3512 |
| Adsorbed gas, toxic, n.o.s. (Inhalation hazard zone B) | **173** | 3512 |
| Adsorbed gas, toxic, n.o.s. (Inhalation hazard zone C) | **173** | 3512 |
| Adsorbed gas, toxic, n.o.s. (Inhalation hazard zone D) | **173** | 3512 |
| Adsorbed gas, toxic, oxidizing, corrosive, n.o.s. | **173** | 3518 |
| Adsorbed gas, toxic, oxidizing, corrosive, n.o.s. (Inhalation hazard zone A) | **173** | 3518 |
| Adsorbed gas, toxic, oxidizing, corrosive, n.o.s. (Inhalation hazard zone B) | **173** | 3518 |
| Adsorbed gas, toxic, oxidizing, corrosive, n.o.s. (Inhalation hazard zone C) | **173** | 3518 |
| Adsorbed gas, toxic, oxidizing, corrosive, n.o.s. (Inhalation hazard zone D) | **173** | 3518 |
| Adsorbed gas, toxic, oxidizing, n.o.s. | **173** | 3515 |

| Name of Material | Guide No. | ID No. |
|---|---|---|
| Adsorbed gas, toxic, oxidizing, n.o.s. (Inhalation hazard zone A) | **173** | 3515 |
| Adsorbed gas, toxic, oxidizing, n.o.s. (Inhalation hazard zone B) | **173** | 3515 |
| Adsorbed gas, toxic, oxidizing, n.o.s. (Inhalation hazard zone C) | **173** | 3515 |
| Adsorbed gas, toxic, oxidizing, n.o.s. (Inhalation hazard zone D) | **173** | 3515 |
| Aerosols | **126** | 1950 |
| Air, compressed | **122** | 1002 |
| Air, refrigerated liquid (cryogenic liquid) | **122** | 1003 |
| Air, refrigerated liquid (cryogenic liquid), non-pressurized | **122** | 1003 |
| Air bag inflators | **171** | 3268 |
| Air bag modules | **171** | 3268 |
| Aircraft hydraulic power unit fuel tank | **131** | 3165 |
| Alcoholates solution, n.o.s., in alcohol | **132** | 3274 |
| Alcoholic beverages | **127** | 3065 |
| Alcohols, flammable, poisonous, n.o.s. | **131** | 1986 |
| Alcohols, flammable, toxic, n.o.s. | **131** | 1986 |
| Alcohols, n.o.s. | **127** | 1987 |
| Aldehydes, flammable, poisonous, n.o.s. | **131** | 1988 |
| Aldehydes, flammable, toxic, n.o.s. | **131** | 1988 |
| Aldehydes, n.o.s. | **129** | 1989 |
| Aldol | **153** | 2839 |
| Alkali metal alcoholates, self-heating, corrosive, n.o.s. | **136** | 3206 |

| Name of Material | Guide No. | ID No. |
|---|---|---|
| Alkali metal alloy, liquid, n.o.s. | **138** | 1421 |
| Alkali metal amalgam | **138** | 1389 |
| Alkali metal amalgam, liquid | **138** | 1389 |
| Alkali metal amalgam, solid | **138** | 3401 |
| Alkali metal amides | **139** | 1390 |
| Alkali metal dispersion | **138** | 1391 |
| Alkali metal dispersion, flammable | **138** | 3482 |
| Alkaline earth metal alcoholates, n.o.s. | **135** | 3205 |
| Alkaline earth metal alloy, n.o.s. | **138** | 1393 |
| Alkaline earth metal amalgam | **138** | 1392 |
| Alkaline earth metal amalgam, liquid | **138** | 1392 |
| Alkaline earth metal amalgam, solid | **138** | 3402 |
| Alkaline earth metal dispersion | **138** | 1391 |
| Alkaline earth metal dispersion, flammable | **138** | 3482 |
| Alkaloids, liquid, n.o.s. (poisonous) | **151** | 3140 |
| Alkaloids, solid, n.o.s. (poisonous) | **151** | 1544 |
| Alkaloid salts, liquid, n.o.s. (poisonous) | **151** | 3140 |
| Alkaloid salts, solid, n.o.s. (poisonous) | **151** | 1544 |
| Alkylphenols, liquid, n.o.s. (including C2-C12 homologues) | **153** | 3145 |
| Alkylphenols, solid, n.o.s. (including C2-C12 homologues) | **153** | 2430 |
| Alkyl sulfonic acids, liquid, with more than 5% free Sulfuric acid | **153** | 2584 |
| Alkyl sulfonic acids, liquid, with not more than 5% free Sulfuric acid | **153** | 2586 |
| Alkyl sulfonic acids, solid, with more than 5% free Sulfuric acid | **153** | 2583 |
| Alkyl sulfonic acids, solid, with not more than 5% free Sulfuric acid | **153** | 2585 |
| Alkylsulfuric acids | **156** | 2571 |
| Alkyl sulphonic acids, liquid, with more than 5% free Sulphuric acid | **153** | 2584 |
| Alkyl sulphonic acids, liquid, with not more than 5% free Sulphuric acid | **153** | 2586 |
| Alkyl sulphonic acids, solid, with more than 5% free Sulphuric acid | **153** | 2583 |
| Alkyl sulphonic acids, solid, with not more than 5% free Sulphuric acid | **153** | 2585 |
| Alkylsulphuric acids | **156** | 2571 |
| Allyl acetate | **131** | 2333 |
| Allyl alcohol | **131** | 1098 |
| Allylamine | **131** | 2334 |
| Allyl bromide | **131** | 1099 |
| Allyl chloride | **131** | 1100 |
| Allyl chlorocarbonate | **155** | 1722 |
| Allyl chloroformate | **155** | 1722 |
| Allyl ethyl ether | **131** | 2335 |
| Allyl formate | **131** | 2336 |
| Allyl glycidyl ether | **129** | 2219 |
| Allyl iodide | **132** | 1723 |
| Allyl isothiocyanate, stabilized | **155** | 1545 |
| Allyltrichlorosilane, stabilized | **155** | 1724 |
| Aluminum, molten | **169** | 9260 |
| Aluminum alkyl halides, liquid | **135** | 3052 |

| Name of Material | Guide No. | ID No. |
|---|---|---|
| Aluminum alkyl halides, solid | **135** | 3052 |
| Aluminum alkyl halides, solid | **135** | 3461 |
| Aluminum alkyl hydrides | **138** | 3076 |
| Aluminum alkyls | **135** | 3051 |
| Aluminum borohydride | **135** | 2870 |
| Aluminum borohydride in devices | **135** | 2870 |
| Aluminum bromide, anhydrous | **137** | 1725 |
| Aluminum bromide, solution | **154** | 2580 |
| Aluminum carbide | **138** | 1394 |
| Aluminum chloride, anhydrous | **137** | 1726 |
| Aluminum chloride, solution | **154** | 2581 |
| Aluminum dross | **138** | 3170 |
| Aluminum ferrosilicon powder | **139** | 1395 |
| Aluminum hydride | **138** | 2463 |
| Aluminum nitrate | **140** | 1438 |
| Aluminum phosphide | **139** | 1397 |
| Aluminum phosphide pesticide | **157** | 3048 |
| Aluminum powder, coated | **170** | 1309 |
| Aluminum powder, pyrophoric | **135** | 1383 |
| Aluminum powder, uncoated | **138** | 1396 |
| Aluminum remelting by-products | **138** | 3170 |
| Aluminum resinate | **133** | 2715 |
| Aluminum silicon powder, uncoated | **138** | 1398 |
| Aluminum smelting by-products | **138** | 3170 |
| Amines, flammable, corrosive, n.o.s. | **132** | 2733 |
| Amines, liquid, corrosive, flammable, n.o.s. | **132** | 2734 |
| Amines, liquid, corrosive, n.o.s. | **153** | 2735 |
| Amines, solid, corrosive, n.o.s. | **154** | 3259 |
| 2-Amino-4-chlorophenol | **151** | 2673 |
| 2-Amino-5-diethylaminopentane | **153** | 2946 |
| 2-Amino-4,6-dinitrophenol, wetted with not less than 20% water | **113** | 3317 |
| 2-(2-Aminoethoxy)ethanol | **154** | 3055 |
| N-Aminoethylpiperazine | **153** | 2815 |
| Aminophenols | **152** | 2512 |
| Aminopyridines | **153** | 2671 |
| Ammonia, anhydrous | **125** | 1005 |
| Ammonia, solution, with more than 10% but not more than 35% Ammonia | **154** | 2672 |
| Ammonia, solution, with more than 35% but not more than 50% Ammonia | **125** | 2073 |
| Ammonia solution, with more than 50% Ammonia | **125** | 3318 |
| Ammonium arsenate | **151** | 1546 |
| Ammonium bifluoride, solid | **154** | 1727 |
| Ammonium bifluoride, solution | **154** | 2817 |
| Ammonium dichromate | **141** | 1439 |
| Ammonium dinitro-o-cresolate | **141** | 1843 |
| Ammonium dinitro-o-cresolate, solid | **141** | 1843 |
| Ammonium dinitro-o-cresolate, solution | **141** | 3424 |
| Ammonium fluoride | **154** | 2505 |
| Ammonium fluorosilicate | **151** | 2854 |
| Ammonium hydrogendifluoride, solid | **154** | 1727 |
| Ammonium hydrogendifluoride, solution | **154** | 2817 |
| Ammonium hydrogen sulfate | **154** | 2506 |
| Ammonium hydrogen sulphate | **154** | 2506 |
| Ammonium hydroxide | **154** | 2672 |

| Name of Material | Guide No. | ID No. |
|---|---|---|
| Ammonium hydroxide, with more than 10% but not more than 35% Ammonia | **154** | 2672 |
| Ammonium metavanadate | **154** | 2859 |
| Ammonium nitrate, liquid (hot concentrated solution) | **140** | 2426 |
| Ammonium nitrate, with not more than 0.2% combustible substances | **140** | 1942 |
| Ammonium nitrate based fertilizer | **140** | 2067 |
| Ammonium nitrate based fertilizer | **140** | 2071 |
| Ammonium nitrate emulsion | **140** | 3375 |
| Ammonium nitrate fertilizer, n.o.s. | **140** | 2072 |
| Ammonium nitrate fertilizers, with Ammonium sulfate | **140** | 2069 |
| Ammonium nitrate fertilizers, with Ammonium sulphate | **140** | 2069 |
| Ammonium nitrate fertilizers, with Calcium carbonate | **140** | 2068 |
| Ammonium nitrate fertilizers, with Phosphate or Potash | **143** | 2070 |
| Ammonium nitrate-fuel oil mixtures | **112** | —— |
| Ammonium nitrate gel | **140** | 3375 |
| Ammonium nitrate suspension | **140** | 3375 |
| Ammonium perchlorate | **143** | 1442 |
| Ammonium persulfate | **140** | 1444 |
| Ammonium persulphate | **140** | 1444 |
| Ammonium picrate, wetted with not less than 10% water | **113** | 1310 |
| Ammonium polysulfide, solution | **154** | 2818 |
| Ammonium polysulphide, solution | **154** | 2818 |
| Ammonium polyvanadate | **151** | 2861 |

| Name of Material | Guide No. | ID No. |
|---|---|---|
| Ammonium silicofluoride | **151** | 2854 |
| Ammonium sulfide, solution | **132** | 2683 |
| Ammonium sulphide, solution | **132** | 2683 |
| Ammunition, poisonous, non-explosive | **151** | 2016 |
| Ammunition, tear-producing, non-explosive | **159** | 2017 |
| Ammunition, toxic, non-explosive | **151** | 2016 |
| Amyl acetates | **129** | 1104 |
| Amyl acid phosphate | **153** | 2819 |
| Amylamine | **132** | 1106 |
| Amyl butyrates | **130** | 2620 |
| Amyl chloride | **129** | 1107 |
| n-Amylene | **128** | 1108 |
| Amyl formates | **129** | 1109 |
| Amyl mercaptan | **130** | 1111 |
| n-Amyl methyl ketone | **127** | 1110 |
| Amyl nitrate | **140** | 1112 |
| Amyl nitrite | **129** | 1113 |
| Amyltrichlorosilane | **155** | 1728 |
| Anhydrous ammonia | **125** | 1005 |
| Aniline | **153** | 1547 |
| Aniline hydrochloride | **153** | 1548 |
| Anisidines | **153** | 2431 |
| Anisidines, liquid | **153** | 2431 |
| Anisidines, solid | **153** | 2431 |
| Anisole | **128** | 2222 |
| Anisoyl chloride | **156** | 1729 |
| Antimony compound, inorganic, liquid, n.o.s. | **157** | 3141 |
| Antimony compound, inorganic, solid, n.o.s. | **157** | 1549 |
| Antimony lactate | **151** | 1550 |

| Name of Material | Guide No. | ID No. |
|---|---|---|
| Antimony pentachloride, liquid | **157** | 1730 |
| Antimony pentachloride, solution | **157** | 1731 |
| Antimony pentafluoride | **157** | 1732 |
| Antimony potassium tartrate | **151** | 1551 |
| Antimony powder | **170** | 2871 |
| Antimony trichloride | **157** | 1733 |
| Antimony trichloride, liquid | **157** | 1733 |
| Antimony trichloride, solid | **157** | 1733 |
| Aqua regia | **157** | 1798 |
| Argon | **121** | 1006 |
| Argon, compressed | **121** | 1006 |
| Argon, refrigerated liquid (cryogenic liquid) | **120** | 1951 |
| Arsenic | **152** | 1558 |
| Arsenic acid, liquid | **154** | 1553 |
| Arsenic acid, solid | **154** | 1554 |
| Arsenical dust | **152** | 1562 |
| Arsenical pesticide, liquid, flammable, poisonous | **131** | 2760 |
| Arsenical pesticide, liquid, flammable, toxic | **131** | 2760 |
| Arsenical pesticide, liquid, poisonous | **151** | 2994 |
| Arsenical pesticide, liquid, poisonous, flammable | **131** | 2993 |
| Arsenical pesticide, liquid, toxic | **151** | 2994 |
| Arsenical pesticide, liquid, toxic, flammable | **131** | 2993 |
| Arsenical pesticide, solid, poisonous | **151** | 2759 |
| Arsenical pesticide, solid, toxic | **151** | 2759 |
| Arsenic bromide | **151** | 1555 |
| Arsenic chloride | **157** | 1560 |
| Arsenic compound, liquid, n.o.s. | **152** | 1556 |
| Arsenic compound, liquid, n.o.s., inorganic | **152** | 1556 |
| Arsenic compound, solid, n.o.s. | **152** | 1557 |
| Arsenic compound, solid, n.o.s., inorganic | **152** | 1557 |
| Arsenic pentoxide | **151** | 1559 |
| Arsenic trichloride | **157** | 1560 |
| Arsenic trioxide | **151** | 1561 |
| Arsine | **119** | 2188 |
| Arsine, adsorbed | **173** | 3522 |
| Articles containing Polychlorinated biphenyls (PCB) | **171** | 2315 |
| Articles, pressurized, hydraulic (containing non-flammable gas) | **126** | 3164 |
| Articles, pressurized, pneumatic (containing non-flammable gas) | **126** | 3164 |
| Aryl sulfonic acids, liquid, with more than 5% free Sulfuric acid | **153** | 2584 |
| Aryl sulfonic acids, liquid, with not more than 5% free Sulfuric acid | **153** | 2586 |
| Aryl sulfonic acids, solid, with more than 5% free Sulfuric acid | **153** | 2583 |
| Aryl sulfonic acids, solid, with not more than 5% free Sulfuric acid | **153** | 2585 |
| Aryl sulphonic acids, liquid, with more than 5% free Sulphuric acid | **153** | 2584 |

| Name of Material | Guide No. | ID No. |
|---|---|---|
| Aryl sulphonic acids, liquid, with not more than 5% free Sulphuric acid | **153** | 2586 |
| Aryl sulphonic acids, solid, with more than 5% free Sulphuric acid | **153** | 2583 |
| Aryl sulphonic acids, solid, with not more than 5% free Sulphuric acid | **153** | 2585 |
| Asbestos | **171** | 2212 |
| Asbestos, amphibole | **171** | 2212 |
| Asbestos, blue | **171** | 2212 |
| Asbestos, brown | **171** | 2212 |
| Asbestos, chrysotile | **171** | 2590 |
| Asbestos, white | **171** | 2590 |
| Asphalt | **130** | 1999 |
| Asphalt, cut back | **130** | 1999 |
| Aviation regulated liquid, n.o.s. | **171** | 3334 |
| Aviation regulated solid, n.o.s. | **171** | 3335 |
| Azodicarbonamide | **149** | 3242 |
| Barium | **138** | 1400 |
| Barium alloys, pyrophoric | **135** | 1854 |
| Barium azide, wetted with not less than 50% water | **113** | 1571 |
| Barium bromate | **141** | 2719 |
| Barium chlorate | **141** | 1445 |
| Barium chlorate, solid | **141** | 1445 |
| Barium chlorate, solution | **141** | 3405 |
| Barium compound, n.o.s. | **154** | 1564 |
| Barium cyanide | **157** | 1565 |
| Barium hypochlorite, with more than 22% available Chlorine | **141** | 2741 |
| Barium nitrate | **141** | 1446 |
| Barium oxide | **157** | 1884 |
| Barium perchlorate | **141** | 1447 |
| Barium perchlorate, solid | **141** | 1447 |
| Barium perchlorate, solution | **141** | 3406 |
| Barium permanganate | **141** | 1448 |
| Barium peroxide | **141** | 1449 |
| Batteries, containing Sodium | **138** | 3292 |
| Batteries, dry, containing Potassium hydroxide solid | **154** | 3028 |
| Batteries, nickel-metal hydride | **171** | 3496 |
| Batteries, wet, filled with acid | **154** | 2794 |
| Batteries, wet, filled with alkali | **154** | 2795 |
| Batteries, wet, non-spillable | **154** | 2800 |
| Battery fluid, acid | **157** | 2796 |
| Battery fluid, alkali | **154** | 2797 |
| Battery-powered equipment (wet battery) | **154** | 3171 |
| Battery-powered equipment (with lithium ion batteries) | **147** | 3171 |
| Battery-powered equipment (with lithium metal batteries) | **138** | 3171 |
| Battery-powered equipment (with sodium batteries) | **138** | 3171 |
| Battery-powered vehicle (wet battery) | **154** | 3171 |
| Battery-powered vehicle (with lithium ion batteries) | **147** | 3171 |
| Battery-powered vehicle (with sodium batteries) | **138** | 3171 |
| Benzaldehyde | **129** | 1990 |
| Benzene | **130** | 1114 |
| Benzene phosphorus dichloride | **137** | 2798 |
| Benzene phosphorus thiodichloride | **137** | 2799 |
| Benzenesulfonyl chloride | **156** | 2225 |

| Name of Material | Guide No. | ID No. |
|---|---|---|
| Benzenesulphonyl chloride | **156** | 2225 |
| Benzidine | **153** | 1885 |
| Benzonitrile | **152** | 2224 |
| Benzoquinone | **153** | 2587 |
| Benzotrichloride | **156** | 2226 |
| Benzotrifluoride | **127** | 2338 |
| Benzoyl chloride | **137** | 1736 |
| Benzyl bromide | **156** | 1737 |
| Benzyl chloride | **156** | 1738 |
| Benzyl chloroformate | **137** | 1739 |
| Benzyldimethylamine | **132** | 2619 |
| Benzylidene chloride | **156** | 1886 |
| Benzyl iodide | **156** | 2653 |
| Beryllium compound, n.o.s. | **154** | 1566 |
| Beryllium nitrate | **141** | 2464 |
| Beryllium powder | **134** | 1567 |
| Bhusa, wet, damp or contaminated with oil | **133** | 1327 |
| Bicyclo[2.2.1]hepta-2,5-diene, stabilized | **128P** | 2251 |
| Biological agents | **158** | —— |
| Biological substance, category B | **158** | 3373 |
| (Bio)Medical waste, n.o.s. | **158** | 3291 |
| Bipyridilium pesticide, liquid, flammable, poisonous | **131** | 2782 |
| Bipyridilium pesticide, liquid, flammable, toxic | **131** | 2782 |
| Bipyridilium pesticide, liquid, poisonous | **151** | 3016 |
| Bipyridilium pesticide, liquid, poisonous, flammable | **131** | 3015 |
| Bipyridilium pesticide, liquid, toxic | **151** | 3016 |
| Bipyridilium pesticide, liquid, toxic, flammable | **131** | 3015 |
| Bipyridilium pesticide, solid, poisonous | **151** | 2781 |
| Bipyridilium pesticide, solid, toxic | **151** | 2781 |
| Bisulfates, aqueous solution | **154** | 2837 |
| Bisulfites, aqueous solution, n.o.s. | **154** | 2693 |
| Bisulphates, aqueous solution | **154** | 2837 |
| Bisulphites, aqueous solution, n.o.s. | **154** | 2693 |
| Blasting agent, n.o.s. | **112** | —— |
| Bleaching powder | **140** | 2208 |
| Blue asbestos | **171** | 2212 |
| Bombs, smoke, non-explosive, with corrosive liquid, without initiating device | **153** | 2028 |
| Borate and Chlorate mixture | **140** | 1458 |
| Borneol | **133** | 1312 |
| Boron tribromide | **157** | 2692 |
| Boron trichloride | **125** | 1741 |
| Boron trifluoride | **125** | 1008 |
| Boron trifluoride, adsorbed | **173** | 3519 |
| Boron trifluoride, compressed | **125** | 1008 |
| Boron trifluoride, dihydrate | **157** | 2851 |
| Boron trifluoride acetic acid complex | **157** | 1742 |
| Boron trifluoride acetic acid complex, liquid | **157** | 1742 |
| Boron trifluoride acetic acid complex, solid | **157** | 3419 |
| Boron trifluoride diethyl etherate | **132** | 2604 |
| Boron trifluoride dimethyl etherate | **139** | 2965 |

| Name of Material | Guide No. | ID No. |
|---|---|---|
| Boron trifluoride propionic acid complex | **157** | 1743 |
| Boron trifluoride propionic acid complex, liquid | **157** | 1743 |
| Boron trifluoride propionic acid complex, solid | **157** | 3420 |
| Bromates, inorganic, aqueous solution, n.o.s. | **140** | 3213 |
| Bromates, inorganic, n.o.s. | **141** | 1450 |
| Bromine | **154** | 1744 |
| Bromine, solution | **154** | 1744 |
| Bromine, solution (Inhalation Hazard Zone A) | **154** | 1744 |
| Bromine, solution (Inhalation Hazard Zone B) | **154** | 1744 |
| Bromine chloride | **124** | 2901 |
| Bromine pentafluoride | **144** | 1745 |
| Bromine trifluoride | **144** | 1746 |
| Bromoacetic acid | **156** | 1938 |
| Bromoacetic acid, solid | **156** | 3425 |
| Bromoacetic acid, solution | **156** | 1938 |
| Bromoacetone | **131** | 1569 |
| Bromoacetyl bromide | **156** | 2513 |
| Bromobenzene | **130** | 2514 |
| Bromobenzyl cyanides, liquid | **159** | 1694 |
| Bromobenzyl cyanides, solid | **159** | 1694 |
| Bromobenzyl cyanides, solid | **159** | 3449 |
| 1-Bromobutane | **130** | 1126 |
| 2-Bromobutane | **130** | 2339 |
| Bromochloromethane | **160** | 1887 |
| 1-Bromo-3-chloropropane | **159** | 2688 |
| 2-Bromoethyl ethyl ether | **130** | 2340 |
| Bromoform | **159** | 2515 |
| 1-Bromo-3-methylbutane | **130** | 2341 |
| Bromomethylpropanes | **130** | 2342 |
| 2-Bromo-2-nitropropane-1,3-diol | **133** | 3241 |
| 2-Bromopentane | **130** | 2343 |
| Bromopropanes | **129** | 2344 |
| 3-Bromopropyne | **130** | 2345 |
| Bromotrifluoroethylene | **116** | 2419 |
| Bromotrifluoromethane | **126** | 1009 |
| Brown asbestos | **171** | 2212 |
| Brucine | **152** | 1570 |
| Butadienes, stabilized | **116P** | 1010 |
| Butadienes and hydrocarbon mixture, stabilized | **116P** | 1010 |
| Butane | **115** | 1011 |
| Butane | **115** | 1075 |
| Butanedione | **127** | 2346 |
| Butanols | **129** | 1120 |
| Butyl acetates | **129** | 1123 |
| Butyl acid phosphate | **153** | 1718 |
| Butyl acrylates, stabilized | **129P** | 2348 |
| n-Butylamine | **132** | 1125 |
| N-Butylaniline | **153** | 2738 |
| Butylbenzenes | **128** | 2709 |
| n-Butyl bromide | **130** | 1126 |
| n-Butyl chloride | **130** | 1127 |
| n-Butyl chloroformate | **155** | 2743 |
| sec-Butyl chloroformate | **155** | 2742 |
| tert-Butylcyclohexyl chloroformate | **156** | 2747 |
| Butylene | **115** | 1012 |
| Butylene | **115** | 1075 |
| 1,2-Butylene oxide, stabilized | **127P** | 3022 |
| Butyl ethers | **128** | 1149 |
| n-Butyl formate | **129** | 1128 |

| Name of Material | Guide No. | ID No. |
|---|---|---|
| tert-Butyl hypochlorite | **135** | 3255 |
| N,n-Butylimidazole | **152** | 2690 |
| n-Butyl isocyanate | **155** | 2485 |
| tert-Butyl isocyanate | **155** | 2484 |
| Butyl mercaptan | **130** | 2347 |
| n-Butyl methacrylate, stabilized | **130P** | 2227 |
| Butyl methyl ether | **127** | 2350 |
| Butyl nitrites | **129** | 2351 |
| Butyl propionates | **130** | 1914 |
| Butyltoluenes | **152** | 2667 |
| Butyltrichlorosilane | **155** | 1747 |
| 5-tert-Butyl-2,4,6-trinitro-m-xylene | **149** | 2956 |
| Butyl vinyl ether, stabilized | **127P** | 2352 |
| 1,4-Butynediol | **153** | 2716 |
| Butyraldehyde | **129** | 1129 |
| Butyraldoxime | **129** | 2840 |
| Butyric acid | **153** | 2820 |
| Butyric anhydride | **156** | 2739 |
| Butyronitrile | **131** | 2411 |
| Butyryl chloride | **132** | 2353 |
| Buzz | **153** | 2810 |
| BZ | **153** | 2810 |
| CA | **159** | 1694 |
| Cacodylic acid | **151** | 1572 |
| Cadmium compound | **154** | 2570 |
| Caesium | **138** | 1407 |
| Caesium hydroxide | **157** | 2682 |
| Caesium hydroxide, solution | **154** | 2681 |
| Caesium nitrate | **140** | 1451 |
| Calcium | **138** | 1401 |
| Calcium, pyrophoric | **135** | 1855 |
| Calcium alloys, pyrophoric | **135** | 1855 |
| Calcium arsenate | **151** | 1573 |
| Calcium arsenate and Calcium arsenite mixture, solid | **151** | 1574 |
| Calcium arsenite and Calcium arsenate mixture, solid | **151** | 1574 |
| Calcium carbide | **138** | 1402 |
| Calcium chlorate | **140** | 1452 |
| Calcium chlorate, aqueous solution | **140** | 2429 |
| Calcium chlorite | **140** | 1453 |
| Calcium cyanamide, with more than 0.1% Calcium carbide | **138** | 1403 |
| Calcium cyanide | **157** | 1575 |
| Calcium dithionite | **135** | 1923 |
| Calcium hydride | **138** | 1404 |
| Calcium hydrosulfite | **135** | 1923 |
| Calcium hydrosulphite | **135** | 1923 |
| Calcium hypochlorite, dry | **140** | 1748 |
| Calcium hypochlorite, dry, corrosive, with more than 39% available chlorine (8.8% available oxygen) | **140** | 3485 |
| Calcium hypochlorite, hydrated, corrosive, with not less than 5.5% but not more than 16% water | **140** | 3487 |
| Calcium hypochlorite, hydrated, with not less than 5.5% but not more than 16% water | **140** | 2880 |
| Calcium hypochlorite, hydrated mixture, corrosive, with not less than 5.5% but not more than 16% water | **140** | 3487 |
| Calcium hypochlorite, hydrated mixture, with not less than 5.5% but not more than 16% water | **140** | 2880 |

| Name of Material | Guide No. | ID No. |
|---|---|---|
| Calcium hypochlorite mixture, dry, corrosive, with more than 10% but not more than 39% available chlorine | **140** | 3486 |
| Calcium hypochlorite mixture, dry, corrosive, with more than 39% available chlorine (8.8% available oxygen) | **140** | 3485 |
| Calcium hypochlorite mixture, dry, with more than 10% but not more than 39% available Chlorine | **140** | 2208 |
| Calcium hypochlorite mixture, dry, with more than 39% available Chlorine (8.8% available Oxygen) | **140** | 1748 |
| Calcium manganese silicon | **138** | 2844 |
| Calcium nitrate | **140** | 1454 |
| Calcium oxide | **157** | 1910 |
| Calcium perchlorate | **140** | 1455 |
| Calcium permanganate | **140** | 1456 |
| Calcium peroxide | **140** | 1457 |
| Calcium phosphide | **139** | 1360 |
| Calcium resinate | **133** | 1313 |
| Calcium resinate, fused | **133** | 1314 |
| Calcium silicide | **138** | 1405 |
| Camphor | **133** | 2717 |
| Camphor, synthetic | **133** | 2717 |
| Camphor oil | **128** | 1130 |
| Capacitor, asymmetric | **171** | 3508 |
| Capacitor, electric double layer | **171** | 3499 |
| Caproic acid | **153** | 2829 |
| Carbamate pesticide, liquid, flammable, poisonous | **131** | 2758 |
| Carbamate pesticide, liquid, flammable, toxic | **131** | 2758 |
| Carbamate pesticide, liquid, poisonous | **151** | 2992 |
| Carbamate pesticide, liquid, poisonous, flammable | **131** | 2991 |
| Carbamate pesticide, liquid, toxic | **151** | 2992 |
| Carbamate pesticide, liquid, toxic, flammable | **131** | 2991 |
| Carbamate pesticide, solid, poisonous | **151** | 2757 |
| Carbamate pesticide, solid, toxic | **151** | 2757 |
| Carbon, activated | **133** | 1362 |
| Carbon, animal or vegetable origin | **133** | 1361 |
| Carbon bisulfide | **131** | 1131 |
| Carbon bisulphide | **131** | 1131 |
| Carbon dioxide | **120** | 1013 |
| Carbon dioxide, compressed | **120** | 1013 |
| Carbon dioxide, refrigerated liquid | **120** | 2187 |
| Carbon dioxide, solid | **120** | 1845 |
| Carbon dioxide and Ethylene oxide mixture, with more than 9% but not more than 87% Ethylene oxide | **115** | 1041 |
| Carbon dioxide and Ethylene oxide mixture, with more than 87% Ethylene oxide | **119P** | 3300 |
| Carbon dioxide and Ethylene oxide mixtures, with not more than 9% Ethylene oxide | **126** | 1952 |
| Carbon dioxide and Nitrous oxide mixture | **126** | 1015 |
| Carbon dioxide and Oxygen mixture, compressed | **122** | 1014 |
| Carbon disulfide | **131** | 1131 |
| Carbon disulphide | **131** | 1131 |
| Carbon monoxide | **119** | 1016 |

| Name of Material | Guide No. | ID No. |
|---|---|---|
| Carbon monoxide, compressed | **119** | 1016 |
| Carbon monoxide, refrigerated liquid (cryogenic liquid) | **168** | 9202 |
| Carbon monoxide and Hydrogen mixture, compressed | **119** | 2600 |
| Carbon tetrabromide | **151** | 2516 |
| Carbon tetrachloride | **151** | 1846 |
| Carbonyl fluoride | **125** | 2417 |
| Carbonyl fluoride, compressed | **125** | 2417 |
| Carbonyl sulfide | **119** | 2204 |
| Carbonyl sulphide | **119** | 2204 |
| Castor beans, meal, pomace or flake | **171** | 2969 |
| Caustic alkali liquid, n.o.s. | **154** | 1719 |
| Caustic potash, solid | **154** | 1813 |
| Caustic potash, solution | **154** | 1814 |
| Caustic soda, solid | **154** | 1823 |
| Caustic soda, solution | **154** | 1824 |
| Cells, containing Sodium | **138** | 3292 |
| Celluloid, in blocks, rods, rolls, sheets, tubes, etc., except scrap | **133** | 2000 |
| Celluloid, scrap | **135** | 2002 |
| Cerium, slabs, ingots or rods | **170** | 1333 |
| Cerium, turnings or gritty powder | **138** | 3078 |
| Cesium | **138** | 1407 |
| Cesium hydroxide | **157** | 2682 |
| Cesium hydroxide, solution | **154** | 2681 |
| Cesium nitrate | **140** | 1451 |
| CG | **125** | 1076 |
| Charcoal | **133** | 1361 |
| Chemical kit | **154** | 1760 |
| Chemical kit | **171** | 3316 |
| Chemical sample, poisonous | **151** | 3315 |
| Chemical sample, toxic | **151** | 3315 |
| Chemical under pressure, corrosive, n.o.s. | **125** | 3503 |
| Chemical under pressure, flammable, corrosive, n.o.s. | **118** | 3505 |
| Chemical under pressure, flammable, n.o.s. | **115** | 3501 |
| Chemical under pressure, flammable, poisonous, n.o.s. | **119** | 3504 |
| Chemical under pressure, flammable, toxic, n.o.s. | **119** | 3504 |
| Chemical under pressure, n.o.s. | **126** | 3500 |
| Chemical under pressure, poisonous, n.o.s. | **123** | 3502 |
| Chemical under pressure, toxic, n.o.s. | **123** | 3502 |
| Chloral, anhydrous, stabilized | **153** | 2075 |
| Chlorate and Borate mixture | **140** | 1458 |
| Chlorate and Magnesium chloride mixture | **140** | 1459 |
| Chlorate and Magnesium chloride mixture, solid | **140** | 1459 |
| Chlorate and Magnesium chloride mixture, solution | **140** | 3407 |
| Chlorates, inorganic, aqueous solution, n.o.s. | **140** | 3210 |
| Chlorates, inorganic, n.o.s. | **140** | 1461 |
| Chloric acid, aqueous solution, with not more than 10% Chloric acid | **140** | 2626 |
| Chlorine | **124** | 1017 |
| Chlorine, adsorbed | **173** | 3520 |
| Chlorine dioxide, hydrate, frozen | **143** | 9191 |

| Name of Material | Guide No. | ID No. |
|---|---|---|
| Chlorine pentafluoride | **124** | 2548 |
| Chlorine trifluoride | **124** | 1749 |
| Chlorite solution | **154** | 1908 |
| Chlorites, inorganic, n.o.s. | **143** | 1462 |
| Chloroacetaldehyde | **153** | 2232 |
| Chloroacetic acid, molten | **153** | 3250 |
| Chloroacetic acid, solid | **153** | 1751 |
| Chloroacetic acid, solution | **153** | 1750 |
| Chloroacetone, stabilized | **131** | 1695 |
| Chloroacetonitrile | **131** | 2668 |
| Chloroacetophenone | **153** | 1697 |
| Chloroacetophenone, liquid | **153** | 3416 |
| Chloroacetophenone, solid | **153** | 1697 |
| Chloroacetyl chloride | **156** | 1752 |
| Chloroanilines, liquid | **152** | 2019 |
| Chloroanilines, solid | **152** | 2018 |
| Chloroanisidines | **152** | 2233 |
| Chlorobenzene | **130** | 1134 |
| Chlorobenzotrifluorides | **130** | 2234 |
| Chlorobenzyl chlorides | **153** | 2235 |
| Chlorobenzyl chlorides, liquid | **153** | 2235 |
| Chlorobenzyl chlorides, solid | **153** | 3427 |
| Chlorobutanes | **130** | 1127 |
| Chlorocresols | **152** | 2669 |
| Chlorocresols, solid | **152** | 3437 |
| Chlorocresols, solution | **152** | 2669 |
| Chlorodifluorobromomethane | **126** | 1974 |
| 1-Chloro-1,1-difluoroethane | **115** | 2517 |
| Chlorodifluoromethane | **126** | 1018 |
| Chlorodifluoromethane and Chloropentafluoroethane mixture | **126** | 1973 |
| Chlorodinitrobenzenes, liquid | **153** | 1577 |
| Chlorodinitrobenzenes, solid | **153** | 1577 |
| Chlorodinitrobenzenes, solid | **153** | 3441 |
| 1-Chloro-2,3-epoxypropane | **131P** | 2023 |
| 2-Chloroethanal | **153** | 2232 |
| Chloroform | **151** | 1888 |
| Chloroformates, poisonous, corrosive, flammable, n.o.s. | **155** | 2742 |
| Chloroformates, poisonous, corrosive, n.o.s. | **154** | 3277 |
| Chloroformates, toxic, corrosive, flammable, n.o.s. | **155** | 2742 |
| Chloroformates, toxic, corrosive, n.o.s. | **154** | 3277 |
| Chloromethyl chloroformate | **157** | 2745 |
| Chloromethyl ethyl ether | **131** | 2354 |
| 3-Chloro-4-methylphenyl isocyanate | **156** | 2236 |
| 3-Chloro-4-methylphenyl isocyanate, liquid | **156** | 2236 |
| 3-Chloro-4-methylphenyl isocyanate, solid | **156** | 3428 |
| Chloronitroanilines | **153** | 2237 |
| Chloronitrobenzenes | **152** | 1578 |
| Chloronitrobenzenes, liquid | **152** | 3409 |
| Chloronitrobenzenes, solid | **152** | 1578 |
| Chloronitrotoluenes, liquid | **152** | 2433 |
| Chloronitrotoluenes, solid | **152** | 2433 |
| Chloronitrotoluenes, solid | **152** | 3457 |
| Chloropentafluoroethane | **126** | 1020 |
| Chloropentafluoroethane and Chlorodifluoromethane mixture | **126** | 1973 |
| Chlorophenolates, liquid | **154** | 2904 |
| Chlorophenolates, solid | **154** | 2905 |
| Chlorophenols, liquid | **153** | 2021 |
| Chlorophenols, solid | **153** | 2020 |

| Name of Material | Guide No. | ID No. |
|---|---|---|
| Chlorophenyltrichlorosilane | **156** | 1753 |
| Chloropicrin | **154** | 1580 |
| Chloropicrin and Methyl bromide mixture | **123** | 1581 |
| Chloropicrin and Methyl chloride mixture | **119** | 1582 |
| Chloropicrin mixture, n.o.s. | **154** | 1583 |
| Chloropivaloyl chloride | **156** | 9263 |
| Chloroplatinic acid, solid | **154** | 2507 |
| Chloroprene, stabilized | **131P** | 1991 |
| 1-Chloropropane | **129** | 1278 |
| 2-Chloropropane | **129** | 2356 |
| 3-Chloropropanol-1 | **153** | 2849 |
| 2-Chloropropene | **130P** | 2456 |
| 2-Chloropropionic acid | **153** | 2511 |
| 2-Chloropropionic acid, solid | **153** | 2511 |
| 2-Chloropropionic acid, solution | **153** | 2511 |
| 2-Chloropyridine | **153** | 2822 |
| Chlorosilanes, corrosive, flammable, n.o.s. | **155** | 2986 |
| Chlorosilanes, corrosive, n.o.s. | **156** | 2987 |
| Chlorosilanes, flammable, corrosive, n.o.s. | **155** | 2985 |
| Chlorosilanes, poisonous, corrosive, flammable, n.o.s. | **155** | 3362 |
| Chlorosilanes, poisonous, corrosive, n.o.s. | **156** | 3361 |
| Chlorosilanes, toxic, corrosive, flammable, n.o.s. | **155** | 3362 |
| Chlorosilanes, toxic, corrosive, n.o.s. | **156** | 3361 |
| Chlorosilanes, water-reactive, flammable, corrosive, n.o.s. | **139** | 2988 |
| Chlorosulfonic acid (with or without sulfur trioxide mixture) | **137** | 1754 |
| Chlorosulphonic acid (with or without sulphur trioxide mixture) | **137** | 1754 |
| 1-Chloro-1,2,2,2-tetrafluoroethane | **126** | 1021 |
| Chlorotetrafluoroethane and Ethylene oxide mixture, with not more than 8.8% Ethylene oxide | **126** | 3297 |
| Chlorotoluenes | **129** | 2238 |
| 4-Chloro-o-toluidine hydrochloride | **153** | 1579 |
| 4-Chloro-o-toluidine hydrochloride, solid | **153** | 1579 |
| 4-Chloro-o-toluidine hydrochloride, solution | **153** | 3410 |
| Chlorotoluidines | **153** | 2239 |
| Chlorotoluidines, liquid | **153** | 3429 |
| Chlorotoluidines, solid | **153** | 2239 |
| 1-Chloro-2,2,2-trifluoroethane | **126** | 1983 |
| Chlorotrifluoromethane | **126** | 1022 |
| Chlorotrifluoromethane and Trifluoromethane azeotropic mixture with approximately 60% Chlorotrifluoromethane | **126** | 2599 |
| Chromic acid, solution | **154** | 1755 |
| Chromic fluoride, solid | **154** | 1756 |
| Chromic fluoride, solution | **154** | 1757 |
| Chromium nitrate | **141** | 2720 |
| Chromium oxychloride | **137** | 1758 |
| Chromium trioxide, anhydrous | **141** | 1463 |
| Chromosulfuric acid | **154** | 2240 |
| Chromosulphuric acid | **154** | 2240 |
| CK | **125** | 1589 |

| Name of Material | Guide No. | ID No. |
|---|---|---|
| Clinical waste, unspecified, n.o.s. | **158** | 3291 |
| CN | **153** | 1697 |
| CN | **153** | 3416 |
| Coal gas | **119** | 1023 |
| Coal gas, compressed | **119** | 1023 |
| Coal tar distillates, flammable | **128** | 1136 |
| Coating solution | **127** | 1139 |
| Cobalt naphthenates, powder | **133** | 2001 |
| Cobalt resinate, precipitated | **133** | 1318 |
| Combustible liquid, n.o.s. | **128** | 1993 |
| Compounds, cleaning liquid (corrosive) | **154** | 1760 |
| Compounds, cleaning liquid (flammable) | **128** | 1993 |
| Compounds, tree or weed killing, liquid (corrosive) | **154** | 1760 |
| Compounds, tree or weed killing, liquid (flammable) | **128** | 1993 |
| Compounds, tree or weed killing, liquid (toxic) | **153** | 2810 |
| Compressed gas, flammable, n.o.s. | **115** | 1954 |
| Compressed gas, n.o.s. | **126** | 1956 |
| Compressed gas, oxidizing, n.o.s. | **122** | 3156 |
| Compressed gas, poisonous, corrosive, n.o.s. | **123** | 3304 |
| Compressed gas, poisonous, corrosive, n.o.s. (Inhalation Hazard Zone A) | **123** | 3304 |
| Compressed gas, poisonous, corrosive, n.o.s. (Inhalation Hazard Zone B) | **123** | 3304 |
| Compressed gas, poisonous, corrosive, n.o.s. (Inhalation Hazard Zone C) | **123** | 3304 |
| Compressed gas, poisonous, corrosive, n.o.s. (Inhalation Hazard Zone D) | **123** | 3304 |
| Compressed gas, poisonous, flammable, corrosive, n.o.s. | **119** | 3305 |
| Compressed gas, poisonous, flammable, corrosive, n.o.s. (Inhalation Hazard Zone A) | **119** | 3305 |
| Compressed gas, poisonous, flammable, corrosive, n.o.s. (Inhalation Hazard Zone B) | **119** | 3305 |
| Compressed gas, poisonous, flammable, corrosive, n.o.s. (Inhalation Hazard Zone C) | **119** | 3305 |
| Compressed gas, poisonous, flammable, corrosive, n.o.s. (Inhalation Hazard Zone D) | **119** | 3305 |
| Compressed gas, poisonous, flammable, n.o.s. | **119** | 1953 |
| Compressed gas, poisonous, flammable, n.o.s. (Inhalation Hazard Zone A) | **119** | 1953 |
| Compressed gas, poisonous, flammable, n.o.s. (Inhalation Hazard Zone B) | **119** | 1953 |
| Compressed gas, poisonous, flammable, n.o.s. (Inhalation Hazard Zone C) | **119** | 1953 |
| Compressed gas, poisonous, flammable, n.o.s. (Inhalation Hazard Zone D) | **119** | 1953 |
| Compressed gas, poisonous, n.o.s. | **123** | 1955 |
| Compressed gas, poisonous, n.o.s. (Inhalation Hazard Zone A) | **123** | 1955 |
| Compressed gas, poisonous, n.o.s. (Inhalation Hazard Zone B) | **123** | 1955 |
| Compressed gas, poisonous, n.o.s. (Inhalation Hazard Zone C) | **123** | 1955 |

| Name of Material | Guide No. | ID No. |
|---|---|---|
| Compressed gas, poisonous, n.o.s. (Inhalation Hazard Zone D) | 123 | 1955 |
| Compressed gas, poisonous, oxidizing, corrosive, n.o.s. | 124 | 3306 |
| Compressed gas, poisonous, oxidizing, corrosive, n.o.s. (Inhalation Hazard Zone A) | 124 | 3306 |
| Compressed gas, poisonous, oxidizing, corrosive, n.o.s. (Inhalation Hazard Zone B) | 124 | 3306 |
| Compressed gas, poisonous, oxidizing, corrosive, n.o.s. (Inhalation Hazard Zone C) | 124 | 3306 |
| Compressed gas, poisonous, oxidizing, corrosive, n.o.s. (Inhalation Hazard Zone D) | 124 | 3306 |
| Compressed gas, poisonous, oxidizing, n.o.s. | 124 | 3303 |
| Compressed gas, poisonous, oxidizing, n.o.s. (Inhalation Hazard Zone A) | 124 | 3303 |
| Compressed gas, poisonous, oxidizing, n.o.s. (Inhalation Hazard Zone B) | 124 | 3303 |
| Compressed gas, poisonous, oxidizing, n.o.s. (Inhalation Hazard Zone C) | 124 | 3303 |
| Compressed gas, poisonous, oxidizing, n.o.s. (Inhalation Hazard Zone D) | 124 | 3303 |
| Compressed gas, toxic, corrosive, n.o.s. | 123 | 3304 |
| Compressed gas, toxic, corrosive, n.o.s. (Inhalation Hazard Zone A) | 123 | 3304 |
| Compressed gas, toxic, corrosive, n.o.s. (Inhalation Hazard Zone B) | 123 | 3304 |
| Compressed gas, toxic, corrosive, n.o.s. (Inhalation Hazard Zone C) | 123 | 3304 |

| Name of Material | Guide No. | ID No. |
|---|---|---|
| Compressed gas, toxic, corrosive, n.o.s. (Inhalation Hazard Zone D) | 123 | 3304 |
| Compressed gas, toxic, flammable, corrosive, n.o.s. | 119 | 3305 |
| Compressed gas, toxic, flammable, corrosive, n.o.s. (Inhalation Hazard Zone A) | 119 | 3305 |
| Compressed gas, toxic, flammable, corrosive, n.o.s. (Inhalation Hazard Zone B) | 119 | 3305 |
| Compressed gas, toxic, flammable, corrosive, n.o.s. (Inhalation Hazard Zone C) | 119 | 3305 |
| Compressed gas, toxic, flammable, corrosive, n.o.s. (Inhalation Hazard Zone D) | 119 | 3305 |
| Compressed gas, toxic, flammable, n.o.s. | 119 | 1953 |
| Compressed gas, toxic, flammable, n.o.s. (Inhalation Hazard Zone A) | 119 | 1953 |
| Compressed gas, toxic, flammable, n.o.s. (Inhalation Hazard Zone B) | 119 | 1953 |
| Compressed gas, toxic, flammable, n.o.s. (Inhalation Hazard Zone C) | 119 | 1953 |
| Compressed gas, toxic, flammable, n.o.s. (Inhalation Hazard Zone D) | 119 | 1953 |
| Compressed gas, toxic, n.o.s. | 123 | 1955 |
| Compressed gas, toxic, n.o.s. (Inhalation Hazard Zone A) | 123 | 1955 |
| Compressed gas, toxic, n.o.s. (Inhalation Hazard Zone B) | 123 | 1955 |
| Compressed gas, toxic, n.o.s. (Inhalation Hazard Zone C) | 123 | 1955 |
| Compressed gas, toxic, n.o.s. (Inhalation Hazard Zone D) | 123 | 1955 |
| Compressed gas, toxic, oxidizing, corrosive, n.o.s. | 124 | 3306 |

| Name of Material | Guide No. | ID No. |
|---|---|---|
| Compressed gas, toxic, oxidizing, corrosive, n.o.s. (Inhalation Hazard Zone A) | **124** | 3306 |
| Compressed gas, toxic, oxidizing, corrosive, n.o.s. (Inhalation Hazard Zone B) | **124** | 3306 |
| Compressed gas, toxic, oxidizing, corrosive, n.o.s. (Inhalation Hazard Zone C) | **124** | 3306 |
| Compressed gas, toxic, oxidizing, corrosive, n.o.s. (Inhalation Hazard Zone D) | **124** | 3306 |
| Compressed gas, toxic, oxidizing, n.o.s. | **124** | 3303 |
| Compressed gas, toxic, oxidizing, n.o.s. (Inhalation Hazard Zone A) | **124** | 3303 |
| Compressed gas, toxic, oxidizing, n.o.s. (Inhalation Hazard Zone B) | **124** | 3303 |
| Compressed gas, toxic, oxidizing, n.o.s. (Inhalation Hazard Zone C) | **124** | 3303 |
| Compressed gas, toxic, oxidizing, n.o.s. (Inhalation Hazard Zone D) | **124** | 3303 |
| Compressed gas and hexaethyl tetraphosphate mixture | **123** | 1612 |
| Consumer commodity | **171** | 8000 |
| Copper acetoarsenite | **151** | 1585 |
| Copper arsenite | **151** | 1586 |
| Copper based pesticide, liquid, flammable, poisonous | **131** | 2776 |
| Copper based pesticide, liquid, flammable, toxic | **131** | 2776 |
| Copper based pesticide, liquid, poisonous | **151** | 3010 |
| Copper based pesticide, liquid, poisonous, flammable | **131** | 3009 |
| Copper based pesticide, liquid, toxic | **151** | 3010 |
| Copper based pesticide, liquid, toxic, flammable | **131** | 3009 |
| Copper based pesticide, solid, poisonous | **151** | 2775 |
| Copper based pesticide, solid, toxic | **151** | 2775 |
| Copper chlorate | **141** | 2721 |
| Copper chloride | **154** | 2802 |
| Copper cyanide | **151** | 1587 |
| Copra | **135** | 1363 |
| Corrosive liquid, acidic, inorganic, n.o.s. | **154** | 3264 |
| Corrosive liquid, acidic, organic, n.o.s. | **153** | 3265 |
| Corrosive liquid, basic, inorganic, n.o.s. | **154** | 3266 |
| Corrosive liquid, basic, organic, n.o.s. | **153** | 3267 |
| Corrosive liquid, flammable, n.o.s. | **132** | 2920 |
| Corrosive liquid, n.o.s. | **154** | 1760 |
| Corrosive liquid, oxidizing, n.o.s. | **140** | 3093 |
| Corrosive liquid, poisonous, n.o.s. | **154** | 2922 |
| Corrosive liquid, self-heating, n.o.s. | **136** | 3301 |
| Corrosive liquid, toxic, n.o.s. | **154** | 2922 |
| Corrosive liquid, water-reactive, n.o.s. | **138** | 3094 |
| Corrosive solid, acidic, inorganic, n.o.s. | **154** | 3260 |
| Corrosive solid, acidic, organic, n.o.s. | **154** | 3261 |
| Corrosive solid, basic, inorganic, n.o.s. | **154** | 3262 |

| Name of Material | Guide No. | ID No. |
|---|---|---|
| Corrosive solid, basic, organic, n.o.s. | **154** | 3263 |
| Corrosive solid, flammable, n.o.s. | **134** | 2921 |
| Corrosive solid, n.o.s. | **154** | 1759 |
| Corrosive solid, oxidizing, n.o.s. | **140** | 3084 |
| Corrosive solid, poisonous, n.o.s. | **154** | 2923 |
| Corrosive solid, self-heating, n.o.s. | **136** | 3095 |
| Corrosive solid, toxic, n.o.s. | **154** | 2923 |
| Corrosive solid, water-reactive, n.o.s. | **138** | 3096 |
| Cotton | **133** | 1365 |
| Cotton, wet | **133** | 1365 |
| Cotton waste, oily | **133** | 1364 |
| Coumarin derivative pesticide, liquid, flammable, poisonous | **131** | 3024 |
| Coumarin derivative pesticide, liquid, flammable, toxic | **131** | 3024 |
| Coumarin derivative pesticide, liquid, poisonous | **151** | 3026 |
| Coumarin derivative pesticide, liquid, poisonous, flammable | **131** | 3025 |
| Coumarin derivative pesticide, liquid, toxic | **151** | 3026 |
| Coumarin derivative pesticide, liquid, toxic, flammable | **131** | 3025 |
| Coumarin derivative pesticide, solid, poisonous | **151** | 3027 |
| Coumarin derivative pesticide, solid, toxic | **151** | 3027 |
| Cresols, liquid | **153** | 2076 |
| Cresols, solid | **153** | 2076 |
| Cresols, solid | **153** | 3455 |

| Name of Material | Guide No. | ID No. |
|---|---|---|
| Cresylic acid | **153** | 2022 |
| Crotonaldehyde | **131P** | 1143 |
| Crotonaldehyde, stabilized | **131P** | 1143 |
| Crotonic acid | **153** | 2823 |
| Crotonic acid, liquid | **153** | 2823 |
| Crotonic acid, liquid | **153** | 3472 |
| Crotonic acid, solid | **153** | 2823 |
| Crotonylene | **128** | 1144 |
| CS | **153** | 2810 |
| Cumene | **130** | 1918 |
| Cupriethylenediamine, solution | **154** | 1761 |
| CX | **154** | 2811 |
| Cyanide solution, n.o.s. | **157** | 1935 |
| Cyanides, inorganic, solid, n.o.s. | **157** | 1588 |
| Cyanogen | **119** | 1026 |
| Cyanogen bromide | **157** | 1889 |
| Cyanogen chloride, stabilized | **125** | 1589 |
| Cyanuric chloride | **157** | 2670 |
| Cyclobutane | **115** | 2601 |
| Cyclobutyl chloroformate | **155** | 2744 |
| 1,5,9-Cyclododecatriene | **153** | 2518 |
| Cycloheptane | **128** | 2241 |
| Cycloheptatriene | **131** | 2603 |
| Cycloheptene | **128** | 2242 |
| Cyclohexane | **128** | 1145 |
| Cyclohexanethiol | **129** | 3054 |
| Cyclohexanone | **127** | 1915 |
| Cyclohexene | **130** | 2256 |
| Cyclohexenyltrichlorosilane | **156** | 1762 |
| Cyclohexyl acetate | **130** | 2243 |
| Cyclohexylamine | **132** | 2357 |

| Name of Material | Guide No. | ID No. |
|---|---|---|
| Cyclohexyl isocyanate | **155** | 2488 |
| Cyclohexyl mercaptan | **129** | 3054 |
| Cyclohexyltrichlorosilane | **156** | 1763 |
| Cyclooctadiene phosphines | **135** | 2940 |
| Cyclooctadienes | **130P** | 2520 |
| Cyclooctatetraene | **128P** | 2358 |
| Cyclopentane | **128** | 1146 |
| Cyclopentanol | **129** | 2244 |
| Cyclopentanone | **128** | 2245 |
| Cyclopentene | **128** | 2246 |
| Cyclopropane | **115** | 1027 |
| Cymenes | **130** | 2046 |
| DA | **151** | 1699 |
| Dangerous goods in apparatus | **171** | 3363 |
| Dangerous goods in machinery | **171** | 3363 |
| DC | **153** | 2810 |
| Decaborane | **134** | 1868 |
| Decahydronaphthalene | **130** | 1147 |
| n-Decane | **128** | 2247 |
| Denatured alcohol | **127** | 1987 |
| Desensitized explosive, liquid, n.o.s. | **128** | 3379 |
| Desensitized explosive, solid, n.o.s. | **133** | 3380 |
| Deuterium | **115** | 1957 |
| Deuterium, compressed | **115** | 1957 |
| Devices, small, hydrocarbon gas powered, with release device | **115** | 3150 |
| Diacetone alcohol | **129** | 1148 |
| Diacetyl | **127** | 2346 |
| Diallylamine | **132** | 2359 |
| Diallyl ether | **131P** | 2360 |
| 4,4'-Diaminodiphenylmethane | **153** | 2651 |

| Name of Material | Guide No. | ID No. |
|---|---|---|
| Di-n-amylamine | **131** | 2841 |
| Dibenzyldichlorosilane | **156** | 2434 |
| Diborane | **119** | 1911 |
| Diborane, compressed | **119** | 1911 |
| Diborane mixtures | **119** | 1911 |
| 1,2-Dibromobutan-3-one | **154** | 2648 |
| Dibromochloropropanes | **159** | 2872 |
| Dibromodifluoromethane | **171** | 1941 |
| Dibromomethane | **160** | 2664 |
| Di-n-butylamine | **132** | 2248 |
| Dibutylaminoethanol | **153** | 2873 |
| Dibutyl ethers | **128** | 1149 |
| Dichloroacetic acid | **153** | 1764 |
| 1,3-Dichloroacetone | **153** | 2649 |
| Dichloroacetyl chloride | **156** | 1765 |
| Dichloroanilines, liquid | **153** | 1590 |
| Dichloroanilines, solid | **153** | 1590 |
| Dichloroanilines, solid | **153** | 3442 |
| o-Dichlorobenzene | **152** | 1591 |
| 2,2'-Dichlorodiethyl ether | **152** | 1916 |
| Dichlorodifluoromethane | **126** | 1028 |
| Dichlorodifluoromethane and Difluoroethane azeotropic mixture with approximately 74% Dichlorodifluoromethane | **126** | 2602 |
| Dichlorodifluoromethane and Ethylene oxide mixture, with not more than 12.5% Ethylene oxide | **126** | 3070 |
| Dichlorodimethyl ether, symmetrical | **131** | 2249 |
| 1,1-Dichloroethane | **130** | 2362 |
| 1,2-Dichloroethylene | **130P** | 1150 |
| Dichloroethyl ether | **152** | 1916 |

| Name of Material | Guide No. | ID No. |
|---|---|---|
| Dichlorofluoromethane | **126** | 1029 |
| Dichloroisocyanuric acid, dry | **140** | 2465 |
| Dichloroisocyanuric acid salts | **140** | 2465 |
| Dichloroisopropyl ether | **153** | 2490 |
| Dichloromethane | **160** | 1593 |
| 1,1-Dichloro-1-nitroethane | **153** | 2650 |
| Dichloropentanes | **130** | 1152 |
| Dichlorophenyl isocyanates | **156** | 2250 |
| Dichlorophenyltrichlorosilane | **156** | 1766 |
| 1,2-Dichloropropane | **130** | 1279 |
| 1,3-Dichloropropanol-2 | **153** | 2750 |
| Dichloropropenes | **129** | 2047 |
| Dichlorosilane | **119** | 2189 |
| 1,2-Dichloro-1,1,2,2-tetrafluoroethane | **126** | 1958 |
| 3,5-Dichloro-2,4,6-trifluoropyridine | **151** | 9264 |
| Dicyclohexylamine | **153** | 2565 |
| Dicyclohexylammonium nitrite | **133** | 2687 |
| Dicyclopentadiene | **130** | 2048 |
| 1,2-Di-(dimethylamino)ethane | **129** | 2372 |
| Didymium nitrate | **140** | 1465 |
| Diesel fuel | **128** | 1202 |
| Diesel fuel | **128** | 1993 |
| Diethoxymethane | **127** | 2373 |
| 3,3-Diethoxypropene | **127** | 2374 |
| Diethylamine | **132** | 1154 |
| 2-Diethylaminoethanol | **132** | 2686 |
| 3-Diethylaminopropylamine | **132** | 2684 |
| Diethylaminopropylamine | **132** | 2684 |
| N,N-Diethylaniline | **153** | 2432 |
| Diethylbenzene | **130** | 2049 |
| Diethyl carbonate | **128** | 2366 |
| Diethyldichlorosilane | **155** | 1767 |
| Diethylenetriamine | **154** | 2079 |
| Diethyl ether | **127** | 1155 |
| N,N-Diethylethylenediamine | **132** | 2685 |
| Diethyl ketone | **127** | 1156 |
| Diethyl sulfate | **152** | 1594 |
| Diethyl sulfide | **129** | 2375 |
| Diethyl sulphate | **152** | 1594 |
| Diethyl sulphide | **129** | 2375 |
| Diethylthiophosphoryl chloride | **155** | 2751 |
| Diethylzinc | **135** | 1366 |
| Difluorochloroethanes | **115** | 2517 |
| 1,1-Difluoroethane | **115** | 1030 |
| Difluoroethane and Dichlorodifluoromethane azeotropic mixture with approximately 74% Dichlorodifluoromethane | **126** | 2602 |
| 1,1-Difluoroethylene | **116P** | 1959 |
| Difluoromethane | **115** | 3252 |
| Difluorophosphoric acid, anhydrous | **154** | 1768 |
| 2,3-Dihydropyran | **127** | 2376 |
| Diisobutylamine | **132** | 2361 |
| Diisobutylene, isomeric compounds | **128** | 2050 |
| Diisobutyl ketone | **128** | 1157 |
| Diisooctyl acid phosphate | **153** | 1902 |
| Diisopropylamine | **132** | 1158 |
| Diisopropyl ether | **127** | 1159 |
| Diketene, stabilized | **131P** | 2521 |
| 1,1-Dimethoxyethane | **127** | 2377 |
| 1,2-Dimethoxyethane | **127** | 2252 |
| Dimethylamine, anhydrous | **118** | 1032 |

| Name of Material | Guide No. | ID No. |
|---|---|---|
| Dimethylamine, aqueous solution | **132** | 1160 |
| Dimethylamine, solution | **132** | 1160 |
| 2-Dimethylaminoacetonitrile | **131** | 2378 |
| 2-Dimethylaminoethanol | **132** | 2051 |
| 2-Dimethylaminoethyl acrylate | **152** | 3302 |
| 2-Dimethylaminoethyl methacrylate | **153P** | 2522 |
| N,N-Dimethylaniline | **153** | 2253 |
| 2,3-Dimethylbutane | **128** | 2457 |
| 1,3-Dimethylbutylamine | **132** | 2379 |
| Dimethylcarbamoyl chloride | **156** | 2262 |
| Dimethyl carbonate | **129** | 1161 |
| Dimethylcyclohexanes | **128** | 2263 |
| N,N-Dimethylcyclohexylamine | **132** | 2264 |
| Dimethylcyclohexylamine | **132** | 2264 |
| Dimethyldichlorosilane | **155** | 1162 |
| Dimethyldiethoxysilane | **127** | 2380 |
| Dimethyldioxanes | **127** | 2707 |
| Dimethyl disulfide | **130** | 2381 |
| Dimethyl disulphide | **130** | 2381 |
| Dimethyl ether | **115** | 1033 |
| N,N-Dimethylformamide | **129** | 2265 |
| 1,1-Dimethylhydrazine | **131** | 1163 |
| Dimethylhydrazine, symmetrical | **131** | 2382 |
| Dimethylhydrazine, unsymmetrical | **131** | 1163 |
| 2,2-Dimethylpropane | **115** | 2044 |
| Dimethyl-N-propylamine | **132** | 2266 |
| Dimethyl sulfate | **156** | 1595 |
| Dimethyl sulfide | **130** | 1164 |
| Dimethyl sulphate | **156** | 1595 |
| Dimethyl sulphide | **130** | 1164 |
| Dimethyl thiophosphoryl chloride | **156** | 2267 |
| Dimethylzinc | **135** | 1370 |
| Dinitroanilines | **153** | 1596 |
| Dinitrobenzenes, liquid | **152** | 1597 |
| Dinitrobenzenes, solid | **152** | 1597 |
| Dinitrobenzenes, solid | **152** | 3443 |
| Dinitrochlorobenzenes | **153** | 1577 |
| Dinitro-o-cresol | **153** | 1598 |
| Dinitrogen tetroxide | **124** | 1067 |
| Dinitrogen tetroxide and Nitric oxide mixture | **124** | 1975 |
| Dinitrophenol, solution | **153** | 1599 |
| Dinitrophenol, wetted with not less than 15% water | **113** | 1320 |
| Dinitrophenolates, wetted with not less than 15% water | **113** | 1321 |
| Dinitroresorcinol, wetted with not less than 15% water | **113** | 1322 |
| Dinitrotoluenes | **152** | 2038 |
| Dinitrotoluenes, liquid | **152** | 2038 |
| Dinitrotoluenes, molten | **152** | 1600 |
| Dinitrotoluenes, solid | **152** | 2038 |
| Dinitrotoluenes, solid | **152** | 3454 |
| Dioxane | **127** | 1165 |
| Dioxolane | **127** | 1166 |
| Dipentene | **128** | 2052 |
| Diphenylamine chloroarsine | **154** | 1698 |
| Diphenylchloroarsine, liquid | **151** | 1699 |
| Diphenylchloroarsine, solid | **151** | 1699 |
| Diphenylchloroarsine, solid | **151** | 3450 |
| Diphenyldichlorosilane | **156** | 1769 |
| Diphenylmethyl bromide | **153** | 1770 |

| Name of Material | Guide No. | ID No. |
|---|---|---|
| Dipicryl sulfide, wetted with not less than 10% water | **113** | 2852 |
| Dipicryl sulphide, wetted with not less than 10% water | **113** | 2852 |
| Dipropylamine | **132** | 2383 |
| Di-n-propyl ether | **127** | 2384 |
| Dipropyl ketone | **128** | 2710 |
| Disinfectant, liquid, corrosive, n.o.s. | **153** | 1903 |
| Disinfectant, liquid, poisonous, n.o.s. | **151** | 3142 |
| Disinfectant, liquid, toxic, n.o.s. | **151** | 3142 |
| Disinfectant, solid, poisonous, n.o.s. | **151** | 1601 |
| Disinfectant, solid, toxic, n.o.s. | **151** | 1601 |
| Disodium trioxosilicate | **154** | 3253 |
| Dispersant gas, n.o.s. | **126** | 1078 |
| Dispersant gases, n.o.s. (flammable) | **115** | 1954 |
| Divinyl ether, stabilized | **128P** | 1167 |
| DM | **154** | 1698 |
| Dodecyltrichlorosilane | **156** | 1771 |
| DP | **125** | 1076 |
| Dry ice | **120** | 1845 |
| Dye, liquid, corrosive, n.o.s. | **154** | 2801 |
| Dye, liquid, poisonous, n.o.s. | **151** | 1602 |
| Dye, liquid, toxic, n.o.s. | **151** | 1602 |
| Dye, solid, corrosive, n.o.s. | **154** | 3147 |
| Dye, solid, poisonous, n.o.s. | **151** | 3143 |
| Dye, solid, toxic, n.o.s. | **151** | 3143 |
| Dye intermediate, liquid, corrosive, n.o.s. | **154** | 2801 |
| Dye intermediate, liquid, poisonous, n.o.s. | **151** | 1602 |
| Dye intermediate, liquid, toxic, n.o.s. | **151** | 1602 |
| Dye intermediate, solid, corrosive, n.o.s. | **154** | 3147 |
| Dye intermediate, solid, poisonous, n.o.s. | **151** | 3143 |
| Dye intermediate, solid, toxic, n.o.s. | **151** | 3143 |
| ED | **151** | 1892 |
| Elevated temperature liquid, flammable, n.o.s., with flash point above 37.8°C (100°F), at or above its flash point | **128** | 3256 |
| Elevated temperature liquid, flammable, n.o.s., with flash point above 60°C (140°F), at or above its flash point | **128** | 3256 |
| Elevated temperature liquid, n.o.s., at or above 100°C (212°F), and below its flash point | **128** | 3257 |
| Elevated temperature solid, n.o.s., at or above 240°C (464°F) | **171** | 3258 |
| Engine, fuel cell, flammable gas powered | **115** | 3166 |
| Engine, fuel cell, flammable gas powered | **115** | 3529 |
| Engine, fuel cell, flammable liquid powered | **128** | 3166 |
| Engine, fuel cell, flammable liquid powered | **128** | 3528 |
| Engine, internal combustion | **128** | 3166 |
| Engine, internal combustion | **171** | 3530 |
| Engine, internal combustion flammable gas powered | **115** | 3529 |
| Engine, internal combustion flammable liquid powered | **128** | 3528 |
| Engines, internal combustion, flammable gas powered | **115** | 3166 |

| Name of Material | Guide No. | ID No. |
|---|---|---|
| Engines, internal combustion, flammable liquid powered | **128** | 3166 |
| Environmentally hazardous substance, liquid, n.o.s. | **171** | 3082 |
| Environmentally hazardous substance, solid, n.o.s. | **171** | 3077 |
| Epibromohydrin | **131** | 2558 |
| Epichlorohydrin | **131P** | 2023 |
| 1,2-Epoxy-3-ethoxypropane | **127** | 2752 |
| Esters, n.o.s. | **127** | 3272 |
| Ethane | **115** | 1035 |
| Ethane, compressed | **115** | 1035 |
| Ethane, refrigerated liquid | **115** | 1961 |
| Ethane-Propane mixture, refrigerated liquid | **115** | 1961 |
| Ethanol | **127** | 1170 |
| Ethanol and gasoline mixture, with more than 10% ethanol | **127** | 3475 |
| Ethanol and motor spirit mixture, with more than 10% ethanol | **127** | 3475 |
| Ethanol and petrol mixture, with more than 10% ethanol | **127** | 3475 |
| Ethanol, solution | **127** | 1170 |
| Ethanolamine | **153** | 2491 |
| Ethanolamine, solution | **153** | 2491 |
| Ethers, n.o.s. | **127** | 3271 |
| Ethyl acetate | **129** | 1173 |
| Ethylacetylene, stabilized | **116P** | 2452 |
| Ethyl acrylate, stabilized | **129P** | 1917 |
| Ethyl alcohol | **127** | 1170 |
| Ethyl alcohol, solution | **127** | 1170 |
| Ethylamine | **118** | 1036 |
| Ethylamine, aqueous solution, with not less than 50% but not more than 70% Ethylamine | **132** | 2270 |
| Ethyl amyl ketone | **128** | 2271 |
| 2-Ethylaniline | **153** | 2273 |
| N-Ethylaniline | **153** | 2272 |
| Ethylbenzene | **130** | 1175 |
| N-Ethyl-N-benzylaniline | **153** | 2274 |
| N-Ethylbenzyltoluidines, liquid | **153** | 2753 |
| N-Ethylbenzyltoluidines, solid | **153** | 2753 |
| N-Ethylbenzyltoluidines, solid | **153** | 3460 |
| Ethyl borate | **129** | 1176 |
| Ethyl bromide | **131** | 1891 |
| Ethyl bromoacetate | **155** | 1603 |
| 2-Ethylbutanol | **129** | 2275 |
| 2-Ethylbutyl acetate | **130** | 1177 |
| Ethylbutyl acetate | **130** | 1177 |
| Ethyl butyl ether | **127** | 1179 |
| 2-Ethylbutyraldehyde | **130** | 1178 |
| Ethyl butyrate | **130** | 1180 |
| Ethyl chloride | **115** | 1037 |
| Ethyl chloroacetate | **155** | 1181 |
| Ethyl chloroformate | **155** | 1182 |
| Ethyl 2-chloropropionate | **129** | 2935 |
| Ethyl chlorothioformate | **155** | 2826 |
| Ethyl crotonate | **130** | 1862 |
| Ethyldichloroarsine | **151** | 1892 |
| Ethyldichlorosilane | **139** | 1183 |
| Ethylene | **116P** | 1962 |

| Name of Material | Guide No. | ID No. |
|---|---|---|
| Ethylene, Acetylene and Propylene in mixture, refrigerated liquid containing at least 71.5% Ethylene with not more than 22.5% Acetylene and not more than 6% Propylene | **115** | 3138 |
| Ethylene, compressed | **116P** | 1962 |
| Ethylene, refrigerated liquid (cryogenic liquid) | **115** | 1038 |
| Ethylene chlorohydrin | **131** | 1135 |
| Ethylenediamine | **132** | 1604 |
| Ethylene dibromide | **154** | 1605 |
| Ethylene dibromide and Methyl bromide mixture, liquid | **151** | 1647 |
| Ethylene dichloride | **131** | 1184 |
| Ethylene glycol diethyl ether | **127** | 1153 |
| Ethylene glycol monoethyl ether | **127** | 1171 |
| Ethylene glycol monoethyl ether acetate | **129** | 1172 |
| Ethylene glycol monomethyl ether | **127** | 1188 |
| Ethylene glycol monomethyl ether acetate | **129** | 1189 |
| Ethyleneimine, stabilized | **131P** | 1185 |
| Ethylene oxide | **119P** | 1040 |
| Ethylene oxide and Carbon dioxide mixture, with more than 9% but not more than 87% Ethylene oxide | **115** | 1041 |
| Ethylene oxide and Carbon dioxide mixture, with more than 87% Ethylene oxide | **119P** | 3300 |
| Ethylene oxide and Carbon dioxide mixtures, with not more than 9% Ethylene oxide | **126** | 1952 |
| Ethylene oxide and Chlorotetrafluoroethane mixture, with not more than 8.8% Ethylene oxide | **126** | 3297 |
| Ethylene oxide and Dichlorodifluoromethane mixture, with not more than 12.5% Ethylene oxide | **126** | 3070 |
| Ethylene oxide and Pentafluoroethane mixture, with not more than 7.9% Ethylene oxide | **126** | 3298 |
| Ethylene oxide and Propylene oxide mixture, with not more than 30% Ethylene oxide | **129P** | 2983 |
| Ethylene oxide and Tetrafluoroethane mixture, with not more than 5.6% Ethylene oxide | **126** | 3299 |
| Ethylene oxide with Nitrogen | **119P** | 1040 |
| Ethyl ether | **127** | 1155 |
| Ethyl fluoride | **115** | 2453 |
| Ethyl formate | **129** | 1190 |
| Ethylhexaldehydes | **129** | 1191 |
| 2-Ethylhexylamine | **132** | 2276 |
| 2-Ethylhexyl chloroformate | **156** | 2748 |
| Ethyl isobutyrate | **129** | 2385 |
| Ethyl isocyanate | **155** | 2481 |
| Ethyl lactate | **129** | 1192 |
| Ethyl mercaptan | **129** | 2363 |
| Ethyl methacrylate | **130P** | 2277 |
| Ethyl methacrylate, stabilized | **130P** | 2277 |
| Ethyl methyl ether | **115** | 1039 |
| Ethyl methyl ketone | **127** | 1193 |
| Ethyl nitrite, solution | **131** | 1194 |
| Ethyl orthoformate | **129** | 2524 |
| Ethyl oxalate | **156** | 2525 |
| Ethylphenyldichlorosilane | **156** | 2435 |

| Name of Material | Guide No. | ID No. |
| --- | --- | --- |
| Ethyl phosphonothioic dichloride, anhydrous | **154** | 2927 |
| Ethyl phosphonous dichloride, anhydrous | **135** | 2845 |
| Ethyl phosphorodichloridate | **154** | 2927 |
| 1-Ethylpiperidine | **132** | 2386 |
| Ethyl propionate | **129** | 1195 |
| Ethyl propyl ether | **127** | 2615 |
| Ethyl silicate | **129** | 1292 |
| N-Ethyltoluidines | **153** | 2754 |
| Ethyltrichlorosilane | **155** | 1196 |
| Explosives, division 1.1, 1.2, 1.3 or 1.5 | **112** | —— |
| Explosives, division 1.4 or 1.6 | **114** | —— |
| Extracts, aromatic, liquid | **127** | 1169 |
| Extracts, flavoring, liquid | **127** | 1197 |
| Extracts, flavouring, liquid | **127** | 1197 |
| Fabrics, animal or vegetable or synthetic, n.o.s. with oil | **133** | 1373 |
| Fabrics impregnated with weakly nitrated Nitrocellulose, n.o.s. | **133** | 1353 |
| Ferric arsenate | **151** | 1606 |
| Ferric arsenite | **151** | 1607 |
| Ferric chloride, anhydrous | **157** | 1773 |
| Ferric chloride, solution | **154** | 2582 |
| Ferric nitrate | **140** | 1466 |
| Ferrocerium | **170** | 1323 |
| Ferrosilicon | **139** | 1408 |
| Ferrous arsenate | **151** | 1608 |
| Ferrous chloride, solid | **154** | 1759 |
| Ferrous chloride, solution | **154** | 1760 |
| Ferrous metal borings, shavings, turnings or cuttings | **170** | 2793 |

| Name of Material | Guide No. | ID No. |
| --- | --- | --- |
| Fertilizer, ammoniating solution, with free Ammonia | **125** | 1043 |
| Fibers, animal or vegetable, burnt, wet or damp | **133** | 1372 |
| Fibers, animal or vegetable or synthetic, n.o.s. with oil | **133** | 1373 |
| Fibers, vegetable, dry | **133** | 3360 |
| Fibers impregnated with weakly nitrated Nitrocellulose, n.o.s. | **133** | 1353 |
| Fibres, animal or vegetable, burnt, wet or damp | **133** | 1372 |
| Fibres, animal or vegetable or synthetic, n.o.s. with oil | **133** | 1373 |
| Fibres, vegetable, dry | **133** | 3360 |
| Fibres impregnated with weakly nitrated Nitrocellulose, n.o.s. | **133** | 1353 |
| Films, nitrocellulose base | **133** | 1324 |
| Fire extinguisher charges, corrosive liquid | **154** | 1774 |
| Fire extinguishers with compressed gas | **126** | 1044 |
| Fire extinguishers with liquefied gas | **126** | 1044 |
| Firelighters, solid, with flammable liquid | **133** | 2623 |
| First aid kit | **171** | 3316 |
| Fish meal, stabilized | **171** | 2216 |
| Fish meal, unstabilized | **133** | 1374 |
| Fish scrap, stabilized | **171** | 2216 |
| Fish scrap, unstabilized | **133** | 1374 |
| Flammable liquid, corrosive, n.o.s | **132** | 2924 |
| Flammable liquid, n.o.s. | **128** | 1993 |
| Flammable liquid, poisonous, corrosive, n.o.s. | **131** | 3286 |

| Name of Material | Guide No. | ID No. |
|---|---|---|
| Flammable liquid, poisonous, n.o.s. | **131** | 1992 |
| Flammable liquid, toxic, corrosive, n.o.s. | **131** | 3286 |
| Flammable liquid, toxic, n.o.s. | **131** | 1992 |
| Flammable solid, corrosive, inorganic, n.o.s. | **134** | 3180 |
| Flammable solid, corrosive, organic, n.o.s. | **134** | 2925 |
| Flammable solid, inorganic, n.o.s. | **133** | 3178 |
| Flammable solid, organic, molten, n.o.s. | **133** | 3176 |
| Flammable solid, organic, n.o.s. | **133** | 1325 |
| Flammable solid, oxidizing, n.o.s. | **140** | 3097 |
| Flammable solid, poisonous, inorganic, n.o.s. | **134** | 3179 |
| Flammable solid, poisonous, organic, n.o.s. | **134** | 2926 |
| Flammable solid, toxic, inorganic, n.o.s. | **134** | 3179 |
| Flammable solid, toxic, organic, n.o.s. | **134** | 2926 |
| Fluorine | **124** | 1045 |
| Fluorine, compressed | **124** | 1045 |
| Fluoroacetic acid | **154** | 2642 |
| Fluoroanilines | **153** | 2941 |
| Fluorobenzene | **130** | 2387 |
| Fluoroboric acid | **154** | 1775 |
| Fluorophosphoric acid, anhydrous | **154** | 1776 |
| Fluorosilicates, n.o.s. | **151** | 2856 |
| Fluorosilicic acid | **154** | 1778 |
| Fluorosulfonic acid | **137** | 1777 |
| Fluorosulphonic acid | **137** | 1777 |

| Name of Material | Guide No. | ID No. |
|---|---|---|
| Fluorotoluenes | **130** | 2388 |
| Formaldehyde, solution (corrosive) | **132** | 2209 |
| Formaldehyde, solution, flammable | **132** | 1198 |
| Formalin (corrosive) | **132** | 2209 |
| Formalin (flammable) | **132** | 1198 |
| Formic acid | **153** | 1779 |
| Formic acid, with more than 85% acid | **153** | 1779 |
| Formic acid, with not less than 5% but less than 10% acid | **153** | 3412 |
| Formic acid, with not less than 10% but not more than 85% acid | **153** | 3412 |
| Fuel, aviation, turbine engine | **128** | 1863 |
| Fuel cell cartridges contained in equipment, containing corrosive substances | **153** | 3477 |
| Fuel cell cartridges contained in equipment, containing flammable liquids | **128** | 3473 |
| Fuel cell cartridges contained in equipment, containing hydrogen in metal hydride | **115** | 3479 |
| Fuel cell cartridges contained in equipment, containing liquefied flammable gas | **115** | 3478 |
| Fuel cell cartridges contained in equipment, containing water-reactive substances | **138** | 3476 |
| Fuel cell cartridges, containing corrosive substances | **153** | 3477 |
| Fuel cell cartridges, containing flammable liquids | **128** | 3473 |
| Fuel cell cartridges, containing hydrogen in metal hydride | **115** | 3479 |

| Name of Material | Guide No. | ID No. |
|---|---|---|
| Fuel cell cartridges, containing liquefied flammable gas | **115** | 3478 |
| Fuel cell cartridges, containing water-reactive substances | **138** | 3476 |
| Fuel cell cartridges packed with equipment, containing corrosive substances | **153** | 3477 |
| Fuel cell cartridges packed with equipment, containing flammable liquids | **128** | 3473 |
| Fuel cell cartridges packed with equipment, containing hydrogen in metal hydride | **115** | 3479 |
| Fuel cell cartridges packed with equipment, containing liquefied flammable gas | **115** | 3478 |
| Fuel cell cartridges packed with equipment, containing water-reactive substances | **138** | 3476 |
| Fuel oil | **128** | 1202 |
| Fuel oil | **128** | 1993 |
| Fumaryl chloride | **156** | 1780 |
| Fumigated cargo transport unit | **171** | 3359 |
| Fumigated unit | **171** | 3359 |
| Furaldehydes | **132P** | 1199 |
| Furan | **128** | 2389 |
| Furfural | **132P** | 1199 |
| Furfuraldehydes | **132P** | 1199 |
| Furfuryl alcohol | **153** | 2874 |
| Furfurylamine | **132** | 2526 |
| Fusee (rail or highway) | **133** | 1325 |
| Fusel oil | **127** | 1201 |
| GA | **153** | 2810 |
| Gallium | **172** | 2803 |
| Gas, refrigerated liquid, flammable, n.o.s. | **115** | 3312 |
| Gas, refrigerated liquid, n.o.s. | **120** | 3158 |
| Gas, refrigerated liquid, oxidizing, n.o.s. | **122** | 3311 |
| Gas cartridges | **115** | 2037 |
| Gas identification set | **123** | 9035 |
| Gasohol | **128** | 1203 |
| Gas oil | **128** | 1202 |
| Gasoline | **128** | 1203 |
| Gasoline and ethanol mixture, with more than 10% ethanol | **127** | 3475 |
| Gas sample, non-pressurized, flammable, n.o.s., not refrigerated liquid | **115** | 3167 |
| Gas sample, non-pressurized, poisonous, flammable, n.o.s., not refrigerated liquid | **119** | 3168 |
| Gas sample, non-pressurized, poisonous, n.o.s., not refrigerated liquid | **123** | 3169 |
| Gas sample, non-pressurized, toxic, flammable, n.o.s., not refrigerated liquid | **119** | 3168 |
| Gas sample, non-pressurized, toxic, n.o.s., not refrigerated liquid | **123** | 3169 |
| GB | **153** | 2810 |
| GD | **153** | 2810 |
| Genetically modified micro-organisms | **171** | 3245 |
| Genetically modified organisms | **171** | 3245 |
| Germane | **119** | 2192 |
| Germane, adsorbed | **173** | 3523 |
| GF | **153** | 2810 |
| Glycerol alpha-monochlorohydrin | **153** | 2689 |
| Glycidaldehyde | **131P** | 2622 |

| Name of Material | Guide No. | ID No. |
|---|---|---|
| Guanidine nitrate | **143** | 1467 |
| H | **153** | 2810 |
| Hafnium powder, dry | **135** | 2545 |
| Hafnium powder, wetted with not less than 25% water | **170** | 1326 |
| Halogenated monomethyldiphenylmethanes, liquid | **171** | 3151 |
| Halogenated monomethyldiphenylmethanes, solid | **171** | 3152 |
| Hay, wet, damp or contaminated with oil | **133** | 1327 |
| Hazardous waste, liquid, n.o.s. | **171** | 3082 |
| Hazardous waste, solid, n.o.s. | **171** | 3077 |
| HD | **153** | 2810 |
| Heating oil, light | **128** | 1202 |
| Helium | **121** | 1046 |
| Helium, compressed | **121** | 1046 |
| Helium, refrigerated liquid (cryogenic liquid) | **120** | 1963 |
| Heptafluoropropane | **126** | 3296 |
| n-Heptaldehyde | **129** | 3056 |
| Heptanes | **128** | 1206 |
| n-Heptene | **128** | 2278 |
| Hexachloroacetone | **153** | 2661 |
| Hexachlorobenzene | **152** | 2729 |
| Hexachlorobutadiene | **151** | 2279 |
| Hexachlorocyclopentadiene | **151** | 2646 |
| Hexachlorophene | **151** | 2875 |
| Hexadecyltrichlorosilane | **156** | 1781 |
| Hexadiene | **130** | 2458 |
| Hexaethyl tetraphosphate | **151** | 1611 |
| Hexaethyl tetraphosphate and compressed gas mixture | **123** | 1612 |

| Name of Material | Guide No. | ID No. |
|---|---|---|
| Hexafluoroacetone | **125** | 2420 |
| Hexafluoroacetone hydrate | **151** | 2552 |
| Hexafluoroacetone hydrate, liquid | **151** | 2552 |
| Hexafluoroacetone hydrate, solid | **151** | 3436 |
| Hexafluoroethane | **126** | 2193 |
| Hexafluoroethane, compressed | **126** | 2193 |
| Hexafluorophosphoric acid | **154** | 1782 |
| Hexafluoropropylene | **126** | 1858 |
| Hexafluoropropylene, compressed | **126** | 1858 |
| Hexaldehyde | **130** | 1207 |
| Hexamethylenediamine, solid | **153** | 2280 |
| Hexamethylenediamine, solution | **153** | 1783 |
| Hexamethylene diisocyanate | **156** | 2281 |
| Hexamethyleneimine | **132** | 2493 |
| Hexamethylenetetramine | **133** | 1328 |
| Hexanes | **128** | 1208 |
| Hexanoic acid | **153** | 2829 |
| Hexanols | **129** | 2282 |
| 1-Hexene | **128** | 2370 |
| Hexyltrichlorosilane | **156** | 1784 |
| HL | **153** | 2810 |
| HN-1 | **153** | 2810 |
| HN-2 | **153** | 2810 |
| HN-3 | **153** | 2810 |
| Hydrazine, anhydrous | **132** | 2029 |
| Hydrazine aqueous solution, flammable, with more than 37% hydrazine, by mass | **132** | 3484 |
| Hydrazine, aqueous solution, with more than 37% Hydrazine | **153** | 2030 |

| Name of Material | Guide No. | ID No. |
|---|---|---|
| Hydrazine, aqueous solution, with not less than 37% but not more than 64% Hydrazine | **153** | 2030 |
| Hydrazine, aqueous solution, with not more than 37% Hydrazine | **152** | 3293 |
| Hydrazine hydrate | **153** | 2030 |
| Hydriodic acid | **154** | 1787 |
| Hydrobromic acid | **154** | 1788 |
| Hydrocarbon and butadienes mixture, stabilized | **116P** | 1010 |
| Hydrocarbon gas mixture, compressed, n.o.s. | **115** | 1964 |
| Hydrocarbon gas mixture, liquefied, n.o.s. | **115** | 1965 |
| Hydrocarbon gas refills for small devices, with release device | **115** | 3150 |
| Hydrocarbons, liquid, n.o.s. | **128** | 3295 |
| Hydrochloric acid | **157** | 1789 |
| Hydrocyanic acid, aqueous solution, with less than 5% Hydrogen cyanide | **154** | 1613 |
| Hydrocyanic acid, aqueous solution, with not more than 20% Hydrogen cyanide | **154** | 1613 |
| Hydrocyanic acid, aqueous solutions, with more than 20% Hydrogen cyanide | **117** | 1051 |
| Hydrofluoric acid | **157** | 1790 |
| Hydrofluoric acid and Sulfuric acid mixture | **157** | 1786 |
| Hydrofluoric acid and Sulphuric acid mixture | **157** | 1786 |
| Hydrofluorosilicic acid | **154** | 1778 |
| Hydrogen | **115** | 1049 |
| Hydrogen absorbed in metal hydride | **115** | 9279 |
| Hydrogen, compressed | **115** | 1049 |
| Hydrogen in a metal hydride storage system | **115** | 3468 |
| Hydrogen in a metal hydride storage system contained in equipment | **115** | 3468 |
| Hydrogen in a metal hydride storage system packed with equipment | **115** | 3468 |
| Hydrogen, refrigerated liquid (cryogenic liquid) | **115** | 1966 |
| Hydrogen and Carbon monoxide mixture, compressed | **119** | 2600 |
| Hydrogen and Methane mixture, compressed | **115** | 2034 |
| Hydrogen bromide, anhydrous | **125** | 1048 |
| Hydrogen chloride, anhydrous | **125** | 1050 |
| Hydrogen chloride, refrigerated liquid | **125** | 2186 |
| Hydrogen cyanide, anhydrous, stabilized | **117** | 1051 |
| Hydrogen cyanide, aqueous solution, with not more than 20% Hydrogen cyanide | **154** | 1613 |
| Hydrogen cyanide, solution in alcohol, with not more than 45% Hydrogen cyanide | **131** | 3294 |
| Hydrogen cyanide, stabilized | **117** | 1051 |
| Hydrogen cyanide, stabilized (absorbed) | **152** | 1614 |
| Hydrogendifluorides, n.o.s. | **154** | 1740 |
| Hydrogendifluorides, solid, n.o.s. | **154** | 1740 |
| Hydrogendifluorides, solution, n.o.s. | **154** | 3471 |
| Hydrogen fluoride, anhydrous | **125** | 1052 |
| Hydrogen iodide, anhydrous | **125** | 2197 |

| Name of Material | Guide No. | ID No. |
|---|---|---|
| Hydrogen peroxide, aqueous solution, stabilized, with more than 60% Hydrogen peroxide | **143** | 2015 |
| Hydrogen peroxide, aqueous solution, with not less than 8% but less than 20% Hydrogen peroxide | **140** | 2984 |
| Hydrogen peroxide, aqueous solution, with not less than 20% but not more than 60% Hydrogen peroxide (stabilized as necessary) | **140** | 2014 |
| Hydrogen peroxide, stabilized | **143** | 2015 |
| Hydrogen peroxide and Peroxyacetic acid mixture, with acid(s), water and not more than 5% Peroxyacetic acid, stabilized | **140** | 3149 |
| Hydrogen selenide, adsorbed | **173** | 3526 |
| Hydrogen selenide, anhydrous | **117** | 2202 |
| Hydrogen sulfide | **117** | 1053 |
| Hydrogen sulphide | **117** | 1053 |
| Hydroquinone | **153** | 2662 |
| Hydroquinone, solution | **153** | 3435 |
| 1-Hydroxybenzotriazole, anhydrous, wetted with not less than 20% water | **113** | 3474 |
| 1-Hydroxybenzotriazole, monohydrate | **113** | 3474 |
| Hydroxylamine sulfate | **154** | 2865 |
| Hydroxylamine sulphate | **154** | 2865 |
| Hypochlorite solution | **154** | 1791 |
| Hypochlorites, inorganic, n.o.s. | **140** | 3212 |
| 3,3'-Iminodipropylamine | **153** | 2269 |
| Infectious substance, affecting animals only | **158** | 2900 |
| Infectious substance, affecting humans | **158** | 2814 |

| Name of Material | Guide No. | ID No. |
|---|---|---|
| Ink, printer's, flammable | **129** | 1210 |
| Insecticide gas, flammable, n.o.s. | **115** | 3354 |
| Insecticide gas, n.o.s. | **126** | 1968 |
| Insecticide gas, poisonous, flammable, n.o.s. | **119** | 3355 |
| Insecticide gas, poisonous, flammable, n.o.s. (Inhalation Hazard Zone A) | **119** | 3355 |
| Insecticide gas, poisonous, flammable, n.o.s. (Inhalation Hazard Zone B) | **119** | 3355 |
| Insecticide gas, poisonous, flammable, n.o.s. (Inhalation Hazard Zone C) | **119** | 3355 |
| Insecticide gas, poisonous, flammable, n.o.s. (Inhalation Hazard Zone D) | **119** | 3355 |
| Insecticide gas, poisonous, n.o.s. | **123** | 1967 |
| Insecticide gas, toxic, flammable, n.o.s. | **119** | 3355 |
| Insecticide gas, toxic, flammable, n.o.s. (Inhalation Hazard Zone A) | **119** | 3355 |
| Insecticide gas, toxic, flammable, n.o.s. (Inhalation Hazard Zone B) | **119** | 3355 |
| Insecticide gas, toxic, flammable, n.o.s. (Inhalation Hazard Zone C) | **119** | 3355 |
| Insecticide gas, toxic, flammable, n.o.s. (Inhalation Hazard Zone D) | **119** | 3355 |
| Insecticide gas, toxic, n.o.s. | **123** | 1967 |
| Iodine | **154** | 3495 |
| Iodine monochloride, liquid | **157** | 3498 |
| Iodine monochloride, solid | **157** | 1792 |
| Iodine pentafluoride | **144** | 2495 |
| 2-Iodobutane | **129** | 2390 |

| Name of Material | Guide No. | ID No. |
|---|---|---|
| Iodomethylpropanes | **129** | 2391 |
| Iodopropanes | **129** | 2392 |
| IPDI | **156** | 2290 |
| Iron oxide, spent | **135** | 1376 |
| Iron pentacarbonyl | **131** | 1994 |
| Iron sponge, spent | **135** | 1376 |
| Isobutane | **115** | 1075 |
| Isobutane | **115** | 1969 |
| Isobutanol | **129** | 1212 |
| Isobutyl acetate | **129** | 1213 |
| Isobutyl acrylate, stabilized | **129P** | 2527 |
| Isobutyl alcohol | **129** | 1212 |
| Isobutyl aldehyde | **130** | 2045 |
| Isobutylamine | **132** | 1214 |
| Isobutyl chloroformate | **155** | 2742 |
| Isobutylene | **115** | 1055 |
| Isobutylene | **115** | 1075 |
| Isobutyl formate | **129** | 2393 |
| Isobutyl isobutyrate | **130** | 2528 |
| Isobutyl isocyanate | **155** | 2486 |
| Isobutyl methacrylate, stabilized | **130P** | 2283 |
| Isobutyl propionate | **129** | 2394 |
| Isobutyraldehyde | **130** | 2045 |
| Isobutyric acid | **132** | 2529 |
| Isobutyronitrile | **131** | 2284 |
| Isobutyryl chloride | **132** | 2395 |
| Isocyanate solution, flammable, poisonous, n.o.s. | **155** | 2478 |
| Isocyanate solution, flammable, toxic, n.o.s. | **155** | 2478 |
| Isocyanate solution, poisonous, flammable, n.o.s. | **155** | 3080 |
| Isocyanate solution, poisonous, n.o.s. | **155** | 2206 |
| Isocyanate solution, toxic, flammable, n.o.s. | **155** | 3080 |
| Isocyanate solution, toxic, n.o.s. | **155** | 2206 |
| Isocyanates, flammable, poisonous, n.o.s. | **155** | 2478 |
| Isocyanates, flammable, toxic, n.o.s. | **155** | 2478 |
| Isocyanates, poisonous, flammable, n.o.s. | **155** | 3080 |
| Isocyanates, poisonous, n.o.s. | **155** | 2206 |
| Isocyanates, toxic, flammable, n.o.s. | **155** | 3080 |
| Isocyanates, toxic, n.o.s. | **155** | 2206 |
| Isocyanatobenzotrifluorides | **156** | 2285 |
| Isoheptenes | **128** | 2287 |
| Isohexenes | **128** | 2288 |
| Isooctane | **128** | 1262 |
| Isooctenes | **128** | 1216 |
| Isopentane | **128** | 1265 |
| Isopentenes | **128** | 2371 |
| Isophoronediamine | **153** | 2289 |
| Isophorone diisocyanate | **156** | 2290 |
| Isoprene, stabilized | **130P** | 1218 |
| Isopropanol | **129** | 1219 |
| Isopropenyl acetate | **129P** | 2403 |
| Isopropenylbenzene | **128** | 2303 |
| Isopropyl acetate | **129** | 1220 |
| Isopropyl acid phosphate | **153** | 1793 |
| Isopropyl alcohol | **129** | 1219 |
| Isopropylamine | **132** | 1221 |

| Name of Material | Guide No. | ID No. |
|---|---|---|
| Isopropylbenzene | **130** | 1918 |
| Isopropyl butyrate | **129** | 2405 |
| Isopropyl chloroacetate | **155** | 2947 |
| Isopropyl chloroformate | **155** | 2407 |
| Isopropyl 2-chloropropionate | **129** | 2934 |
| Isopropyl isobutyrate | **127** | 2406 |
| Isopropyl isocyanate | **155** | 2483 |
| Isopropyl nitrate | **130** | 1222 |
| Isopropyl propionate | **129** | 2409 |
| Isosorbide dinitrate mixture | **133** | 2907 |
| Isosorbide-5-mononitrate | **133** | 3251 |
| Kerosene | **128** | 1223 |
| Ketones, liquid, n.o.s. | **127** | 1224 |
| Krill meal | **133** | 3497 |
| Krypton | **121** | 1056 |
| Krypton, compressed | **121** | 1056 |
| Krypton, refrigerated liquid (cryogenic liquid) | **120** | 1970 |
| L (Lewisite) | **153** | 2810 |
| Lead acetate | **151** | 1616 |
| Lead arsenates | **151** | 1617 |
| Lead arsenites | **151** | 1618 |
| Lead compound, soluble, n.o.s. | **151** | 2291 |
| Lead cyanide | **151** | 1620 |
| Lead dioxide | **141** | 1872 |
| Lead nitrate | **141** | 1469 |
| Lead perchlorate | **141** | 1470 |
| Lead perchlorate, solid | **141** | 1470 |
| Lead perchlorate, solution | **141** | 3408 |
| Lead phosphite, dibasic | **133** | 2989 |
| Lead sulfate, with more than 3% free acid | **154** | 1794 |
| Lead sulphate, with more than 3% free acid | **154** | 1794 |
| Lewisite | **153** | 2810 |
| Life-saving appliances, not self-inflating | **171** | 3072 |
| Life-saving appliances, self-inflating | **171** | 2990 |
| Lighter refills (cigarettes) (flammable gas) | **115** | 1057 |
| Lighters (cigarettes) (flammable gas) | **115** | 1057 |
| Lighters, non-pressurized, containing flammable liquid | **128** | 1057 |
| Liquefied gas, flammable, n.o.s. | **115** | 3161 |
| Liquefied gas, n.o.s. | **126** | 3163 |
| Liquefied gas, oxidizing, n.o.s. | **122** | 3157 |
| Liquefied gas, poisonous, corrosive, n.o.s. | **123** | 3308 |
| Liquefied gas, poisonous, corrosive, n.o.s. (Inhalation Hazard Zone A) | **123** | 3308 |
| Liquefied gas, poisonous, corrosive, n.o.s. (Inhalation Hazard Zone B) | **123** | 3308 |
| Liquefied gas, poisonous, corrosive, n.o.s. (Inhalation Hazard Zone C) | **123** | 3308 |
| Liquefied gas, poisonous, corrosive, n.o.s. (Inhalation Hazard Zone D) | **123** | 3308 |
| Liquefied gas, poisonous, flammable, corrosive, n.o.s. | **119** | 3309 |
| Liquefied gas, poisonous, flammable, corrosive, n.o.s. (Inhalation Hazard Zone A) | **119** | 3309 |
| Liquefied gas, poisonous, flammable, corrosive, n.o.s. (Inhalation Hazard Zone B) | **119** | 3309 |

| Name of Material | Guide No. | ID No. |
| --- | --- | --- |
| Liquefied gas, poisonous, flammable, corrosive, n.o.s. (Inhalation Hazard Zone C) | **119** | 3309 |
| Liquefied gas, poisonous, flammable, corrosive, n.o.s. (Inhalation Hazard Zone D) | **119** | 3309 |
| Liquefied gas, poisonous, flammable, n.o.s. | **119** | 3160 |
| Liquefied gas, poisonous, flammable, n.o.s. (Inhalation Hazard Zone A) | **119** | 3160 |
| Liquefied gas, poisonous, flammable, n.o.s. (Inhalation Hazard Zone B) | **119** | 3160 |
| Liquefied gas, poisonous, flammable, n.o.s. (Inhalation Hazard Zone C) | **119** | 3160 |
| Liquefied gas, poisonous, flammable, n.o.s. (Inhalation Hazard Zone D) | **119** | 3160 |
| Liquefied gas, poisonous, n.o.s. | **123** | 3162 |
| Liquefied gas, poisonous, n.o.s. (Inhalation Hazard Zone A) | **123** | 3162 |
| Liquefied gas, poisonous, n.o.s. (Inhalation Hazard Zone B) | **123** | 3162 |
| Liquefied gas, poisonous, n.o.s. (Inhalation Hazard Zone C) | **123** | 3162 |
| Liquefied gas, poisonous, n.o.s. (Inhalation Hazard Zone D) | **123** | 3162 |
| Liquefied gas, poisonous, oxidizing, corrosive, n.o.s. | **124** | 3310 |
| Liquefied gas, poisonous, oxidizing, corrosive, n.o.s. (Inhalation Hazard Zone A) | **124** | 3310 |
| Liquefied gas, poisonous, oxidizing, corrosive, n.o.s. (Inhalation Hazard Zone B) | **124** | 3310 |

| Name of Material | Guide No. | ID No. |
| --- | --- | --- |
| Liquefied gas, poisonous, oxidizing, corrosive, n.o.s. (Inhalation Hazard Zone C) | **124** | 3310 |
| Liquefied gas, poisonous, oxidizing, corrosive, n.o.s. (Inhalation Hazard Zone D) | **124** | 3310 |
| Liquefied gas, poisonous, oxidizing, n.o.s. | **124** | 3307 |
| Liquefied gas, poisonous, oxidizing, n.o.s. (Inhalation Hazard Zone A) | **124** | 3307 |
| Liquefied gas, poisonous, oxidizing, n.o.s. (Inhalation Hazard Zone B) | **124** | 3307 |
| Liquefied gas, poisonous, oxidizing, n.o.s. (Inhalation Hazard Zone C) | **124** | 3307 |
| Liquefied gas, poisonous, oxidizing, n.o.s. (Inhalation Hazard Zone D) | **124** | 3307 |
| Liquefied gas, toxic, corrosive, n.o.s. | **123** | 3308 |
| Liquefied gas, toxic, corrosive, n.o.s. (Inhalation Hazard Zone A) | **123** | 3308 |
| Liquefied gas, toxic, corrosive, n.o.s. (Inhalation Hazard Zone B) | **123** | 3308 |
| Liquefied gas, toxic, corrosive, n.o.s. (Inhalation Hazard Zone C) | **123** | 3308 |
| Liquefied gas, toxic, corrosive, n.o.s. (Inhalation Hazard Zone D) | **123** | 3308 |
| Liquefied gas, toxic, flammable, corrosive, n.o.s. | **119** | 3309 |
| Liquefied gas, toxic, flammable, corrosive, n.o.s. (Inhalation Hazard Zone A) | **119** | 3309 |
| Liquefied gas, toxic, flammable, corrosive, n.o.s. (Inhalation Hazard Zone B) | **119** | 3309 |

| Name of Material | Guide No. | ID No. |
|---|---|---|
| Liquefied gas, toxic, flammable, corrosive, n.o.s. (Inhalation Hazard Zone C) | **119** | 3309 |
| Liquefied gas, toxic, flammable, corrosive, n.o.s. (Inhalation Hazard Zone D) | **119** | 3309 |
| Liquefied gas, toxic, flammable, n.o.s. | **119** | 3160 |
| Liquefied gas, toxic, flammable, n.o.s. (Inhalation Hazard Zone A) | **119** | 3160 |
| Liquefied gas, toxic, flammable, n.o.s. (Inhalation Hazard Zone B) | **119** | 3160 |
| Liquefied gas, toxic, flammable, n.o.s. (Inhalation Hazard Zone C) | **119** | 3160 |
| Liquefied gas, toxic, flammable, n.o.s. (Inhalation Hazard Zone D) | **119** | 3160 |
| Liquefied gas, toxic, n.o.s. | **123** | 3162 |
| Liquefied gas, toxic, n.o.s. (Inhalation Hazard Zone A) | **123** | 3162 |
| Liquefied gas, toxic, n.o.s. (Inhalation Hazard Zone B) | **123** | 3162 |
| Liquefied gas, toxic, n.o.s. (Inhalation Hazard Zone C) | **123** | 3162 |
| Liquefied gas, toxic, n.o.s. (Inhalation Hazard Zone D) | **123** | 3162 |
| Liquefied gas, toxic, oxidizing, corrosive, n.o.s. | **124** | 3310 |
| Liquefied gas, toxic, oxidizing, corrosive, n.o.s. (Inhalation Hazard Zone A) | **124** | 3310 |
| Liquefied gas, toxic, oxidizing, corrosive, n.o.s. (Inhalation Hazard Zone B) | **124** | 3310 |
| Liquefied gas, toxic, oxidizing, corrosive, n.o.s. (Inhalation Hazard Zone C) | **124** | 3310 |
| Liquefied gas, toxic, oxidizing, corrosive, n.o.s. (Inhalation Hazard Zone D) | **124** | 3310 |
| Liquefied gas, toxic, oxidizing, n.o.s. | **124** | 3307 |
| Liquefied gas, toxic, oxidizing, n.o.s. (Inhalation Hazard Zone A) | **124** | 3307 |
| Liquefied gas, toxic, oxidizing, n.o.s. (Inhalation Hazard Zone B) | **124** | 3307 |
| Liquefied gas, toxic, oxidizing, n.o.s. (Inhalation Hazard Zone C) | **124** | 3307 |
| Liquefied gas, toxic, oxidizing, n.o.s. (Inhalation Hazard Zone D) | **124** | 3307 |
| Liquefied gases, non-flammable, charged with Nitrogen, Carbon dioxide or Air | **120** | 1058 |
| Liquefied natural gas (cryogenic liquid) | **115** | 1972 |
| Liquefied petroleum gas | **115** | 1075 |
| Lithium | **138** | 1415 |
| Lithium alkyls | **135** | 2445 |
| Lithium alkyls, liquid | **135** | 2445 |
| Lithium alkyls, solid | **135** | 3433 |
| Lithium aluminum hydride | **138** | 1410 |
| Lithium aluminum hydride, ethereal | **138** | 1411 |
| Lithium batteries | **138** | 3090 |
| Lithium batteries contained in equipment | **138** | 3091 |
| Lithium batteries packed with equipment | **138** | 3091 |
| Lithium borohydride | **138** | 1413 |
| Lithium ferrosilicon | **139** | 2830 |
| Lithium hydride | **138** | 1414 |

| Name of Material | Guide No. | ID No. |
|---|---|---|
| Lithium hydride, fused solid | **138** | 2805 |
| Lithium hydroxide | **154** | 2680 |
| Lithium hydroxide, monohydrate | **154** | 2680 |
| Lithium hydroxide, solution | **154** | 2679 |
| Lithium hypochlorite, dry | **140** | 1471 |
| Lithium hypochlorite mixture | **140** | 1471 |
| Lithium hypochlorite mixtures, dry | **140** | 1471 |
| Lithium ion batteries (including lithium ion polymer batteries) | **147** | 3480 |
| Lithium ion batteries contained in equipment (including lithium ion polymer batteries) | **147** | 3481 |
| Lithium ion batteries packed with equipment (including lithium ion polymer batteries) | **147** | 3481 |
| Lithium metal batteries (including lithium alloy batteries) | **138** | 3090 |
| Lithium metal batteries contained in equipment (including lithium alloy batteries) | **138** | 3091 |
| Lithium metal batteries packed with equipment (including lithium alloy batteries) | **138** | 3091 |
| Lithium nitrate | **140** | 2722 |
| Lithium nitride | **138** | 2806 |
| Lithium peroxide | **143** | 1472 |
| Lithium silicon | **138** | 1417 |
| LNG (cryogenic liquid) | **115** | 1972 |
| London purple | **151** | 1621 |
| LPG | **115** | 1075 |
| Machinery, fuel cell, flammable gas powered | **115** | 3529 |
| Machinery, fuel cell, flammable liquid powered | **128** | 3528 |
| Machinery, internal combustion | **171** | 3530 |
| Machinery, internal combustion, flammable gas powered | **115** | 3529 |
| Machinery, internal combustion, flammable liquid powered | **128** | 3528 |
| Magnesium | **138** | 1869 |
| Magnesium, in pellets, turnings or ribbons | **138** | 1869 |
| Magnesium alkyls | **135** | 3053 |
| Magnesium alloys, with more than 50% Magnesium, in pellets, turnings or ribbons | **138** | 1869 |
| Magnesium alloys powder | **138** | 1418 |
| Magnesium aluminum phosphide | **139** | 1419 |
| Magnesium arsenate | **151** | 1622 |
| Magnesium bromate | **140** | 1473 |
| Magnesium chlorate | **140** | 2723 |
| Magnesium chloride and Chlorate mixture | **140** | 1459 |
| Magnesium chloride and Chlorate mixture, solid | **140** | 1459 |
| Magnesium chloride and Chlorate mixture, solution | **140** | 3407 |
| Magnesium diamide | **135** | 2004 |
| Magnesium diphenyl | **135** | 2005 |
| Magnesium fluorosilicate | **151** | 2853 |
| Magnesium granules, coated | **138** | 2950 |
| Magnesium hydride | **138** | 2010 |
| Magnesium nitrate | **140** | 1474 |
| Magnesium perchlorate | **140** | 1475 |
| Magnesium peroxide | **140** | 1476 |

| Name of Material | Guide No. | ID No. |
|---|---|---|
| Magnesium phosphide | **139** | 2011 |
| Magnesium powder | **138** | 1418 |
| Magnesium silicide | **138** | 2624 |
| Magnesium silicofluoride | **151** | 2853 |
| Magnetized material | **171** | 2807 |
| Maleic anhydride | **156** | 2215 |
| Maleic anhydride, molten | **156** | 2215 |
| Malononitrile | **153** | 2647 |
| Maneb | **135** | 2210 |
| Maneb, stabilized | **135** | 2968 |
| Maneb preparation, stabilized | **135** | 2968 |
| Maneb preparation, with not less than 60% Maneb | **135** | 2210 |
| Manganese nitrate | **140** | 2724 |
| Manganese resinate | **133** | 1330 |
| Matches, fusee | **133** | 2254 |
| Matches, safety | **133** | 1944 |
| Matches, "strike anywhere" | **133** | 1331 |
| Matches, wax "vesta" | **133** | 1945 |
| MD | **152** | 1556 |
| Medical waste, n.o.s. | **158** | 3291 |
| Medicine, liquid, flammable, poisonous, n.o.s. | **131** | 3248 |
| Medicine, liquid, flammable, toxic, n.o.s. | **131** | 3248 |
| Medicine, liquid, poisonous, n.o.s. | **151** | 1851 |
| Medicine, liquid, toxic, n.o.s. | **151** | 1851 |
| Medicine, solid, poisonous, n.o.s. | **151** | 3249 |
| Medicine, solid, toxic, n.o.s. | **151** | 3249 |
| Mercaptan mixture, liquid, flammable, n.o.s. | **130** | 3336 |
| Mercaptan mixture, liquid, flammable, poisonous, n.o.s. | **131** | 1228 |
| Mercaptan mixture, liquid, flammable, toxic, n.o.s. | **131** | 1228 |
| Mercaptan mixture, liquid, poisonous, flammable, n.o.s. | **131** | 3071 |
| Mercaptan mixture, liquid, toxic, flammable, n.o.s. | **131** | 3071 |
| Mercaptans, liquid, flammable, n.o.s. | **130** | 3336 |
| Mercaptans, liquid, flammable, poisonous, n.o.s. | **131** | 1228 |
| Mercaptans, liquid, flammable, toxic, n.o.s. | **131** | 1228 |
| Mercaptans, liquid, poisonous, flammable, n.o.s. | **131** | 3071 |
| Mercaptans, liquid, toxic, flammable, n.o.s. | **131** | 3071 |
| Mercuric arsenate | **151** | 1623 |
| Mercuric bromide | **154** | 1634 |
| Mercuric chloride | **154** | 1624 |
| Mercuric cyanide | **154** | 1636 |
| Mercuric nitrate | **141** | 1625 |
| Mercuric oxycyanide | **151** | 1642 |
| Mercuric potassium cyanide | **157** | 1626 |
| Mercuric sulfate | **151** | 1645 |
| Mercuric sulphate | **151** | 1645 |
| Mercurous bromide | **154** | 1634 |
| Mercurous nitrate | **141** | 1627 |
| Mercury | **172** | 2809 |
| Mercury acetate | **151** | 1629 |
| Mercury ammonium chloride | **151** | 1630 |
| Mercury based pesticide, liquid, flammable, poisonous | **131** | 2778 |

| Name of Material | Guide No. | ID No. |
|---|---|---|
| Mercury based pesticide, liquid, flammable, toxic | **131** | 2778 |
| Mercury based pesticide, liquid, poisonous | **151** | 3012 |
| Mercury based pesticide, liquid, poisonous, flammable | **131** | 3011 |
| Mercury based pesticide, liquid, toxic | **151** | 3012 |
| Mercury based pesticide, liquid, toxic, flammable | **131** | 3011 |
| Mercury based pesticide, solid, poisonous | **151** | 2777 |
| Mercury based pesticide, solid, toxic | **151** | 2777 |
| Mercury benzoate | **154** | 1631 |
| Mercury bromides | **154** | 1634 |
| Mercury compound, liquid, n.o.s. | **151** | 2024 |
| Mercury compound, solid, n.o.s. | **151** | 2025 |
| Mercury contained in manufactured articles | **172** | 3506 |
| Mercury cyanide | **154** | 1636 |
| Mercury gluconate | **151** | 1637 |
| Mercury iodide | **151** | 1638 |
| Mercury metal | **172** | 2809 |
| Mercury nucleate | **151** | 1639 |
| Mercury oleate | **151** | 1640 |
| Mercury oxide | **151** | 1641 |
| Mercury oxycyanide, desensitized | **151** | 1642 |
| Mercury potassium iodide | **151** | 1643 |
| Mercury salicylate | **151** | 1644 |
| Mercury sulfate | **151** | 1645 |
| Mercury sulphate | **151** | 1645 |
| Mercury thiocyanate | **151** | 1646 |

| Name of Material | Guide No. | ID No. |
|---|---|---|
| Mesityl oxide | **129** | 1229 |
| Metal alkyl halides, water-reactive, n.o.s. | **138** | 3049 |
| Metal alkyl hydrides, water-reactive, n.o.s. | **138** | 3050 |
| Metal alkyls, water-reactive, n.o.s. | **135** | 2003 |
| Metal aryl halides, water-reactive, n.o.s. | **138** | 3049 |
| Metal aryl hydrides, water-reactive, n.o.s. | **138** | 3050 |
| Metal aryls, water-reactive, n.o.s. | **135** | 2003 |
| Metal carbonyls, liquid, n.o.s. | **151** | 3281 |
| Metal carbonyls, n.o.s. | **151** | 3281 |
| Metal carbonyls, solid, n.o.s. | **151** | 3466 |
| Metal catalyst, dry | **135** | 2881 |
| Metal catalyst, wetted | **170** | 1378 |
| Metaldehyde | **133** | 1332 |
| Metal hydrides, flammable, n.o.s. | **170** | 3182 |
| Metal hydrides, water-reactive, n.o.s. | **138** | 1409 |
| Metallic substance, water-reactive, n.o.s. | **138** | 3208 |
| Metallic substance, water-reactive, self-heating, n.o.s. | **138** | 3209 |
| Metal powder, flammable, n.o.s. | **170** | 3089 |
| Metal powder, self-heating, n.o.s. | **135** | 3189 |
| Metal salts of organic compounds, flammable, n.o.s. | **133** | 3181 |
| Methacrylaldehyde, stabilized | **131P** | 2396 |
| Methacrylic acid, stabilized | **153P** | 2531 |
| Methacrylonitrile, stabilized | **131P** | 3079 |
| Methallyl alcohol | **129** | 2614 |

| Name of Material | Guide No. | ID No. |
|---|---|---|
| Methane | **115** | 1971 |
| Methane, compressed | **115** | 1971 |
| Methane, refrigerated liquid (cryogenic liquid) | **115** | 1972 |
| Methane and Hydrogen mixture, compressed | **115** | 2034 |
| Methanesulfonyl chloride | **156** | 3246 |
| Methanesulphonyl chloride | **156** | 3246 |
| Methanol | **131** | 1230 |
| Methoxymethyl isocyanate | **155** | 2605 |
| 4-Methoxy-4-methylpentan-2-one | **128** | 2293 |
| 1-Methoxy-2-propanol | **129** | 3092 |
| Methyl acetate | **129** | 1231 |
| Methylacetylene and Propadiene mixture, stabilized | **116P** | 1060 |
| Methyl acrylate, stabilized | **129P** | 1919 |
| Methylal | **127** | 1234 |
| Methyl alcohol | **131** | 1230 |
| Methylallyl chloride | **130P** | 2554 |
| Methylamine, anhydrous | **118** | 1061 |
| Methylamine, aqueous solution | **132** | 1235 |
| Methylamyl acetate | **130** | 1233 |
| Methylamyl alcohol | **129** | 2053 |
| Methyl amyl ketone | **127** | 1110 |
| N-Methylaniline | **153** | 2294 |
| alpha-Methylbenzyl alcohol | **153** | 2937 |
| alpha-Methylbenzyl alcohol, liquid | **153** | 2937 |
| alpha-Methylbenzyl alcohol, solid | **153** | 3438 |
| Methylbenzyl alcohol (alpha) | **153** | 2937 |
| Methyl bromide | **123** | 1062 |
| Methyl bromide and Chloropicrin mixture | **123** | 1581 |
| Methyl bromide and Ethylene dibromide mixture, liquid | **151** | 1647 |
| Methyl bromoacetate | **155** | 2643 |
| 2-Methylbutanal | **129** | 3371 |
| 3-Methylbutan-2-one | **127** | 2397 |
| 2-Methyl-1-butene | **128** | 2459 |
| 2-Methyl-2-butene | **128** | 2460 |
| 3-Methyl-1-butene | **128** | 2561 |
| N-Methylbutylamine | **132** | 2945 |
| Methyl tert-butyl ether | **127** | 2398 |
| Methyl butyrate | **129** | 1237 |
| Methyl chloride | **115** | 1063 |
| Methyl chloride and Chloropicrin mixture | **119** | 1582 |
| Methyl chloride and Methylene chloride mixture | **115** | 1912 |
| Methyl chloroacetate | **155** | 2295 |
| Methyl chloroformate | **155** | 1238 |
| Methyl chloromethyl ether | **131** | 1239 |
| Methyl 2-chloropropionate | **129** | 2933 |
| Methylchlorosilane | **119** | 2534 |
| Methylcyclohexane | **128** | 2296 |
| Methylcyclohexanols | **129** | 2617 |
| Methylcyclohexanone | **128** | 2297 |
| Methylcyclopentane | **128** | 2298 |
| Methyl dichloroacetate | **155** | 2299 |
| Methyldichloroarsine | **152** | 1556 |
| Methyldichlorosilane | **139** | 1242 |
| Methylene chloride | **160** | 1593 |
| Methylene chloride and Methyl chloride mixture | **115** | 1912 |
| Methyl ethyl ether | **115** | 1039 |

| Name of Material | Guide No. | ID No. |
|---|---|---|
| Methyl ethyl ketone | **127** | 1193 |
| 2-Methyl-5-ethylpyridine | **153** | 2300 |
| Methyl fluoride | **115** | 2454 |
| Methyl formate | **129** | 1243 |
| 2-Methylfuran | **128** | 2301 |
| 2-Methyl-2-heptanethiol | **131** | 3023 |
| 5-Methylhexan-2-one | **127** | 2302 |
| Methylhydrazine | **131** | 1244 |
| Methyl iodide | **151** | 2644 |
| Methyl isobutyl carbinol | **129** | 2053 |
| Methyl isobutyl ketone | **127** | 1245 |
| Methyl isocyanate | **155** | 2480 |
| Methyl isopropenyl ketone, stabilized | **127P** | 1246 |
| Methyl isothiocyanate | **131** | 2477 |
| Methyl isovalerate | **130** | 2400 |
| Methyl magnesium bromide in Ethyl ether | **135** | 1928 |
| Methyl mercaptan | **117** | 1064 |
| Methyl methacrylate monomer, stabilized | **129P** | 1247 |
| 4-Methylmorpholine | **132** | 2535 |
| N-Methylmorpholine | **132** | 2535 |
| Methyl nitrite | **116** | 2455 |
| Methyl orthosilicate | **155** | 2606 |
| Methylpentadiene | **128** | 2461 |
| 2-Methylpentan-2-ol | **129** | 2560 |
| Methylphenyldichlorosilane | **156** | 2437 |
| Methyl phosphonic dichloride | **137** | 9206 |
| Methyl phosphonous dichloride | **135** | 2845 |
| 1-Methylpiperidine | **132** | 2399 |
| Methyl propionate | **129** | 1248 |
| Methyl propyl ether | **127** | 2612 |
| Methyl propyl ketone | **127** | 1249 |
| Methyltetrahydrofuran | **127** | 2536 |
| Methyl trichloroacetate | **156** | 2533 |
| Methyltrichlorosilane | **155** | 1250 |
| alpha-Methylvaleraldehyde | **130** | 2367 |
| Methyl valeraldehyde (alpha) | **130** | 2367 |
| Methyl vinyl ketone, stabilized | **131P** | 1251 |
| M.I.B.C. | **129** | 2053 |
| Molten sulfur | **133** | 2448 |
| Molten sulphur | **133** | 2448 |
| Molybdenum pentachloride | **156** | 2508 |
| Monoethanolamine | **153** | 2491 |
| Mononitrotoluidines | **153** | 2660 |
| Morpholine | **132** | 2054 |
| Motor fuel anti-knock mixture | **131** | 1649 |
| Motor fuel anti-knock mixture, flammable | **131** | 3483 |
| Motor spirit | **128** | 1203 |
| Motor spirit and ethanol mixture, with more than 10% ethanol | **127** | 3475 |
| Muriatic acid | **157** | 1789 |
| Musk xylene | **149** | 2956 |
| Mustard | **153** | 2810 |
| Mustard Lewisite | **153** | 2810 |
| Naphthalene, crude | **133** | 1334 |
| Naphthalene, molten | **133** | 2304 |
| Naphthalene, refined | **133** | 1334 |
| alpha-Naphthylamine | **153** | 2077 |
| beta-Naphthylamine | **153** | 1650 |
| beta-Naphthylamine, solid | **153** | 1650 |
| beta-Naphthylamine, solution | **153** | 3411 |
| Naphthylamine (alpha) | **153** | 2077 |

| Name of Material | Guide No. | ID No. |
|---|---|---|
| Naphthylamine (beta) | **153** | 1650 |
| Naphthylamine (beta), solid | **153** | 1650 |
| Naphthylamine (beta), solution | **153** | 3411 |
| Naphthylthiourea | **153** | 1651 |
| Naphthylurea | **153** | 1652 |
| Natural gas, compressed | **115** | 1971 |
| Natural gas, refrigerated liquid (cryogenic liquid) | **115** | 1972 |
| Neohexane | **128** | 1208 |
| Neon | **121** | 1065 |
| Neon, compressed | **121** | 1065 |
| Neon, refrigerated liquid (cryogenic liquid) | **120** | 1913 |
| Nickel carbonyl | **131** | 1259 |
| Nickel catalyst, dry | **135** | 2881 |
| Nickel cyanide | **151** | 1653 |
| Nickel nitrate | **140** | 2725 |
| Nickel nitrite | **140** | 2726 |
| Nicotine | **151** | 1654 |
| Nicotine compound, liquid, n.o.s. | **151** | 3144 |
| Nicotine compound, solid, n.o.s. | **151** | 1655 |
| Nicotine hydrochloride | **151** | 1656 |
| Nicotine hydrochloride, liquid | **151** | 1656 |
| Nicotine hydrochloride, solid | **151** | 3444 |
| Nicotine hydrochloride, solution | **151** | 1656 |
| Nicotine preparation, liquid, n.o.s. | **151** | 3144 |
| Nicotine preparation, solid, n.o.s. | **151** | 1655 |
| Nicotine salicylate | **151** | 1657 |
| Nicotine sulfate, solid | **151** | 1658 |
| Nicotine sulfate, solid | **151** | 3445 |
| Nicotine sulfate, solution | **151** | 1658 |
| Nicotine sulphate, solid | **151** | 1658 |
| Nicotine sulphate, solid | **151** | 3445 |
| Nicotine sulphate, solution | **151** | 1658 |
| Nicotine tartrate | **151** | 1659 |
| Nitrates, inorganic, aqueous solution, n.o.s. | **140** | 3218 |
| Nitrates, inorganic, n.o.s. | **140** | 1477 |
| Nitrating acid mixture with more than 50% nitric acid | **157** | 1796 |
| Nitrating acid mixture with not more than 50% nitric acid | **157** | 1796 |
| Nitrating acid mixture, spent, with more than 50% nitric acid | **157** | 1826 |
| Nitrating acid mixture, spent, with not more than 50% nitric acid | **157** | 1826 |
| Nitric acid, other than red fuming, with more than 70% nitric acid | **157** | 2031 |
| Nitric acid, other than red fuming, with not more than 70% nitric acid | **157** | 2031 |
| Nitric acid, red fuming | **157** | 2032 |
| Nitric oxide | **124** | 1660 |
| Nitric oxide, compressed | **124** | 1660 |
| Nitric oxide and Dinitrogen tetroxide mixture | **124** | 1975 |
| Nitric oxide and Nitrogen dioxide mixture | **124** | 1975 |
| Nitric oxide and Nitrogen tetroxide mixture | **124** | 1975 |
| Nitriles, flammable, poisonous, n.o.s. | **131** | 3273 |
| Nitriles, flammable, toxic, n.o.s. | **131** | 3273 |

| Name of Material | Guide No. | ID No. |
|---|---|---|
| Nitriles, liquid, poisonous, n.o.s. | **151** | 3276 |
| Nitriles, liquid, toxic, n.o.s. | **151** | 3276 |
| Nitriles, poisonous, flammable, n.o.s. | **131** | 3275 |
| Nitriles, poisonous, liquid, n.o.s. | **151** | 3276 |
| Nitriles, poisonous, n.o.s. | **151** | 3276 |
| Nitriles, poisonous, solid, n.o.s. | **151** | 3439 |
| Nitriles, solid, poisonous, n.o.s. | **151** | 3439 |
| Nitriles, solid, toxic, n.o.s. | **151** | 3439 |
| Nitriles, toxic, flammable, n.o.s. | **131** | 3275 |
| Nitriles, toxic, liquid, n.o.s. | **151** | 3276 |
| Nitriles, toxic, n.o.s. | **151** | 3276 |
| Nitriles, toxic, solid, n.o.s. | **151** | 3439 |
| Nitrites, inorganic, aqueous solution, n.o.s. | **140** | 3219 |
| Nitrites, inorganic, n.o.s. | **140** | 2627 |
| Nitroanilines | **153** | 1661 |
| Nitroanisoles, liquid | **152** | 2730 |
| Nitroanisoles, solid | **152** | 2730 |
| Nitroanisoles, solid | **152** | 3458 |
| Nitrobenzene | **152** | 1662 |
| Nitrobenzenesulfonic acid | **153** | 2305 |
| Nitrobenzenesulphonic acid | **153** | 2305 |
| Nitrobenzotrifluorides | **152** | 2306 |
| Nitrobenzotrifluorides, liquid | **152** | 2306 |
| Nitrobenzotrifluorides, solid | **152** | 3431 |
| Nitrobromobenzenes, liquid | **152** | 2732 |
| Nitrobromobenzenes, solid | **152** | 2732 |
| Nitrobromobenzenes, solid | **152** | 3459 |
| Nitrocellulose membrane filters | **133** | 3270 |
| Nitrocellulose mixture, without pigment | **133** | 2557 |
| Nitrocellulose mixture, without plasticizer | **133** | 2557 |
| Nitrocellulose mixture, with pigment | **133** | 2557 |
| Nitrocellulose mixture, with plasticizer | **133** | 2557 |
| Nitrocellulose, solution, flammable | **127** | 2059 |
| Nitrocellulose with alcohol | **113** | 2556 |
| Nitrocellulose with not less than 25% alcohol | **113** | 2556 |
| Nitrocellulose with water, not less than 25% water | **113** | 2555 |
| 3-Nitro-4-chlorobenzotrifluoride | **152** | 2307 |
| Nitrocresols | **153** | 2446 |
| Nitrocresols, liquid | **153** | 3434 |
| Nitrocresols, solid | **153** | 2446 |
| Nitroethane | **129** | 2842 |
| Nitrogen | **121** | 1066 |
| Nitrogen, compressed | **121** | 1066 |
| Nitrogen, refrigerated liquid (cryogenic liquid) | **120** | 1977 |
| Nitrogen and Rare gases mixture, compressed | **121** | 1981 |
| Nitrogen dioxide | **124** | 1067 |
| Nitrogen dioxide and Nitric oxide mixture | **124** | 1975 |
| Nitrogen tetroxide and Nitric oxide mixture | **124** | 1975 |
| Nitrogen trifluoride | **122** | 2451 |
| Nitrogen trifluoride, compressed | **122** | 2451 |
| Nitrogen trioxide | **124** | 2421 |

| Name of Material | Guide No. | ID No. |
|---|---|---|
| Nitroglycerin, solution in alcohol, with more than 1% but not more than 5% Nitroglycerin | **127** | 3064 |
| Nitroglycerin, solution in alcohol, with not more than 1% Nitroglycerin | **127** | 1204 |
| Nitroglycerin mixture, desensitized, liquid, flammable, n.o.s., with not more than 30% Nitroglycerin | **113** | 3343 |
| Nitroglycerin mixture, desensitized, liquid, n.o.s., with not more than 30% Nitroglycerin | **113** | 3357 |
| Nitroglycerin mixture, desensitized, solid, n.o.s., with more than 2% but not more than 10% Nitroglycerin | **113** | 3319 |
| Nitroguanidine, wetted with not less than 20% water | **113** | 1336 |
| Nitrohydrochloric acid | **157** | 1798 |
| Nitromethane | **129** | 1261 |
| Nitronaphthalene | **133** | 2538 |
| Nitrophenols | **153** | 1663 |
| 4-Nitrophenylhydrazine, with not less than 30% water | **113** | 3376 |
| Nitropropanes | **129** | 2608 |
| p-Nitrosodimethylaniline | **135** | 1369 |
| Nitrostarch, wetted with not less than 20% water | **113** | 1337 |
| Nitrosyl chloride | **125** | 1069 |
| Nitrosylsulfuric acid, liquid | **157** | 2308 |
| Nitrosylsulfuric acid, solid | **157** | 2308 |
| Nitrosylsulfuric acid, solid | **157** | 3456 |
| Nitrosylsulphuric acid, liquid | **157** | 2308 |
| Nitrosylsulphuric acid, solid | **157** | 2308 |
| Nitrosylsulphuric acid, solid | **157** | 3456 |
| Nitrotoluenes, liquid | **152** | 1664 |
| Nitrotoluenes, solid | **152** | 1664 |
| Nitrotoluenes, solid | **152** | 3446 |
| Nitrotoluidines (mono) | **153** | 2660 |
| Nitrous oxide | **122** | 1070 |
| Nitrous oxide, compressed | **122** | 1070 |
| Nitrous oxide, refrigerated liquid | **122** | 2201 |
| Nitrous oxide and Carbon dioxide mixture | **126** | 1015 |
| Nitroxylenes, liquid | **152** | 1665 |
| Nitroxylenes, solid | **152** | 1665 |
| Nitroxylenes, solid | **152** | 3447 |
| Nonanes | **128** | 1920 |
| Nonyltrichlorosilane | **156** | 1799 |
| 2,5-Norbornadiene, stabilized | **128P** | 2251 |
| Octadecyltrichlorosilane | **156** | 1800 |
| Octadiene | **128P** | 2309 |
| Octafluorobut-2-ene | **126** | 2422 |
| Octafluorocyclobutane | **126** | 1976 |
| Octafluoropropane | **126** | 2424 |
| Octanes | **128** | 1262 |
| Octyl aldehydes | **129** | 1191 |
| Octyltrichlorosilane | **156** | 1801 |
| Oil, petroleum | **128** | 1270 |
| Oil gas | **119** | 1071 |
| Oil gas, compressed | **119** | 1071 |
| Organic peroxide type B, liquid | **146** | 3101 |
| Organic peroxide type B, liquid, temperature controlled | **148** | 3111 |
| Organic peroxide type B, solid | **146** | 3102 |
| Organic peroxide type B, solid, temperature controlled | **148** | 3112 |

| Name of Material | Guide No. | ID No. |
|---|---|---|
| Organic peroxide type C, liquid | **146** | 3103 |
| Organic peroxide type C, liquid, temperature controlled | **148** | 3113 |
| Organic peroxide type C, solid | **146** | 3104 |
| Organic peroxide type C, solid, temperature controlled | **148** | 3114 |
| Organic peroxide type D, liquid | **145** | 3105 |
| Organic peroxide type D, liquid, temperature controlled | **148** | 3115 |
| Organic peroxide type D, solid | **145** | 3106 |
| Organic peroxide type D, solid, temperature controlled | **148** | 3116 |
| Organic peroxide type E, liquid | **145** | 3107 |
| Organic peroxide type E, liquid, temperature controlled | **148** | 3117 |
| Organic peroxide type E, solid | **145** | 3108 |
| Organic peroxide type E, solid, temperature controlled | **148** | 3118 |
| Organic peroxide type F, liquid | **145** | 3109 |
| Organic peroxide type F, liquid, temperature controlled | **148** | 3119 |
| Organic peroxide type F, solid | **145** | 3110 |
| Organic peroxide type F, solid, temperature controlled | **148** | 3120 |
| Organic phosphate compound mixed with compressed gas | **123** | 1955 |
| Organic phosphate mixed with compressed gas | **123** | 1955 |
| Organic phosphorus compound mixed with compressed gas | **123** | 1955 |
| Organic pigments, self-heating | **135** | 3313 |
| Organoarsenic compound, liquid, n.o.s. | **151** | 3280 |
| Organoarsenic compound, n.o.s. | **151** | 3280 |
| Organoarsenic compound, solid, n.o.s. | **151** | 3465 |
| Organochlorine pesticide, liquid, flammable, poisonous | **131** | 2762 |
| Organochlorine pesticide, liquid, flammable, toxic | **131** | 2762 |
| Organochlorine pesticide, liquid, poisonous | **151** | 2996 |
| Organochlorine pesticide, liquid, poisonous, flammable | **131** | 2995 |
| Organochlorine pesticide, liquid, toxic | **151** | 2996 |
| Organochlorine pesticide, liquid, toxic, flammable | **131** | 2995 |
| Organochlorine pesticide, solid, poisonous | **151** | 2761 |
| Organochlorine pesticide, solid, toxic | **151** | 2761 |
| Organometallic compound, liquid, poisonous, n.o.s. | **151** | 3282 |
| Organometallic compound, liquid, toxic, n.o.s. | **151** | 3282 |
| Organometallic compound, poisonous, liquid, n.o.s. | **151** | 3282 |
| Organometallic compound, poisonous, n.o.s. | **151** | 3282 |
| Organometallic compound, poisonous, solid, n.o.s. | **151** | 3467 |
| Organometallic compound, solid, poisonous, n.o.s. | **151** | 3467 |
| Organometallic compound, solid, toxic, n.o.s. | **151** | 3467 |

| Name of Material | Guide No. | ID No. |
|---|---|---|
| Organometallic compound, toxic, liquid, n.o.s. | **151** | 3282 |
| Organometallic compound, toxic, n.o.s. | **151** | 3282 |
| Organometallic compound, toxic, solid, n.o.s. | **151** | 3467 |
| Organometallic compound, water-reactive, flammable, n.o.s. | **138** | 3207 |
| Organometallic compound dispersion, water-reactive, flammable, n.o.s. | **138** | 3207 |
| Organometallic compound solution, water-reactive, flammable, n.o.s. | **138** | 3207 |
| Organometallic substance, liquid, pyrophoric | **135** | 3392 |
| Organometallic substance, liquid, pyrophoric, water-reactive | **135** | 3394 |
| Organometallic substance, liquid, water-reactive | **135** | 3398 |
| Organometallic substance, liquid, water-reactive, flammable | **138** | 3399 |
| Organometallic substance, solid, pyrophoric | **135** | 3391 |
| Organometallic substance, solid, pyrophoric, water-reactive | **135** | 3393 |
| Organometallic substance, solid, self-heating | **138** | 3400 |
| Organometallic substance, solid, water-reactive | **135** | 3395 |
| Organometallic substance, solid, water-reactive, flammable | **138** | 3396 |
| Organometallic substance, solid, water-reactive, self-heating | **138** | 3397 |
| Organophosphorus compound, liquid, poisonous, n.o.s. | **151** | 3278 |
| Organophosphorus compound, liquid, toxic, n.o.s. | **151** | 3278 |
| Organophosphorus compound, poisonous, flammable, n.o.s. | **131** | 3279 |
| Organophosphorus compound, poisonous, liquid, n.o.s. | **151** | 3278 |
| Organophosphorus compound, poisonous, n.o.s. | **151** | 3278 |
| Organophosphorus compound, poisonous, solid, n.o.s. | **151** | 3464 |
| Organophosphorus compound, solid, poisonous, n.o.s. | **151** | 3464 |
| Organophosphorus compound, solid, toxic, n.o.s. | **151** | 3464 |
| Organophosphorus compound, toxic, flammable, n.o.s. | **131** | 3279 |
| Organophosphorus compound, toxic, liquid, n.o.s. | **151** | 3278 |
| Organophosphorus compound, toxic, n.o.s. | **151** | 3278 |
| Organophosphorus compound, toxic, solid, n.o.s. | **151** | 3464 |
| Organophosphorus pesticide, liquid, flammable, poisonous | **131** | 2784 |
| Organophosphorus pesticide, liquid, flammable, toxic | **131** | 2784 |
| Organophosphorus pesticide, liquid, poisonous | **152** | 3018 |
| Organophosphorus pesticide, liquid, poisonous, flammable | **131** | 3017 |
| Organophosphorus pesticide, liquid, toxic | **152** | 3018 |
| Organophosphorus pesticide, liquid, toxic, flammable | **131** | 3017 |
| Organophosphorus pesticide, solid, poisonous | **152** | 2783 |
| Organophosphorus pesticide, solid, toxic | **152** | 2783 |

| Name of Material | Guide No. | ID No. |
|---|---|---|
| Organotin compound, liquid, n.o.s. | **153** | 2788 |
| Organotin compound, solid, n.o.s. | **153** | 3146 |
| Organotin pesticide, liquid, flammable, poisonous | **131** | 2787 |
| Organotin pesticide, liquid, flammable, toxic | **131** | 2787 |
| Organotin pesticide, liquid, poisonous | **153** | 3020 |
| Organotin pesticide, liquid, poisonous, flammable | **131** | 3019 |
| Organotin pesticide, liquid, toxic | **153** | 3020 |
| Organotin pesticide, liquid, toxic, flammable | **131** | 3019 |
| Organotin pesticide, solid, poisonous | **153** | 2786 |
| Organotin pesticide, solid, toxic | **153** | 2786 |
| Osmium tetroxide | **154** | 2471 |
| Other regulated substances, liquid, n.o.s. | **171** | 3082 |
| Other regulated substances, solid, n.o.s. | **171** | 3077 |
| Oxidizing liquid, corrosive, n.o.s. | **140** | 3098 |
| Oxidizing liquid, n.o.s. | **140** | 3139 |
| Oxidizing liquid, poisonous, n.o.s. | **142** | 3099 |
| Oxidizing liquid, toxic, n.o.s. | **142** | 3099 |
| Oxidizing solid, corrosive, n.o.s. | **140** | 3085 |
| Oxidizing solid, flammable, n.o.s. | **140** | 3137 |
| Oxidizing solid, n.o.s. | **140** | 1479 |
| Oxidizing solid, poisonous, n.o.s. | **141** | 3087 |
| Oxidizing solid, self-heating, n.o.s. | **135** | 3100 |
| Oxidizing solid, toxic, n.o.s. | **141** | 3087 |
| Oxidizing solid, water-reactive, n.o.s. | **144** | 3121 |
| Oxygen | **122** | 1072 |
| Oxygen, compressed | **122** | 1072 |
| Oxygen, refrigerated liquid (cryogenic liquid) | **122** | 1073 |
| Oxygen and Carbon dioxide mixture, compressed | **122** | 1014 |
| Oxygen and Rare gases mixture, compressed | **121** | 1980 |
| Oxygen difluoride | **124** | 2190 |
| Oxygen difluoride, compressed | **124** | 2190 |
| Oxygen generator, chemical | **140** | 3356 |
| Oxygen generator, chemical, spent | **140** | 3356 |
| Packaging discarded, empty, uncleaned | **171** | 3509 |
| Paint (corrosive) | **153** | 3066 |
| Paint, corrosive, flammable | **132** | 3470 |
| Paint (flammable) | **128** | 1263 |
| Paint, flammable, corrosive | **132** | 3469 |
| Paint related material (corrosive) | **153** | 3066 |
| Paint related material, corrosive, flammable | **132** | 3470 |
| Paint related material (flammable) | **128** | 1263 |
| Paint related material, flammable, corrosive | **132** | 3469 |
| Paper, unsaturated oil treated | **133** | 1379 |
| Paraformaldehyde | **133** | 2213 |
| Paraldehyde | **129** | 1264 |

| Name of Material | Guide No. | ID No. |
|---|---|---|
| Parathion and compressed gas mixture | **123** | 1967 |
| PCB | **171** | 2315 |
| PD | **152** | 1556 |
| Pentaborane | **135** | 1380 |
| Pentachloroethane | **151** | 1669 |
| Pentachlorophenol | **154** | 3155 |
| Pentaerythrite tetranitrate mixture, desensitized, solid, n.o.s., with more than 10% but not more than 20% PETN | **113** | 3344 |
| Pentaerythritol tetranitrate mixture, desensitized, solid, n.o.s., with more than 10% but not more than 20% PETN | **113** | 3344 |
| Pentafluoroethane | **126** | 3220 |
| Pentafluoroethane and Ethylene oxide mixture, with not more than 7.9% Ethylene oxide | **126** | 3298 |
| Pentamethylheptane | **128** | 2286 |
| Pentane-2,4-dione | **131** | 2310 |
| Pentanes | **128** | 1265 |
| Pentanols | **129** | 1105 |
| 1-Pentene | **128** | 1108 |
| 1-Pentol | **153P** | 2705 |
| Perchlorates, inorganic, aqueous solution, n.o.s. | **140** | 3211 |
| Perchlorates, inorganic, n.o.s. | **140** | 1481 |
| Perchloric acid, with more than 50% but not more than 72% acid | **143** | 1873 |
| Perchloric acid, with not more than 50% acid | **140** | 1802 |
| Perchloroethylene | **160** | 1897 |
| Perchloromethyl mercaptan | **157** | 1670 |
| Perchloryl fluoride | **124** | 3083 |
| Perfluoro(ethyl vinyl ether) | **115** | 3154 |
| Perfluoro(methyl vinyl ether) | **115** | 3153 |
| Perfumery products, with flammable solvents | **127** | 1266 |
| Permanganates, inorganic, aqueous solution, n.o.s. | **140** | 3214 |
| Permanganates, inorganic, n.o.s. | **140** | 1482 |
| Peroxides, inorganic, n.o.s. | **140** | 1483 |
| Peroxyacetic acid and hydrogen peroxide mixture, with acid(s), water and not more than 5% Peroxyacetic acid, stabilized | **140** | 3149 |
| Persulfates, inorganic, aqueous solution, n.o.s. | **140** | 3216 |
| Persulfates, inorganic, n.o.s. | **140** | 3215 |
| Persulphates, inorganic, aqueous solution, n.o.s. | **140** | 3216 |
| Persulphates, inorganic, n.o.s. | **140** | 3215 |
| Pesticide, liquid, flammable, poisonous, n.o.s. | **131** | 3021 |
| Pesticide, liquid, flammable, toxic, n.o.s. | **131** | 3021 |
| Pesticide, liquid, poisonous, flammable, n.o.s. | **131** | 2903 |
| Pesticide, liquid, poisonous, n.o.s. | **151** | 2902 |
| Pesticide, liquid, toxic, flammable, n.o.s. | **131** | 2903 |
| Pesticide, liquid, toxic, n.o.s. | **151** | 2902 |
| Pesticide, solid, poisonous, n.o.s. | **151** | 2588 |
| Pesticide, solid, toxic, n.o.s. | **151** | 2588 |
| PETN mixture, desensitized, solid, n.o.s., with more than 10% but not more than 20% PETN | **113** | 3344 |

| Name of Material | Guide No. | ID No. |
|---|---|---|
| Petrol | **128** | 1203 |
| Petrol and ethanol mixture, with more than 10% ethanol | **127** | 3475 |
| Petroleum crude oil | **128** | 1267 |
| Petroleum distillates, n.o.s. | **128** | 1268 |
| Petroleum gases, liquefied | **115** | 1075 |
| Petroleum oil | **128** | 1270 |
| Petroleum products, n.o.s. | **128** | 1268 |
| Petroleum sour crude oil, flammable, poisonous | **131** | 3494 |
| Petroleum sour crude oil, flammable, toxic | **131** | 3494 |
| Phenacyl bromide | **153** | 2645 |
| Phenetidines | **153** | 2311 |
| Phenol, molten | **153** | 2312 |
| Phenol, solid | **153** | 1671 |
| Phenol solution | **153** | 2821 |
| Phenolates, liquid | **154** | 2904 |
| Phenolates, solid | **154** | 2905 |
| Phenolsulfonic acid, liquid | **153** | 1803 |
| Phenolsulphonic acid, liquid | **153** | 1803 |
| Phenoxyacetic acid derivative pesticide, liquid, flammable, poisonous | **131** | 3346 |
| Phenoxyacetic acid derivative pesticide, liquid, flammable, toxic | **131** | 3346 |
| Phenoxyacetic acid derivative pesticide, liquid, poisonous | **153** | 3348 |
| Phenoxyacetic acid derivative pesticide, liquid, poisonous, flammable | **131** | 3347 |
| Phenoxyacetic acid derivative pesticide, liquid, toxic | **153** | 3348 |
| Phenoxyacetic acid derivative pesticide, liquid, toxic, flammable | **131** | 3347 |
| Phenoxyacetic acid derivative pesticide, solid, poisonous | **153** | 3345 |
| Phenoxyacetic acid derivative pesticide, solid, toxic | **153** | 3345 |
| Phenylacetonitrile, liquid | **152** | 2470 |
| Phenylacetyl chloride | **156** | 2577 |
| Phenylcarbylamine chloride | **151** | 1672 |
| Phenyl chloroformate | **156** | 2746 |
| Phenylenediamines | **153** | 1673 |
| Phenylhydrazine | **153** | 2572 |
| Phenyl isocyanate | **155** | 2487 |
| Phenyl mercaptan | **131** | 2337 |
| Phenylmercuric acetate | **151** | 1674 |
| Phenylmercuric compound, n.o.s. | **151** | 2026 |
| Phenylmercuric hydroxide | **151** | 1894 |
| Phenylmercuric nitrate | **151** | 1895 |
| Phenylphosphorus dichloride | **137** | 2798 |
| Phenylphosphorus thiodichloride | **137** | 2799 |
| Phenyltrichlorosilane | **156** | 1804 |
| Phenyl urea pesticide, liquid, poisonous | **151** | 3002 |
| Phenyl urea pesticide, liquid, toxic | **151** | 3002 |
| Phosgene | **125** | 1076 |
| 9-Phosphabicyclononanes | **135** | 2940 |
| Phosphine | **119** | 2199 |
| Phosphine, adsorbed | **173** | 3525 |
| Phosphoric acid, liquid | **154** | 1805 |
| Phosphoric acid, solid | **154** | 1805 |
| Phosphoric acid, solid | **154** | 3453 |
| Phosphoric acid, solution | **154** | 1805 |
| Phosphorous acid | **154** | 2834 |

| Name of Material | Guide No. | ID No. |
|---|---|---|
| Phosphorus, amorphous | **133** | 1338 |
| Phosphorus, white, dry or under water or in solution | **136** | 1381 |
| Phosphorus, white, molten | **136** | 2447 |
| Phosphorus, yellow, dry or under water or in solution | **136** | 1381 |
| Phosphorus heptasulfide, free from yellow and white Phosphorus | **139** | 1339 |
| Phosphorus heptasulphide, free from yellow and white Phosphorus | **139** | 1339 |
| Phosphorus oxybromide | **137** | 1939 |
| Phosphorus oxybromide, molten | **137** | 2576 |
| Phosphorus oxybromide, solid | **137** | 1939 |
| Phosphorus oxychloride | **137** | 1810 |
| Phosphorus pentabromide | **137** | 2691 |
| Phosphorus pentachloride | **137** | 1806 |
| Phosphorus pentafluoride | **125** | 2198 |
| Phosphorus pentafluoride, adsorbed | **173** | 3524 |
| Phosphorus pentafluoride, compressed | **125** | 2198 |
| Phosphorus pentasulfide, free from yellow and white Phosphorus | **139** | 1340 |
| Phosphorus pentasulphide, free from yellow and white Phosphorus | **139** | 1340 |
| Phosphorus pentoxide | **137** | 1807 |
| Phosphorus sesquisulfide, free from yellow and white Phosphorus | **139** | 1341 |
| Phosphorus sesquisulphide, free from yellow and white Phosphorus | **139** | 1341 |
| Phosphorus tribromide | **137** | 1808 |
| Phosphorus trichloride | **137** | 1809 |
| Phosphorus trioxide | **157** | 2578 |
| Phosphorus trisulfide, free from yellow and white Phosphorus | **139** | 1343 |
| Phosphorus trisulphide, free from yellow and white Phosphorus | **139** | 1343 |
| Phthalic anhydride | **156** | 2214 |
| Picolines | **129** | 2313 |
| Picric acid, wetted with not less than 10% water | **113** | 3364 |
| Picric acid, wetted with not less than 30% water | **113** | 1344 |
| Picrite, wetted with not less than 20% water | **113** | 1336 |
| Picryl chloride, wetted with not less than 10% water | **113** | 3365 |
| alpha-Pinene | **128** | 2368 |
| Pinene (alpha) | **128** | 2368 |
| Pine oil | **129** | 1272 |
| Piperazine | **153** | 2579 |
| Piperidine | **132** | 2401 |
| Plastic molding compound | **171** | 3314 |
| Plastics moulding compound | **171** | 3314 |
| Plastics, nitrocellulose-based, self-heating, n.o.s. | **135** | 2006 |
| Poisonous by inhalation liquid, corrosive, flammable, n.o.s. (Inhalation Hazard Zone A) | **131** | 3492 |
| Poisonous by inhalation liquid, corrosive, flammable, n.o.s. (Inhalation Hazard Zone B) | **131** | 3493 |
| Poisonous by inhalation liquid, corrosive, n.o.s. (Inhalation Hazard Zone A) | **154** | 3389 |
| Poisonous by inhalation liquid, corrosive, n.o.s. (Inhalation Hazard Zone B) | **154** | 3390 |

| Name of Material | Guide No. | ID No. |
|---|---|---|
| Poisonous by inhalation liquid, flammable, corrosive, n.o.s. (Inhalation Hazard Zone A) | **131** | 3488 |
| Poisonous by inhalation liquid, flammable, corrosive, n.o.s. (Inhalation Hazard Zone B) | **131** | 3489 |
| Poisonous by inhalation liquid, flammable, n.o.s. (Inhalation Hazard Zone A) | **131** | 3383 |
| Poisonous by inhalation liquid, flammable, n.o.s. (Inhalation Hazard Zone B) | **131** | 3384 |
| Poisonous by inhalation liquid, n.o.s. (Inhalation Hazard Zone A) | **151** | 3381 |
| Poisonous by inhalation liquid, n.o.s. (Inhalation Hazard Zone B) | **151** | 3382 |
| Poisonous by inhalation liquid, oxidizing, n.o.s. (Inhalation Hazard Zone A) | **142** | 3387 |
| Poisonous by inhalation liquid, oxidizing, n.o.s. (Inhalation Hazard Zone B) | **142** | 3388 |
| Poisonous by inhalation liquid, water-reactive, flammable, n.o.s. (Inhalation Hazard Zone A) | **155** | 3490 |
| Poisonous by inhalation liquid, water-reactive, flammable, n.o.s. (Inhalation Hazard Zone B) | **155** | 3491 |
| Poisonous by inhalation liquid, water-reactive, n.o.s. (Inhalation Hazard Zone A) | **139** | 3385 |
| Poisonous by inhalation liquid, water-reactive, n.o.s. (Inhalation Hazard Zone B) | **139** | 3386 |
| Poisonous liquid, corrosive, inorganic, n.o.s. | **154** | 3289 |
| Poisonous liquid, corrosive, organic, n.o.s. | **154** | 2927 |
| Poisonous liquid, flammable, organic, n.o.s. | **131** | 2929 |
| Poisonous liquid, inorganic, n.o.s. | **151** | 3287 |
| Poisonous liquid, organic, n.o.s. | **153** | 2810 |
| Poisonous liquid, oxidizing, n.o.s. | **142** | 3122 |
| Poisonous liquid, water-reactive, n.o.s. | **139** | 3123 |
| Poisonous solid, corrosive, inorganic, n.o.s. | **154** | 3290 |
| Poisonous solid, corrosive, organic, n.o.s. | **154** | 2928 |
| Poisonous solid, flammable, organic, n.o.s. | **134** | 2930 |
| Poisonous solid, inorganic, n.o.s. | **151** | 3288 |
| Poisonous solid, organic, n.o.s. | **154** | 2811 |
| Poisonous solid, oxidizing, n.o.s. | **141** | 3086 |
| Poisonous solid, self-heating, n.o.s. | **136** | 3124 |
| Poisonous solid, water-reactive, n.o.s. | **139** | 3125 |
| Polyalkylamines, n.o.s. | **132** | 2733 |
| Polyalkylamines, n.o.s. | **132** | 2734 |
| Polyalkylamines, n.o.s. | **153** | 2735 |
| Polyamines, flammable, corrosive, n.o.s. | **132** | 2733 |
| Polyamines, liquid, corrosive, flammable, n.o.s. | **132** | 2734 |
| Polyamines, liquid, corrosive, n.o.s. | **153** | 2735 |
| Polyamines, solid, corrosive, n.o.s. | **154** | 3259 |
| Polychlorinated biphenyls | **171** | 2315 |
| Polychlorinated biphenyls, liquid | **171** | 2315 |

| Name of Material | Guide No. | ID No. |
|---|---|---|
| Polychlorinated biphenyls, solid | **171** | 3432 |
| Polyester resin kit | **128** | 3269 |
| Polyester resin kit, liquid base material | **128** | 3269 |
| Polyester resin kit, solid base material | **128P** | 3527 |
| Polyhalogenated biphenyls, liquid | **171** | 3151 |
| Polyhalogenated biphenyls, solid | **171** | 3152 |
| Polyhalogenated terphenyls, liquid | **171** | 3151 |
| Polyhalogenated terphenyls, solid | **171** | 3152 |
| Polymeric beads, expandable | **133** | 2211 |
| Polymerizing substance, liquid, stabilized, n.o.s. | **149P** | 3532 |
| Polymerizing substance, liquid, temperature controlled, n.o.s. | **150P** | 3534 |
| Polymerizing substance, solid, stabilized, n.o.s. | **149P** | 3531 |
| Polymerizing substance, solid, temperature controlled, n.o.s. | **150P** | 3533 |
| Polystyrene beads, expandable | **133** | 2211 |
| Potassium | **138** | 2257 |
| Potassium, metal | **138** | 2257 |
| Potassium, metal alloys | **138** | 1420 |
| Potassium, metal alloys, liquid | **138** | 1420 |
| Potassium, metal alloys, solid | **138** | 3403 |
| Potassium arsenate | **151** | 1677 |
| Potassium arsenite | **154** | 1678 |
| Potassium borohydride | **138** | 1870 |
| Potassium bromate | **140** | 1484 |
| Potassium chlorate | **140** | 1485 |
| Potassium chlorate, aqueous solution | **140** | 2427 |
| Potassium cuprocyanide | **157** | 1679 |
| Potassium cyanide | **157** | 1680 |
| Potassium cyanide, solid | **157** | 1680 |
| Potassium cyanide, solution | **157** | 3413 |
| Potassium dithionite | **135** | 1929 |
| Potassium fluoride | **154** | 1812 |
| Potassium fluoride, solid | **154** | 1812 |
| Potassium fluoride, solution | **154** | 3422 |
| Potassium fluoroacetate | **151** | 2628 |
| Potassium fluorosilicate | **151** | 2655 |
| Potassium hydrogendifluoride | **154** | 1811 |
| Potassium hydrogen difluoride, solid | **154** | 1811 |
| Potassium hydrogen difluoride, solution | **154** | 3421 |
| Potassium hydrogen sulfate | **154** | 2509 |
| Potassium hydrogen sulphate | **154** | 2509 |
| Potassium hydrosulfite | **135** | 1929 |
| Potassium hydrosulphite | **135** | 1929 |
| Potassium hydroxide, solid | **154** | 1813 |
| Potassium hydroxide, solution | **154** | 1814 |
| Potassium metavanadate | **151** | 2864 |
| Potassium monoxide | **154** | 2033 |
| Potassium nitrate | **140** | 1486 |
| Potassium nitrate and Sodium nitrate mixture | **140** | 1499 |
| Potassium nitrate and Sodium nitrite mixture | **140** | 1487 |
| Potassium nitrite | **140** | 1488 |
| Potassium perchlorate | **140** | 1489 |
| Potassium permanganate | **140** | 1490 |
| Potassium peroxide | **144** | 1491 |

| Name of Material | Guide No. | ID No. |
|---|---|---|
| Potassium persulfate | **140** | 1492 |
| Potassium persulphate | **140** | 1492 |
| Potassium phosphide | **139** | 2012 |
| Potassium silicofluoride | **151** | 2655 |
| Potassium sodium alloys | **138** | 1422 |
| Potassium sodium alloys, liquid | **138** | 1422 |
| Potassium sodium alloys, solid | **138** | 3404 |
| Potassium sulfide, anhydrous | **135** | 1382 |
| Potassium sulfide, hydrated, with not less than 30% water of crystallization | **153** | 1847 |
| Potassium sulfide, with less than 30% water of crystallization | **135** | 1382 |
| Potassium sulphide, anhydrous | **135** | 1382 |
| Potassium sulphide, hydrated, with not less than 30% water of crystallization | **153** | 1847 |
| Potassium sulphide, with less than 30% water of crystallization | **135** | 1382 |
| Potassium superoxide | **143** | 2466 |
| Printing ink, flammable | **129** | 1210 |
| Printing ink related material | **129** | 1210 |
| Propadiene, stabilized | **116P** | 2200 |
| Propadiene and Methylacetylene mixture, stabilized | **116P** | 1060 |
| Propane | **115** | 1075 |
| Propane | **115** | 1978 |
| Propane-Ethane mixture, refrigerated liquid | **115** | 1961 |
| Propanethiols | **130** | 2402 |
| n-Propanol | **129** | 1274 |
| Propionaldehyde | **129** | 1275 |

| Name of Material | Guide No. | ID No. |
|---|---|---|
| Propionic acid | **132** | 1848 |
| Propionic acid, with not less than 10% and less than 90% acid | **132** | 1848 |
| Propionic acid, with not less than 90% acid | **132** | 3463 |
| Propionic anhydride | **156** | 2496 |
| Propionitrile | **131** | 2404 |
| Propionyl chloride | **132** | 1815 |
| n-Propyl acetate | **129** | 1276 |
| Propyl alcohol, normal | **129** | 1274 |
| Propylamine | **132** | 1277 |
| n-Propyl benzene | **128** | 2364 |
| Propyl chloride | **129** | 1278 |
| n-Propyl chloroformate | **155** | 2740 |
| Propylene | **115** | 1075 |
| Propylene | **115** | 1077 |
| Propylene, Ethylene and Acetylene in mixture, refrigerated liquid containing at least 71.5% Ethylene with not more than 22.5% Acetylene and not more than 6% Propylene | **115** | 3138 |
| Propylene chlorohydrin | **131** | 2611 |
| 1,2-Propylenediamine | **132** | 2258 |
| Propyleneimine, stabilized | **131P** | 1921 |
| Propylene oxide | **127P** | 1280 |
| Propylene oxide and Ethylene oxide mixture, with not more than 30% Ethylene oxide | **129P** | 2983 |
| Propylene tetramer | **128** | 2850 |
| Propyl formates | **129** | 1281 |
| n-Propyl isocyanate | **155** | 2482 |
| n-Propyl nitrate | **131** | 1865 |
| Propyltrichlorosilane | **155** | 1816 |

| Name of Material | Guide No. | ID No. |
|---|---|---|
| Pyrethroid pesticide, liquid, flammable, poisonous | **131** | 3350 |
| Pyrethroid pesticide, liquid, flammable, toxic | **131** | 3350 |
| Pyrethroid pesticide, liquid, poisonous | **151** | 3352 |
| Pyrethroid pesticide, liquid, poisonous, flammable | **131** | 3351 |
| Pyrethroid pesticide, liquid, toxic | **151** | 3352 |
| Pyrethroid pesticide, liquid, toxic, flammable | **131** | 3351 |
| Pyrethroid pesticide, solid, poisonous | **151** | 3349 |
| Pyrethroid pesticide, solid, toxic | **151** | 3349 |
| Pyridine | **129** | 1282 |
| Pyrophoric alloy, n.o.s. | **135** | 1383 |
| Pyrophoric liquid, inorganic, n.o.s. | **135** | 3194 |
| Pyrophoric liquid, organic, n.o.s. | **135** | 2845 |
| Pyrophoric metal, n.o.s. | **135** | 1383 |
| Pyrophoric organometallic compound, water-reactive, n.o.s. | **135** | 3203 |
| Pyrophoric solid, inorganic, n.o.s. | **135** | 3200 |
| Pyrophoric solid, organic, n.o.s. | **135** | 2846 |
| Pyrosulfuryl chloride | **137** | 1817 |
| Pyrosulphuryl chloride | **137** | 1817 |
| Pyrrolidine | **132** | 1922 |
| Quinoline | **154** | 2656 |
| Radioactive material, excepted package, articles manufactured from depleted Uranium | **161** | 2909 |
| Radioactive material, excepted package, articles manufactured from natural Thorium | **161** | 2909 |
| Radioactive material, excepted package, articles manufactured from natural Uranium | **161** | 2909 |
| Radioactive material, excepted package, empty packaging | **161** | 2908 |
| Radioactive material, excepted package, instruments or articles | **161** | 2911 |
| Radioactive material, excepted package, limited quantity of material | **161** | 2910 |
| Radioactive material, low specific activity (LSA-I), non fissile or fissile-excepted | **162** | 2912 |
| Radioactive material, low specific activity (LSA-II), fissile | **165** | 3324 |
| Radioactive material, low specific activity (LSA-II), non fissile or fissile-excepted | **162** | 3321 |
| Radioactive material, low specific activity (LSA-III), fissile | **165** | 3325 |
| Radioactive material, low specific activity (LSA-III), non fissile or fissile-excepted | **162** | 3322 |
| Radioactive material, surface contaminated objects (SCO-I), fissile | **165** | 3326 |
| Radioactive material, surface contaminated objects (SCO-I), non fissile or fissile-excepted | **162** | 2913 |
| Radioactive material, surface contaminated objects (SCO-II), fissile | **165** | 3326 |

| Name of Material | Guide No. | ID No. |
|---|---|---|
| Radioactive material, surface contaminated objects (SCO-II), non fissile or fissile-excepted | **162** | 2913 |
| Radioactive material, transported under special arrangement, fissile | **165** | 3331 |
| Radioactive material, transported under special arrangement, non fissile or fissile-excepted | **163** | 2919 |
| Radioactive material, Type A package, fissile, non-special form | **165** | 3327 |
| Radioactive material, Type A package, non-special form, non fissile or fissile-excepted | **163** | 2915 |
| Radioactive material, Type A package, special form, fissile | **165** | 3333 |
| Radioactive material, Type A package, special form, non fissile or fissile-excepted | **164** | 3332 |
| Radioactive material, Type B(M) package, fissile | **165** | 3329 |
| Radioactive material, Type B(M) package, non fissile or fissile-excepted | **163** | 2917 |
| Radioactive material, Type B(U) package, fissile | **165** | 3328 |
| Radioactive material, Type B(U) package, non fissile or fissile-excepted | **163** | 2916 |
| Radioactive material, Type C package, fissile | **165** | 3330 |
| Radioactive material, Type C package, non fissile or fissile excepted | **163** | 3323 |
| Radioactive material, Uranium hexafluoride, fissile | **166** | 2977 |
| Radioactive material, Uranium hexafluoride, non fissile or fissile-excepted | **166** | 2978 |
| Rags, oily | **133** | 1856 |
| Rare gases and Nitrogen mixture, compressed | **121** | 1981 |
| Rare gases and Oxygen mixture, compressed | **121** | 1980 |
| Rare gases mixture, compressed | **121** | 1979 |
| Receptacles, small, containing gas | **115** | 2037 |
| Red phosphorus | **133** | 1338 |
| Refrigerant gas, n.o.s. | **126** | 1078 |
| Refrigerant gases, n.o.s. (flammable) | **115** | 1954 |
| Refrigerant gas R-12 | **126** | 1028 |
| Refrigerant gas R-12B1 | **126** | 1974 |
| Refrigerant gas R-12B2 | **171** | 1941 |
| Refrigerant gas R-13 | **126** | 1022 |
| Refrigerant gas R-13B1 | **126** | 1009 |
| Refrigerant gas R-14 | **126** | 1982 |
| Refrigerant gas R-14, compressed | **126** | 1982 |
| Refrigerant gas R-21 | **126** | 1029 |
| Refrigerant gas R-22 | **126** | 1018 |
| Refrigerant gas R-23 | **126** | 1984 |
| Refrigerant gas R-32 | **115** | 3252 |
| Refrigerant gas R-40 | **115** | 1063 |
| Refrigerant gas R-41 | **115** | 2454 |
| Refrigerant gas R-114 | **126** | 1958 |
| Refrigerant gas R-115 | **126** | 1020 |
| Refrigerant gas R-116 | **126** | 2193 |
| Refrigerant gas R-116, compressed | **126** | 2193 |
| Refrigerant gas R-124 | **126** | 1021 |
| Refrigerant gas R-125 | **126** | 3220 |
| Refrigerant gas R-133a | **126** | 1983 |

| Name of Material | Guide No. | ID No. |
|---|---|---|
| Refrigerant gas R-134a | **126** | 3159 |
| Refrigerant gas R-142b | **115** | 2517 |
| Refrigerant gas R-143a | **115** | 2035 |
| Refrigerant gas R-152a | **115** | 1030 |
| Refrigerant gas R-161 | **115** | 2453 |
| Refrigerant gas R-218 | **126** | 2424 |
| Refrigerant gas R-227 | **126** | 3296 |
| Refrigerant gas R-404A | **126** | 3337 |
| Refrigerant gas R-407A | **126** | 3338 |
| Refrigerant gas R-407B | **126** | 3339 |
| Refrigerant gas R-407C | **126** | 3340 |
| Refrigerant gas R-500 | **126** | 2602 |
| Refrigerant gas R-502 | **126** | 1973 |
| Refrigerant gas R-503 | **126** | 2599 |
| Refrigerant gas R-1113 | **119P** | 1082 |
| Refrigerant gas R-1132a | **116P** | 1959 |
| Refrigerant gas R-1216 | **126** | 1858 |
| Refrigerant gas R-1318 | **126** | 2422 |
| Refrigerant gas RC-318 | **126** | 1976 |
| Refrigerating machines, containing Ammonia solutions (UN2672) | **126** | 2857 |
| Refrigerating machines, containing flammable, non-poisonous, liquefied gas | **115** | 3358 |
| Refrigerating machines, containing flammable, non-toxic, liquefied gas | **115** | 3358 |
| Refrigerating machines, containing non-flammable, non-poisonous gases | **126** | 2857 |
| Refrigerating machines, containing non-flammable, non-toxic gases | **126** | 2857 |
| Regulated medical waste, n.o.s. | **158** | 3291 |
| Resin solution | **127** | 1866 |
| Resorcinol | **153** | 2876 |
| Rosin oil | **127** | 1286 |
| Rubber scrap, powdered or granulated | **133** | 1345 |
| Rubber shoddy, powdered or granulated | **133** | 1345 |
| Rubber solution | **127** | 1287 |
| Rubidium | **138** | 1423 |
| Rubidium hydroxide | **154** | 2678 |
| Rubidium hydroxide, solid | **154** | 2678 |
| Rubidium hydroxide, solution | **154** | 2677 |
| Rubidium metal | **138** | 1423 |
| SA | **119** | 2188 |
| Safety devices | **171** | 3268 |
| Sarin | **153** | 2810 |
| Seat-belt pre-tensioners | **171** | 3268 |
| Seed cake, with more than 1.5% oil and not more than 11% moisture | **135** | 1386 |
| Seed cake, with not more than 1.5% oil and not more than 11% moisture | **135** | 2217 |
| Selenates | **151** | 2630 |
| Selenic acid | **154** | 1905 |
| Selenites | **151** | 2630 |
| Selenium compound, liquid, n.o.s. | **151** | 3440 |
| Selenium compound, n.o.s. | **151** | 3283 |
| Selenium compound, solid, n.o.s. | **151** | 3283 |
| Selenium disulfide | **153** | 2657 |
| Selenium disulphide | **153** | 2657 |
| Selenium hexafluoride | **125** | 2194 |
| Selenium oxychloride | **157** | 2879 |

| Name of Material | Guide No. | ID No. |
|---|---|---|
| Self-defense spray, non-pressurized | **171** | 3334 |
| Self-heating liquid, corrosive, inorganic, n.o.s. | **136** | 3188 |
| Self-heating liquid, corrosive, organic, n.o.s. | **136** | 3185 |
| Self-heating liquid, inorganic, n.o.s. | **135** | 3186 |
| Self-heating liquid, organic, n.o.s. | **135** | 3183 |
| Self-heating liquid, poisonous, inorganic, n.o.s. | **136** | 3187 |
| Self-heating liquid, poisonous, organic, n.o.s. | **136** | 3184 |
| Self-heating liquid, toxic, inorganic, n.o.s. | **136** | 3187 |
| Self-heating liquid, toxic, organic, n.o.s. | **136** | 3184 |
| Self-heating solid, corrosive, inorganic, n.o.s. | **136** | 3192 |
| Self-heating solid, corrosive, organic, n.o.s. | **136** | 3126 |
| Self-heating solid, inorganic, n.o.s. | **135** | 3190 |
| Self-heating solid, organic, n.o.s. | **135** | 3088 |
| Self-heating solid, oxidizing, n.o.s. | **135** | 3127 |
| Self-heating solid, poisonous, inorganic, n.o.s. | **136** | 3191 |
| Self-heating solid, poisonous, organic, n.o.s. | **136** | 3128 |
| Self-heating solid, toxic, inorganic, n.o.s. | **136** | 3191 |
| Self-heating solid, toxic, organic, n.o.s. | **136** | 3128 |
| Self-reactive liquid type B | **149** | 3221 |
| Self-reactive liquid type B, temperature controlled | **150** | 3231 |
| Self-reactive liquid type C | **149** | 3223 |
| Self-reactive liquid type C, temperature controlled | **150** | 3233 |
| Self-reactive liquid type D | **149** | 3225 |
| Self-reactive liquid type D, temperature controlled | **150** | 3235 |
| Self-reactive liquid type E | **149** | 3227 |
| Self-reactive liquid type E, temperature controlled | **150** | 3237 |
| Self-reactive liquid type F | **149** | 3229 |
| Self-reactive liquid type F, temperature controlled | **150** | 3239 |
| Self-reactive solid type B | **149** | 3222 |
| Self-reactive solid type B, temperature controlled | **150** | 3232 |
| Self-reactive solid type C | **149** | 3224 |
| Self-reactive solid type C, temperature controlled | **150** | 3234 |
| Self-reactive solid type D | **149** | 3226 |
| Self-reactive solid type D, temperature controlled | **150** | 3236 |
| Self-reactive solid type E | **149** | 3228 |
| Self-reactive solid type E, temperature controlled | **150** | 3238 |
| Self-reactive solid type F | **149** | 3230 |
| Self-reactive solid type F, temperature controlled | **150** | 3240 |
| Shale oil | **128** | 1288 |
| Silane | **116** | 2203 |
| Silane, compressed | **116** | 2203 |
| Silicofluorides, n.o.s. | **151** | 2856 |
| Silicon powder, amorphous | **170** | 1346 |
| Silicon tetrachloride | **157** | 1818 |
| Silicon tetrafluoride | **125** | 1859 |
| Silicon tetrafluoride, adsorbed | **173** | 3521 |
| Silicon tetrafluoride, compressed | **125** | 1859 |

| Name of Material | Guide No. | ID No. |
|---|---|---|
| Silver arsenite | **151** | 1683 |
| Silver cyanide | **151** | 1684 |
| Silver nitrate | **140** | 1493 |
| Silver picrate, wetted with not less than 30% water | **113** | 1347 |
| Sludge acid | **153** | 1906 |
| Smokeless powder for small arms | **133** | 3178 |
| Soda lime, with more than 4% Sodium hydroxide | **154** | 1907 |
| Sodium | **138** | 1428 |
| Sodium aluminate, solid | **154** | 2812 |
| Sodium aluminate, solution | **154** | 1819 |
| Sodium aluminum hydride | **138** | 2835 |
| Sodium ammonium vanadate | **154** | 2863 |
| Sodium arsanilate | **154** | 2473 |
| Sodium arsenate | **151** | 1685 |
| Sodium arsenite, aqueous solution | **154** | 1686 |
| Sodium arsenite, solid | **151** | 2027 |
| Sodium azide | **153** | 1687 |
| Sodium, batteries containing | **138** | 3292 |
| Sodium bisulfate, solution | **154** | 2837 |
| Sodium bisulphate, solution | **154** | 2837 |
| Sodium borohydride | **138** | 1426 |
| Sodium borohydride and Sodium hydroxide solution, with not more than 12% Sodium borohydride and not more than 40% Sodium hydroxide | **157** | 3320 |
| Sodium bromate | **141** | 1494 |
| Sodium cacodylate | **152** | 1688 |
| Sodium carbonate peroxyhydrate | **140** | 3378 |
| Sodium chlorate | **140** | 1495 |

| Name of Material | Guide No. | ID No. |
|---|---|---|
| Sodium chlorate, aqueous solution | **140** | 2428 |
| Sodium chlorite | **143** | 1496 |
| Sodium chloroacetate | **151** | 2659 |
| Sodium cuprocyanide, solid | **157** | 2316 |
| Sodium cuprocyanide, solution | **157** | 2317 |
| Sodium cyanide | **157** | 1689 |
| Sodium cyanide, solid | **157** | 1689 |
| Sodium cyanide, solution | **157** | 3414 |
| Sodium dichloroisocyanurate | **140** | 2465 |
| Sodium dichloro-s-triazinetrione | **140** | 2465 |
| Sodium dinitro-o-cresolate, wetted with not less than 10% water | **113** | 3369 |
| Sodium dinitro-o-cresolate, wetted with not less than 15% water | **113** | 1348 |
| Sodium dithionite | **135** | 1384 |
| Sodium fluoride | **154** | 1690 |
| Sodium fluoride, solid | **154** | 1690 |
| Sodium fluoride, solution | **154** | 3415 |
| Sodium fluoroacetate | **151** | 2629 |
| Sodium fluorosilicate | **154** | 2674 |
| Sodium hydride | **138** | 1427 |
| Sodium hydrogendifluoride | **154** | 2439 |
| Sodium hydrosulfide, hydrated, with not less than 25% water of crystallization | **154** | 2949 |
| Sodium hydrosulfide, with less than 25% water of crystallization | **135** | 2318 |
| Sodium hydrosulfide, with not less than 25% water of crystallization | **154** | 2949 |
| Sodium hydrosulfite | **135** | 1384 |

| Name of Material | Guide No. | ID No. |
|---|---|---|
| Sodium hydrosulphide, hydrated, with not less than 25% water of crystallization | **154** | 2949 |
| Sodium hydrosulphide, with less than 25% water of crystallization | **135** | 2318 |
| Sodium hydrosulphide, with not less than 25% water of crystallization | **154** | 2949 |
| Sodium hydrosulphite | **135** | 1384 |
| Sodium hydroxide, solid | **154** | 1823 |
| Sodium hydroxide, solution | **154** | 1824 |
| Sodium hypochlorite | **154** | 1791 |
| Sodium methylate | **138** | 1431 |
| Sodium methylate, dry | **138** | 1431 |
| Sodium methylate, solution in alcohol | **132** | 1289 |
| Sodium monoxide | **157** | 1825 |
| Sodium nitrate | **140** | 1498 |
| Sodium nitrate and Potassium nitrate mixture | **140** | 1499 |
| Sodium nitrite | **140** | 1500 |
| Sodium nitrite and Potassium nitrate mixture | **140** | 1487 |
| Sodium pentachlorophenate | **154** | 2567 |
| Sodium perborate monohydrate | **140** | 3377 |
| Sodium perchlorate | **140** | 1502 |
| Sodium permanganate | **140** | 1503 |
| Sodium peroxide | **144** | 1504 |
| Sodium peroxoborate, anhydrous | **140** | 3247 |
| Sodium persulfate | **140** | 1505 |
| Sodium persulphate | **140** | 1505 |
| Sodium phosphide | **139** | 1432 |
| Sodium picramate, wetted with not less than 20% water | **113** | 1349 |
| Sodium potassium alloys | **138** | 1422 |
| Sodium potassium alloys, liquid | **138** | 1422 |
| Sodium potassium alloys, solid | **138** | 3404 |
| Sodium silicofluoride | **154** | 2674 |
| Sodium sulfide, anhydrous | **135** | 1385 |
| Sodium sulfide, hydrated, with not less than 30% water | **153** | 1849 |
| Sodium sulfide, with less than 30% water of crystallization | **135** | 1385 |
| Sodium sulphide, anhydrous | **135** | 1385 |
| Sodium sulphide, hydrated, with not less than 30% water | **153** | 1849 |
| Sodium sulphide, with less than 30% water of crystallization | **135** | 1385 |
| Sodium superoxide | **143** | 2547 |
| Solids containing corrosive liquid, n.o.s. | **154** | 3244 |
| Solids containing flammable liquid, n.o.s. | **133** | 3175 |
| Solids containing poisonous liquid, n.o.s. | **151** | 3243 |
| Solids containing toxic liquid, n.o.s. | **151** | 3243 |
| Soman | **153** | 2810 |
| Stannic chloride, anhydrous | **137** | 1827 |
| Stannic chloride, pentahydrate | **154** | 2440 |
| Stannic phosphides | **139** | 1433 |
| Stibine | **119** | 2676 |
| Straw, wet, damp or contaminated with oil | **133** | 1327 |
| Strontium arsenite | **151** | 1691 |
| Strontium chlorate | **143** | 1506 |
| Strontium nitrate | **140** | 1507 |
| Strontium perchlorate | **140** | 1508 |

| Name of Material | Guide No. | ID No. |
|---|---|---|
| Strontium peroxide | **143** | 1509 |
| Strontium phosphide | **139** | 2013 |
| Strychnine | **151** | 1692 |
| Strychnine salts | **151** | 1692 |
| Styrene monomer, stabilized | **128P** | 2055 |
| Substituted nitrophenol pesticide, liquid, flammable, poisonous | **131** | 2780 |
| Substituted nitrophenol pesticide, liquid, flammable, toxic | **131** | 2780 |
| Substituted nitrophenol pesticide, liquid, poisonous | **153** | 3014 |
| Substituted nitrophenol pesticide, liquid, poisonous, flammable | **131** | 3013 |
| Substituted nitrophenol pesticide, liquid, toxic | **153** | 3014 |
| Substituted nitrophenol pesticide, liquid, toxic, flammable | **131** | 3013 |
| Substituted nitrophenol pesticide, solid, poisonous | **153** | 2779 |
| Substituted nitrophenol pesticide, solid, toxic | **153** | 2779 |
| Sulfamic acid | **154** | 2967 |
| Sulfur | **133** | 1350 |
| Sulfur, molten | **133** | 2448 |
| Sulfur chlorides | **137** | 1828 |
| Sulfur dioxide | **125** | 1079 |
| Sulfur hexafluoride | **126** | 1080 |
| Sulfuric acid | **137** | 1830 |
| Sulfuric acid, fuming | **137** | 1831 |
| Sulfuric acid, fuming, with less than 30% free Sulfur trioxide | **137** | 1831 |

| Name of Material | Guide No. | ID No. |
|---|---|---|
| Sulfuric acid, fuming, with not less than 30% free Sulfur trioxide | **137** | 1831 |
| Sulfuric acid, spent | **137** | 1832 |
| Sulfuric acid, with more than 51% acid | **137** | 1830 |
| Sulfuric acid, with not more than 51% acid | **157** | 2796 |
| Sulfuric acid and Hydrofluoric acid mixture | **157** | 1786 |
| Sulfurous acid | **154** | 1833 |
| Sulfur tetrafluoride | **125** | 2418 |
| Sulfur trioxide, stabilized | **137** | 1829 |
| Sulfuryl chloride | **137** | 1834 |
| Sulfuryl fluoride | **123** | 2191 |
| Sulphamic acid | **154** | 2967 |
| Sulphur | **133** | 1350 |
| Sulphur, molten | **133** | 2448 |
| Sulphur chlorides | **137** | 1828 |
| Sulphur dioxide | **125** | 1079 |
| Sulphur hexafluoride | **126** | 1080 |
| Sulphuric acid | **137** | 1830 |
| Sulphuric acid, fuming | **137** | 1831 |
| Sulphuric acid, fuming, with less than 30% free Sulphur trioxide | **137** | 1831 |
| Sulphuric acid, fuming, with not less than 30% free Sulphur trioxide | **137** | 1831 |
| Sulphuric acid, spent | **137** | 1832 |
| Sulphuric acid, with more than 51% acid | **137** | 1830 |
| Sulphuric acid, with not more than 51% acid | **157** | 2796 |
| Sulphuric acid and Hydrofluoric acid mixture | **157** | 1786 |
| Sulphurous acid | **154** | 1833 |

| Name of Material | Guide No. | ID No. |
|---|---|---|
| Sulphur tetrafluoride | **125** | 2418 |
| Sulphur trioxide, stabilized | **137** | 1829 |
| Sulphuryl chloride | **137** | 1834 |
| Sulphuryl fluoride | **123** | 2191 |
| Tabun | **153** | 2810 |
| Tars, liquid | **130** | 1999 |
| Tear gas candles | **159** | 1700 |
| Tear gas devices | **159** | 1693 |
| Tear gas grenades | **159** | 1700 |
| Tear gas substance, liquid, n.o.s. | **159** | 1693 |
| Tear gas substance, solid, n.o.s. | **159** | 1693 |
| Tear gas substance, solid, n.o.s. | **159** | 3448 |
| Tellurium compound, n.o.s. | **151** | 3284 |
| Tellurium hexafluoride | **125** | 2195 |
| Terpene hydrocarbons, n.o.s. | **128** | 2319 |
| Terpinolene | **128** | 2541 |
| Tetrabromoethane | **159** | 2504 |
| 1,1,2,2-Tetrachloroethane | **151** | 1702 |
| Tetrachloroethane | **151** | 1702 |
| Tetrachloroethylene | **160** | 1897 |
| Tetraethyl dithiopyrophosphate | **153** | 1704 |
| Tetraethylenepentamine | **153** | 2320 |
| Tetraethyl silicate | **129** | 1292 |
| 1,1,1,2-Tetrafluoroethane | **126** | 3159 |
| Tetrafluoroethane and Ethylene oxide mixture, with not more than 5.6% Ethylene oxide | **126** | 3299 |
| Tetrafluoroethylene, stabilized | **116P** | 1081 |
| Tetrafluoromethane | **126** | 1982 |
| Tetrafluoromethane, compressed | **126** | 1982 |
| 1,2,3,6-Tetrahydrobenzaldehyde | **129** | 2498 |
| Tetrahydrofuran | **127** | 2056 |
| Tetrahydrofurfurylamine | **129** | 2943 |
| Tetrahydrophthalic anhydrides | **156** | 2698 |
| 1,2,3,6-Tetrahydropyridine | **129** | 2410 |
| Tetrahydrothiophene | **130** | 2412 |
| Tetramethylammonium hydroxide | **153** | 1835 |
| Tetramethylammonium hydroxide, solid | **153** | 3423 |
| Tetramethylammonium hydroxide, solution | **153** | 1835 |
| Tetramethylsilane | **130** | 2749 |
| Tetranitromethane | **143** | 1510 |
| Tetrapropyl orthotitanate | **128** | 2413 |
| Textile waste, wet | **133** | 1857 |
| Thallium chlorate | **141** | 2573 |
| Thallium compound, n.o.s. | **151** | 1707 |
| Thallium nitrate | **141** | 2727 |
| 4-Thiapentanal | **152** | 2785 |
| Thickened GD | **153** | 2810 |
| Thioacetic acid | **129** | 2436 |
| Thiocarbamate pesticide, liquid, flammable, poisonous | **131** | 2772 |
| Thiocarbamate pesticide, liquid, flammable, toxic | **131** | 2772 |
| Thiocarbamate pesticide, liquid, poisonous | **151** | 3006 |
| Thiocarbamate pesticide, liquid, poisonous, flammable | **131** | 3005 |
| Thiocarbamate pesticide, liquid, toxic | **151** | 3006 |

| Name of Material | Guide No. | ID No. |
| --- | --- | --- |
| Thiocarbamate pesticide, liquid, toxic, flammable | **131** | 3005 |
| Thiocarbamate pesticide, solid, poisonous | **151** | 2771 |
| Thiocarbamate pesticide, solid, toxic | **151** | 2771 |
| Thioglycol | **153** | 2966 |
| Thioglycolic acid | **153** | 1940 |
| Thiolactic acid | **153** | 2936 |
| Thionyl chloride | **137** | 1836 |
| Thiophene | **130** | 2414 |
| Thiophosgene | **157** | 2474 |
| Thiophosphoryl chloride | **157** | 1837 |
| Thiourea dioxide | **135** | 3341 |
| Tinctures, medicinal | **127** | 1293 |
| Tin tetrachloride | **137** | 1827 |
| Titanium disulfide | **135** | 3174 |
| Titanium disulphide | **135** | 3174 |
| Titanium hydride | **170** | 1871 |
| Titanium powder, dry | **135** | 2546 |
| Titanium powder, wetted with not less than 25% water | **170** | 1352 |
| Titanium sponge granules | **170** | 2878 |
| Titanium sponge powders | **170** | 2878 |
| Titanium tetrachloride | **137** | 1838 |
| Titanium trichloride, pyrophoric | **135** | 2441 |
| Titanium trichloride mixture | **157** | 2869 |
| Titanium trichloride mixture, pyrophoric | **135** | 2441 |
| TNT, wetted with not less than 10% water | **113** | 3366 |
| TNT, wetted with not less than 30% water | **113** | 1356 |
| Toluene | **130** | 1294 |
| 2,4-Toluenediamine, solid | **151** | 1709 |
| 2,4-Toluenediamine, solution | **151** | 3418 |
| Toluene diisocyanate | **156** | 2078 |
| Toluidines, liquid | **153** | 1708 |
| Toluidines, solid | **153** | 1708 |
| Toluidines, solid | **153** | 3451 |
| 2,4-Toluylenediamine | **151** | 1709 |
| 2,4-Toluylenediamine, solid | **151** | 1709 |
| 2,4-Toluylenediamine, solution | **151** | 3418 |
| Toxic by inhalation liquid, corrosive, flammable, n.o.s. (Inhalation Hazard Zone A) | **131** | 3492 |
| Toxic by inhalation liquid, corrosive, flammable, n.o.s. (Inhalation Hazard Zone B) | **131** | 3493 |
| Toxic by inhalation liquid, corrosive, n.o.s. (Inhalation Hazard Zone A) | **154** | 3389 |
| Toxic by inhalation liquid, corrosive, n.o.s. (Inhalation Hazard Zone B) | **154** | 3390 |
| Toxic by inhalation liquid, flammable, corrosive, n.o.s. (Inhalation Hazard Zone A) | **131** | 3488 |
| Toxic by inhalation liquid, flammable, corrosive, n.o.s. (Inhalation Hazard Zone B) | **131** | 3489 |
| Toxic by inhalation liquid, flammable, n.o.s. (Inhalation Hazard Zone A) | **131** | 3383 |
| Toxic by inhalation liquid, flammable, n.o.s. (Inhalation Hazard Zone B) | **131** | 3384 |
| Toxic by inhalation liquid, n.o.s. (Inhalation Hazard Zone A) | **151** | 3381 |
| Toxic by inhalation liquid, n.o.s. (Inhalation Hazard Zone B) | **151** | 3382 |

| Name of Material | Guide No. | ID No. |
|---|---|---|
| Toxic by inhalation liquid, oxidizing, n.o.s. (Inhalation Hazard Zone A) | **142** | 3387 |
| Toxic by inhalation liquid, oxidizing, n.o.s. (Inhalation Hazard Zone B) | **142** | 3388 |
| Toxic by inhalation liquid, water-reactive, flammable, n.o.s. (Inhalation Hazard Zone A) | **155** | 3490 |
| Toxic by inhalation liquid, water-reactive, flammable, n.o.s. (Inhalation Hazard Zone B) | **155** | 3491 |
| Toxic by inhalation liquid, water-reactive, n.o.s. (Inhalation Hazard Zone A) | **139** | 3385 |
| Toxic by inhalation liquid, water-reactive, n.o.s. (Inhalation Hazard Zone B) | **139** | 3386 |
| Toxic liquid, corrosive, inorganic, n.o.s. | **154** | 3289 |
| Toxic liquid, corrosive, organic, n.o.s. | **154** | 2927 |
| Toxic liquid, flammable, organic, n.o.s. | **131** | 2929 |
| Toxic liquid, inorganic, n.o.s. | **151** | 3287 |
| Toxic liquid, organic, n.o.s. | **153** | 2810 |
| Toxic liquid, oxidizing, n.o.s. | **142** | 3122 |
| Toxic liquid, water-reactive, n.o.s. | **139** | 3123 |
| Toxic solid, corrosive, inorganic, n.o.s. | **154** | 3290 |
| Toxic solid, corrosive, organic, n.o.s. | **154** | 2928 |
| Toxic solid, flammable, organic, n.o.s. | **134** | 2930 |
| Toxic solid, inorganic, n.o.s. | **151** | 3288 |
| Toxic solid, organic, n.o.s. | **154** | 2811 |
| Toxic solid, oxidizing, n.o.s. | **141** | 3086 |

| Name of Material | Guide No. | ID No. |
|---|---|---|
| Toxic solid, self-heating, n.o.s. | **136** | 3124 |
| Toxic solid, water-reactive, n.o.s. | **139** | 3125 |
| Toxins | **153** | —— |
| Toxins, extracted from living sources, liquid, n.o.s. | **153** | 3172 |
| Toxins, extracted from living sources, solid, n.o.s. | **153** | 3172 |
| Toxins, extracted from living sources, solid, n.o.s. | **153** | 3462 |
| Triallylamine | **132** | 2610 |
| Triallyl borate | **156** | 2609 |
| Triazine pesticide, liquid, flammable, poisonous | **131** | 2764 |
| Triazine pesticide, liquid, flammable, toxic | **131** | 2764 |
| Triazine pesticide, liquid, poisonous | **151** | 2998 |
| Triazine pesticide, liquid, poisonous, flammable | **131** | 2997 |
| Triazine pesticide, liquid, toxic | **151** | 2998 |
| Triazine pesticide, liquid, toxic, flammable | **131** | 2997 |
| Triazine pesticide, solid, poisonous | **151** | 2763 |
| Triazine pesticide, solid, toxic | **151** | 2763 |
| Tributylamine | **153** | 2542 |
| Tributylphosphane | **135** | 3254 |
| Trichloroacetic acid | **153** | 1839 |
| Trichloroacetic acid, solution | **153** | 2564 |
| Trichloroacetyl chloride | **156** | 2442 |
| Trichlorobenzenes, liquid | **153** | 2321 |
| Trichlorobutene | **152** | 2322 |
| 1,1,1-Trichloroethane | **160** | 2831 |
| Trichloroethylene | **160** | 1710 |

| Name of Material | Guide No. | ID No. |
|---|---|---|
| Trichloroisocyanuric acid, dry | **140** | 2468 |
| Trichlorosilane | **139** | 1295 |
| Tricresyl phosphate | **151** | 2574 |
| Triethylamine | **132** | 1296 |
| Triethylenetetramine | **153** | 2259 |
| Triethyl phosphite | **130** | 2323 |
| Trifluoroacetic acid | **154** | 2699 |
| Trifluoroacetyl chloride | **125** | 3057 |
| Trifluorochloroethylene, stabilized | **119P** | 1082 |
| 1,1,1-Trifluoroethane | **115** | 2035 |
| Trifluoromethane | **126** | 1984 |
| Trifluoromethane, refrigerated liquid | **120** | 3136 |
| Trifluoromethane and Chlorotrifluoromethane azeotropic mixture with approximately 60% Chlorotrifluoromethane | **126** | 2599 |
| 2-Trifluoromethylaniline | **153** | 2942 |
| 3-Trifluoromethylaniline | **153** | 2948 |
| Triisobutylene | **128** | 2324 |
| Triisopropyl borate | **129** | 2616 |
| Trimethoxysilane | **132** | 9269 |
| Trimethylacetyl chloride | **132** | 2438 |
| Trimethylamine, anhydrous | **118** | 1083 |
| Trimethylamine, aqueous solution | **132** | 1297 |
| 1,3,5-Trimethylbenzene | **129** | 2325 |
| Trimethyl borate | **129** | 2416 |
| Trimethylchlorosilane | **155** | 1298 |
| Trimethylcyclohexylamine | **153** | 2326 |
| Trimethylhexamethylenediamines | **153** | 2327 |
| Trimethylhexamethylene diisocyanate | **156** | 2328 |

| Name of Material | Guide No. | ID No. |
|---|---|---|
| Trimethyl phosphite | **130** | 2329 |
| Trinitrobenzene, wetted with not less than 10% water | **113** | 3367 |
| Trinitrobenzene, wetted with not less than 30% water | **113** | 1354 |
| Trinitrobenzoic acid, wetted with not less than 10% water | **113** | 3368 |
| Trinitrobenzoic acid, wetted with not less than 30% water | **113** | 1355 |
| Trinitrochlorobenzene, wetted with not less than 10% water | **113** | 3365 |
| Trinitrophenol, wetted with not less than 10% water | **113** | 3364 |
| Trinitrophenol, wetted with not less than 30% water | **113** | 1344 |
| Trinitrotoluene, wetted with not less than 10% water | **113** | 3366 |
| Trinitrotoluene, wetted with not less than 30% water | **113** | 1356 |
| Tripropylamine | **132** | 2260 |
| Tripropylene | **128** | 2057 |
| Tris-(1-aziridinyl)phosphine oxide, solution | **152** | 2501 |
| Tungsten hexafluoride | **125** | 2196 |
| Turpentine | **128** | 1299 |
| Turpentine substitute | **128** | 1300 |
| Undecane | **128** | 2330 |
| Uranium hexafluoride, radioactive material, excepted package, less than 0.1 kg per package, non-fissile or fissile-excepted | **166** | 3507 |
| Uranium hexafluoride, radioactive material, fissile | **166** | 2977 |
| Uranium hexafluoride, radioactive material, non fissile or fissile-excepted | **166** | 2978 |
| Urea hydrogen peroxide | **140** | 1511 |
| Urea nitrate, wetted with not less than 10% water | **113** | 3370 |

| Name of Material | Guide No. | ID No. |
|---|---|---|
| Urea nitrate, wetted with not less than 20% water | **113** | 1357 |
| Valeraldehyde | **129** | 2058 |
| Valeryl chloride | **132** | 2502 |
| Vanadium compound, n.o.s. | **151** | 3285 |
| Vanadium oxytrichloride | **137** | 2443 |
| Vanadium pentoxide | **151** | 2862 |
| Vanadium tetrachloride | **137** | 2444 |
| Vanadium trichloride | **157** | 2475 |
| Vanadyl sulfate | **151** | 2931 |
| Vanadyl sulphate | **151** | 2931 |
| Vehicle, flammable gas powered | **115** | 3166 |
| Vehicle, flammable liquid powered | **128** | 3166 |
| Vehicle, fuel cell, flammable gas powered | **115** | 3166 |
| Vehicle, fuel cell, flammable liquid powered | **128** | 3166 |
| Vinyl acetate, stabilized | **129P** | 1301 |
| Vinyl bromide, stabilized | **116P** | 1085 |
| Vinyl butyrate, stabilized | **129P** | 2838 |
| Vinyl chloride, stabilized | **116P** | 1086 |
| Vinyl chloroacetate | **155** | 2589 |
| Vinyl ethyl ether, stabilized | **127P** | 1302 |
| Vinyl fluoride, stabilized | **116P** | 1860 |
| Vinylidene chloride, stabilized | **130P** | 1303 |
| Vinyl isobutyl ether, stabilized | **127P** | 1304 |
| Vinyl methyl ether, stabilized | **116P** | 1087 |
| Vinylpyridines, stabilized | **131P** | 3073 |
| Vinyltoluenes, stabilized | **130P** | 2618 |
| Vinyltrichlorosilane | **155P** | 1305 |
| Vinyltrichlorosilane, stabilized | **155P** | 1305 |
| VX | **153** | 2810 |
| Water-reactive liquid, corrosive, n.o.s. | **138** | 3129 |
| Water-reactive liquid, n.o.s. | **138** | 3148 |
| Water-reactive liquid, poisonous, n.o.s. | **139** | 3130 |
| Water-reactive liquid, toxic, n.o.s. | **139** | 3130 |
| Water-reactive solid, corrosive, n.o.s. | **138** | 3131 |
| Water-reactive solid, flammable, n.o.s. | **138** | 3132 |
| Water-reactive solid, n.o.s. | **138** | 2813 |
| Water-reactive solid, oxidizing, n.o.s. | **138** | 3133 |
| Water-reactive solid, poisonous, n.o.s. | **139** | 3134 |
| Water-reactive solid, self-heating, n.o.s. | **138** | 3135 |
| Water-reactive solid, toxic, n.o.s. | **139** | 3134 |
| Wheelchair, electric, with batteries | **154** | 3171 |
| White asbestos | **171** | 2590 |
| White phosphorus, dry | **136** | 1381 |
| White phosphorus, in solution | **136** | 1381 |
| White phosphorus, molten | **136** | 2447 |
| White phosphorus, under water | **136** | 1381 |
| Wood preservatives, liquid | **129** | 1306 |
| Wool waste, wet | **133** | 1387 |
| Xanthates | **135** | 3342 |
| Xenon | **121** | 2036 |
| Xenon, compressed | **121** | 2036 |
| Xenon, refrigerated liquid (cryogenic liquid) | **120** | 2591 |
| Xylenes | **130** | 1307 |
| Xylenols | **153** | 2261 |

| Name of Material | Guide No. | ID No. |
|---|---|---|
| Xylenols, liquid | **153** | 3430 |
| Xylenols, solid | **153** | 2261 |
| Xylidines, liquid | **153** | 1711 |
| Xylidines, solid | **153** | 1711 |
| Xylidines, solid | **153** | 3452 |
| Xylyl bromide | **152** | 1701 |
| Xylyl bromide, liquid | **152** | 1701 |
| Xylyl bromide, solid | **152** | 3417 |
| Yellow phosphorus, dry | **136** | 1381 |
| Yellow phosphorus, in solution | **136** | 1381 |
| Yellow phosphorus, under water | **136** | 1381 |
| Zinc ammonium nitrite | **140** | 1512 |
| Zinc arsenate | **151** | 1712 |
| Zinc arsenate and Zinc arsenite mixture | **151** | 1712 |
| Zinc arsenite | **151** | 1712 |
| Zinc arsenite and Zinc arsenate mixture | **151** | 1712 |
| Zinc ashes | **138** | 1435 |
| Zinc bromate | **140** | 2469 |
| Zinc chlorate | **140** | 1513 |
| Zinc chloride, anhydrous | **154** | 2331 |
| Zinc chloride, solution | **154** | 1840 |
| Zinc cyanide | **151** | 1713 |
| Zinc dithionite | **171** | 1931 |
| Zinc dross | **138** | 1435 |
| Zinc dust | **138** | 1436 |
| Zinc fluorosilicate | **151** | 2855 |
| Zinc hydrosulfite | **171** | 1931 |
| Zinc hydrosulphite | **171** | 1931 |
| Zinc nitrate | **140** | 1514 |
| Zinc permanganate | **140** | 1515 |
| Zinc peroxide | **143** | 1516 |
| Zinc phosphide | **139** | 1714 |
| Zinc powder | **138** | 1436 |
| Zinc residue | **138** | 1435 |
| Zinc resinate | **133** | 2714 |
| Zinc silicofluoride | **151** | 2855 |
| Zinc skimmings | **138** | 1435 |
| Zirconium, dry, coiled wire, finished metal sheets or strip | **170** | 2858 |
| Zirconium, dry, finished sheets, strips or coiled wire | **135** | 2009 |
| Zirconium hydride | **138** | 1437 |
| Zirconium nitrate | **140** | 2728 |
| Zirconium picramate, wetted with not less than 20% water | **113** | 1517 |
| Zirconium powder, dry | **135** | 2008 |
| Zirconium powder, wetted with not less than 25% water | **170** | 1358 |
| Zirconium scrap | **135** | 1932 |
| Zirconium suspended in a flammable liquid | **170** | 1308 |
| Zirconium suspended in a liquid (flammable) | **170** | 1308 |
| Zirconium tetrachloride | **137** | 2503 |

# GUIDES

## POTENTIAL HAZARDS

### FIRE OR EXPLOSION

- May explode from heat, shock, friction or contamination.
- May react violently or explosively on contact with air, water or foam.
- May be ignited by heat, sparks or flames.
- Vapors may travel to source of ignition and flash back.
- Containers may explode when heated.
- Ruptured cylinders may rocket.

### HEALTH

- Inhalation, ingestion or contact with substance may cause severe injury, infection, disease or death.
- High concentration of gas may cause asphyxiation without warning.
- Contact may cause burns to skin and eyes.
- Fire or contact with water may produce irritating, toxic and/or corrosive gases.
- Runoff from fire control may cause pollution.

## PUBLIC SAFETY

- **CALL EMERGENCY RESPONSE Telephone Number on Shipping Paper first. If Shipping Paper not available or no answer, refer to appropriate telephone number listed on the inside back cover.**
- As an immediate precautionary measure, isolate spill or leak area for at least 100 meters (330 feet) in all directions.
- Keep unauthorized personnel away.
- Stay upwind, uphill and/or upstream.

### PROTECTIVE CLOTHING

- Wear positive pressure self-contained breathing apparatus (SCBA).
- Structural firefighters' protective clothing provides limited protection in fire situations ONLY; it may not be effective in spill situations.

### EVACUATION

**Fire**

- If tank, rail car or tank truck is involved in a fire, ISOLATE for 800 meters (1/2 mile) in all directions; also, consider initial evacuation for 800 meters (1/2 mile) in all directions.

## EMERGENCY RESPONSE

### FIRE

**CAUTION: Material may react with extinguishing agent.**

**Small Fire**

- Dry chemical, $CO_2$, water spray or regular foam.

**Large Fire**

- Water spray, fog or regular foam.
- Move containers from fire area if you can do it without risk.

**Fire involving Tanks**

- Cool containers with flooding quantities of water until well after fire is out.
- Do not get water inside containers.
- Withdraw immediately in case of rising sound from venting safety devices or discoloration of tank.
- ALWAYS stay away from tanks engulfed in fire.

### SPILL OR LEAK

- Do not touch or walk through spilled material.
- ELIMINATE all ignition sources (no smoking, flares, sparks or flames in immediate area).
- All equipment used when handling the product must be grounded.
- Keep combustibles (wood, paper, oil, etc.) away from spilled material.
- Use water spray to reduce vapors or divert vapor cloud drift. Avoid allowing water runoff to contact spilled material.
- Prevent entry into waterways, sewers, basements or confined areas.

**Small Spill**

- Pick up with sand or other non-combustible absorbent material and place into containers for later disposal.

**Large Spill**

- Dike far ahead of liquid spill for later disposal.

### FIRST AID

- Ensure that medical personnel are aware of the material(s) involved and take precautions to protect themselves.
- Move victim to fresh air.
- Call 911 or emergency medical service.
- Give artificial respiration if victim is not breathing.
- **Do not use mouth-to-mouth method if victim ingested or inhaled the substance; give artificial respiration with the aid of a pocket mask equipped with a one-way valve or other proper respiratory medical device.**
- Administer oxygen if breathing is difficult.
- Remove and isolate contaminated clothing and shoes.
- In case of contact with substance, immediately flush skin or eyes with running water for at least 20 minutes.
- Shower and wash with soap and water.
- Keep victim calm and warm.
- Effects of exposure (inhalation, ingestion or skin contact) to substance may be delayed.

# GUIDE 112 EXPLOSIVES* - DIVISION 1.1, 1.2, 1.3 OR 1.5

## POTENTIAL HAZARDS

### FIRE OR EXPLOSION

- **MAY EXPLODE AND THROW FRAGMENTS 1600 METERS (1 MILE) OR MORE IF FIRE REACHES CARGO.**
- **For information on "Compatibility Group" letters, refer to Glossary section.**

### HEALTH

- Fire may produce irritating, corrosive and/or toxic gases.

## PUBLIC SAFETY

- **CALL EMERGENCY RESPONSE Telephone Number on Shipping Paper first. If Shipping Paper not available or no answer, refer to appropriate telephone number listed on the inside back cover.**
- Isolate spill or leak area immediately for at least 500 meters (1/3 mile) in all directions.
- Move people out of line of sight of the scene and away from windows.
- Keep unauthorized personnel away.
- Stay upwind, uphill and/or upstream.
- Ventilate closed spaces before entering.

### PROTECTIVE CLOTHING

- Wear positive pressure self-contained breathing apparatus (SCBA).
- Structural firefighters' protective clothing will only provide limited protection.

### EVACUATION

**Large Spill**

- **Consider initial EVACUATION for 800 meters (1/2 mile) in all directions.**

**Fire**

- If rail car or trailer is involved in a fire, ISOLATE for 1600 meters (1 mile) in all directions; also, initiate evacuation including emergency responders for 1600 meters (1 mile) in all directions.

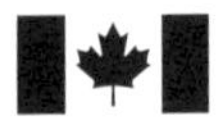

In Canada, an Emergency Response Assistance Plan (ERAP) may be required for this product. Please consult the shipping document and/or the ERAP Program Section (page 391).

* FOR INFORMATION ON "COMPATIBILITY GROUP" LETTERS, REFER TO THE GLOSSARY SECTION.

## EMERGENCY RESPONSE

### FIRE

**CARGO Fire**

- **DO NOT fight fire when fire reaches cargo! Cargo may EXPLODE!**
- Stop all traffic and clear the area for at least 1600 meters (1 mile) in all directions and let burn.
- **Do not move cargo or vehicle if cargo has been exposed to heat.**

**TIRE or VEHICLE Fire**

- **Use plenty of water - FLOOD it! If water is not available, use $CO_2$, dry chemical or dirt.**
- If possible, and WITHOUT RISK, use unmanned hose holders or monitor nozzles from maximum distance to prevent fire from spreading to cargo area.
- Pay special attention to tire fires as re-ignition may occur. Stand by, at a safe distance, with extinguisher ready for possible re-ignition.

### SPILL OR LEAK

- ELIMINATE all ignition sources (no smoking, flares, sparks or flames in immediate area).
- All equipment used when handling the product must be grounded.
- Do not touch or walk through spilled material.
- DO NOT OPERATE RADIO TRANSMITTERS WITHIN 100 METERS (330 FEET) OF ELECTRIC DETONATORS.
- **DO NOT CLEAN-UP OR DISPOSE OF, EXCEPT UNDER SUPERVISION OF A SPECIALIST.**

### FIRST AID

- Ensure that medical personnel are aware of the material(s) involved and take precautions to protect themselves.
- Move victim to fresh air.
- Call 911 or emergency medical service.
- Give artificial respiration if victim is not breathing.
- Administer oxygen if breathing is difficult.
- Remove and isolate contaminated clothing and shoes.
- In case of contact with substance, immediately flush skin or eyes with running water for at least 20 minutes.

* FOR INFORMATION ON "COMPATIBILITY GROUP" LETTERS, REFER TO THE GLOSSARY SECTION.

# GUIDE 113 FLAMMABLE SOLIDS - TOXIC (WET/DESENSITIZED EXPLOSIVE)

## POTENTIAL HAZARDS

### FIRE OR EXPLOSION

- Flammable/combustible material.
- May be ignited by heat, sparks or flames.
- **DRIED OUT material may explode if exposed to heat, flame, friction or shock; treat as an explosive (GUIDE 112).**
- **Keep material wet with water or treat as an explosive (GUIDE 112).**
- Runoff to sewer may create fire or explosion hazard.

### HEALTH

- Some are toxic and may be fatal if inhaled, swallowed or absorbed through skin.
- Contact may cause burns to skin and eyes.
- Fire may produce irritating, corrosive and/or toxic gases.
- Runoff from fire control or dilution water may cause pollution.

## PUBLIC SAFETY

- **CALL EMERGENCY RESPONSE Telephone Number on Shipping Paper first. If Shipping Paper not available or no answer, refer to appropriate telephone number listed on the inside back cover.**
- Isolate spill or leak area immediately for at least 100 meters (330 feet) in all directions.
- Keep unauthorized personnel away.
- Stay upwind, uphill and/or upstream.
- Ventilate closed spaces before entering.

### PROTECTIVE CLOTHING

- Wear positive pressure self-contained breathing apparatus (SCBA).
- Structural firefighters' protective clothing will only provide limited protection.

### EVACUATION

**Large Spill**

- **Consider initial EVACUATION for 500 meters (1/3 mile) in all directions.**

**Fire**

- If tank, rail car or tank truck is involved in a fire, ISOLATE for 800 meters (1/2 mile) in all directions; also, consider initial evacuation for 800 meters (1/2 mile) in all directions.

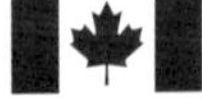

In Canada, an Emergency Response Assistance Plan (ERAP) may be required for this product. Please consult the shipping document and/or the ERAP Program Section (page 391).

## EMERGENCY RESPONSE

### FIRE

**CARGO Fire**

- **DO NOT fight fire when fire reaches cargo! Cargo may EXPLODE!**
- Stop all traffic and clear the area for at least 1600 meters (1 mile) in all directions and let burn.
- **Do not move cargo or vehicle if cargo has been exposed to heat.**

**TIRE or VEHICLE Fire**

- **Use plenty of water - FLOOD it! If water is not available, use $CO_2$, dry chemical or dirt.**
- If possible, and WITHOUT RISK, use unmanned hose holders or monitor nozzles from maximum distance to prevent fire from spreading to cargo area.
- Pay special attention to tire fires as re-ignition may occur. Stand by, at a safe distance, with extinguisher ready for possible re-ignition.

### SPILL OR LEAK

- ELIMINATE all ignition sources (no smoking, flares, sparks or flames in immediate area).
- All equipment used when handling the product must be grounded.
- Do not touch or walk through spilled material.

**Small Spill**

- Flush area with flooding quantities of water.

**Large Spill**

- Wet down with water and dike for later disposal.
- KEEP "WETTED" PRODUCT WET BY SLOWLY ADDING FLOODING QUANTITIES OF WATER.

### FIRST AID

- Ensure that medical personnel are aware of the material(s) involved and take precautions to protect themselves.
- Move victim to fresh air.
- Call 911 or emergency medical service.
- Give artificial respiration if victim is not breathing.
- Administer oxygen if breathing is difficult.
- Remove and isolate contaminated clothing and shoes.
- In case of contact with substance, immediately flush skin or eyes with running water for at least 20 minutes.

# GUIDE 114 EXPLOSIVES* - DIVISION 1.4 OR 1.6

## POTENTIAL HAZARDS

### FIRE OR EXPLOSION

- **MAY EXPLODE AND THROW FRAGMENTS 500 METERS (1/3 MILE) OR MORE IF FIRE REACHES CARGO.**
- **For information on "Compatibility Group" letters, refer to Glossary section.**

### HEALTH

- Fire may produce irritating, corrosive and/or toxic gases.

## PUBLIC SAFETY

- **CALL EMERGENCY RESPONSE Telephone Number on Shipping Paper first. If Shipping Paper not available or no answer, refer to appropriate telephone number listed on the inside back cover.**
- Isolate spill or leak area immediately for at least 100 meters (330 feet) in all directions.
- Move people out of line of sight of the scene and away from windows.
- Keep unauthorized personnel away.
- Stay upwind, uphill and/or upstream.
- Ventilate closed spaces before entering.

### PROTECTIVE CLOTHING

- Wear positive pressure self-contained breathing apparatus (SCBA).
- Structural firefighters' protective clothing will only provide limited protection.

### EVACUATION

**Large Spill**

- **Consider initial EVACUATION for 250 meters (800 feet) in all directions.**

**Fire**

- If rail car or trailer is involved in a fire, ISOLATE for 500 meters (1/3 mile) in all directions; also initiate evacuation including emergency responders for 500 meters (1/3 mile) in all directions.

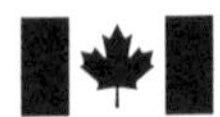

In Canada, an Emergency Response Assistance Plan (ERAP) may be required for this product. Please consult the shipping document and/or the ERAP Program Section (page 391).

* FOR INFORMATION ON "COMPATIBILITY GROUP" LETTERS, REFER TO THE GLOSSARY SECTION.

## EMERGENCY RESPONSE

### FIRE

**CARGO Fire**

- **DO NOT fight fire when fire reaches cargo! Cargo may EXPLODE!**
- Stop all traffic and clear the area for at least 500 meters (1/3 mile) in all directions and let burn.
- **Do not move cargo or vehicle if cargo has been exposed to heat.**

**TIRE or VEHICLE Fire**

- **Use plenty of water - FLOOD it! If water is not available, use $CO_2$, dry chemical or dirt.**
- If possible, and WITHOUT RISK, use unmanned hose holders or monitor nozzles from maximum distance to prevent fire from spreading to cargo area.
- Pay special attention to tire fires as re-ignition may occur. Stand by, at a safe distance, with extinguisher ready for possible re-ignition.

### SPILL OR LEAK

- ELIMINATE all ignition sources (no smoking, flares, sparks or flames in immediate area).
- All equipment used when handling the product must be grounded.
- Do not touch or walk through spilled material.
- DO NOT OPERATE RADIO TRANSMITTERS WITHIN 100 METERS (330 FEET) OF ELECTRIC DETONATORS.
- **DO NOT CLEAN-UP OR DISPOSE OF, EXCEPT UNDER SUPERVISION OF A SPECIALIST.**

### FIRST AID

- Ensure that medical personnel are aware of the material(s) involved and take precautions to protect themselves.
- Move victim to fresh air.
- Call 911 or emergency medical service.
- Give artificial respiration if victim is not breathing.
- Administer oxygen if breathing is difficult.
- Remove and isolate contaminated clothing and shoes.
- In case of contact with substance, immediately flush skin or eyes with running water for at least 20 minutes.

## SUPPLEMENTAL INFORMATION

- Packages bearing the 1.4S label or packages containing material classified as 1.4S are designed or packaged in such a manner that when involved in a fire, they may burn vigorously with localized detonations and projection of fragments.
- Effects are usually confined to immediate vicinity of packages.
- If fire threatens cargo area containing packages bearing the 1.4S label or packages containing material classified as 1.4S, consider isolating at least 15 meters (50 feet) in all directions. Fight fire with normal precautions from a reasonable distance.

* FOR INFORMATION ON "COMPATIBILITY GROUP" LETTERS, REFER TO THE GLOSSARY SECTION.

# GUIDE 115 GASES - FLAMMABLE (INCLUDING REFRIGERATED LIQUIDS)

## POTENTIAL HAZARDS

### FIRE OR EXPLOSION

- **EXTREMELY FLAMMABLE.**
- Will be easily ignited by heat, sparks or flames.
- Will form explosive mixtures with air.
- Vapors from liquefied gas are initially heavier than air and spread along ground.

**CAUTION: Hydrogen (UN1049), Deuterium (UN1957), Hydrogen, refrigerated liquid (UN1966) and Methane (UN1971) are lighter than air and will rise. Hydrogen and Deuterium fires are difficult to detect since they burn with an invisible flame. Use an alternate method of detection (thermal camera, broom handle, etc.)**

- Vapors may travel to source of ignition and flash back.
- Cylinders exposed to fire may vent and release flammable gas through pressure relief devices.
- Containers may explode when heated.
- Ruptured cylinders may rocket.

### HEALTH

- Vapors may cause dizziness or asphyxiation without warning.
- Some may be irritating if inhaled at high concentrations.
- Contact with gas or liquefied gas may cause burns, severe injury and/or frostbite.
- Fire may produce irritating and/or toxic gases.

## PUBLIC SAFETY

- **CALL EMERGENCY RESPONSE Telephone Number on Shipping Paper first. If Shipping Paper not available or no answer, refer to appropriate telephone number listed on the inside back cover.**
- As an immediate precautionary measure, isolate spill or leak area for at least 100 meters (330 feet) in all directions.
- Keep unauthorized personnel away.
- Stay upwind, uphill and/or upstream.
- Many gases are heavier than air and will spread along ground and collect in low or confined areas (sewers, basements, tanks).

### PROTECTIVE CLOTHING

- Wear positive pressure self-contained breathing apparatus (SCBA).
- Structural firefighters' protective clothing will only provide limited protection.
- Always wear thermal protective clothing when handling refrigerated/cryogenic liquids.

### EVACUATION

**Large Spill**

- Consider initial downwind evacuation for at least 800 meters (1/2 mile).

**Fire**

- If tank, rail car or tank truck is involved in a fire, ISOLATE for 1600 meters (1 mile) in all directions; also, consider initial evacuation for 1600 meters (1 mile) in all directions.
- In fires involving Liquefied Petroleum Gases (LPG) (UN1075); Butane, (UN1011); Butylene, (UN1012); Isobutylene, (UN1055); Propylene, (UN1077); Isobutane, (UN1969); and Propane, (UN1978), also refer to BLEVE – SAFETY PRECAUTIONS (Page 368)

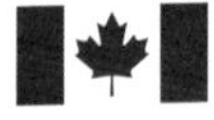

In Canada, an Emergency Response Assistance Plan (ERAP) may be required for this product. Please consult the shipping document and/or the ERAP Program Section (page 391).

## EMERGENCY RESPONSE

### FIRE

- **DO NOT EXTINGUISH A LEAKING GAS FIRE UNLESS LEAK CAN BE STOPPED.**

**CAUTION: Hydrogen (UN1049), Deuterium (UN1957) and Hydrogen, refrigerated liquid (UN1966) burn with an invisible flame. Hydrogen and Methane mixture, compressed (UN2034) may burn with an invisible flame.**

**Small Fire**

- Dry chemical or $CO_2$.

**Large Fire**

- Water spray or fog.
- Move containers from fire area if you can do it without risk.

**Fire involving Tanks**

- Fight fire from maximum distance or use unmanned hose holders or monitor nozzles.
- Cool containers with flooding quantities of water until well after fire is out.
- Do not direct water at source of leak or safety devices; icing may occur.
- Withdraw immediately in case of rising sound from venting safety devices or discoloration of tank.
- ALWAYS stay away from tanks engulfed in fire.
- For massive fire, use unmanned hose holders or monitor nozzles; if this is impossible, withdraw from area and let fire burn.

### SPILL OR LEAK

- ELIMINATE all ignition sources (no smoking, flares, sparks or flames in immediate area).
- All equipment used when handling the product must be grounded.
- Do not touch or walk through spilled material.
- Stop leak if you can do it without risk.
- If possible, turn leaking containers so that gas escapes rather than liquid.
- Use water spray to reduce vapors or divert vapor cloud drift. Avoid allowing water runoff to contact spilled material.
- Do not direct water at spill or source of leak.
- Prevent spreading of vapors through sewers, ventilation systems and confined areas.
- Isolate area until gas has dispersed.

**CAUTION: When in contact with refrigerated/cryogenic liquids, many materials become brittle and are likely to break without warning.**

### FIRST AID

- Ensure that medical personnel are aware of the material(s) involved and take precautions to protect themselves.
- Move victim to fresh air.
- Call 911 or emergency medical service.
- Give artificial respiration if victim is not breathing.
- Administer oxygen if breathing is difficult.
- Remove and isolate contaminated clothing and shoes.
- Clothing frozen to the skin should be thawed before being removed.
- In case of contact with liquefied gas, thaw frosted parts with lukewarm water.
- In case of burns, immediately cool affected skin for as long as possible with cold water. Do not remove clothing if adhering to skin.
- Keep victim calm and warm.

# GUIDE 116 GASES - FLAMMABLE (UNSTABLE)

## POTENTIAL HAZARDS

### FIRE OR EXPLOSION

- **EXTREMELY FLAMMABLE.**
- Will be easily ignited by heat, sparks or flames.
- Will form explosive mixtures with air.
- Silane (UN2203) will ignite spontaneously in air.
- Those substances designated with a **(P)** may polymerize explosively when heated or involved in a fire.
- Vapors from liquefied gas are initially heavier than air and spread along ground.
- Vapors may travel to source of ignition and flash back.
- Cylinders exposed to fire may vent and release flammable gas through pressure relief devices.
- Containers may explode when heated.
- Ruptured cylinders may rocket.

### HEALTH

- Vapors may cause dizziness or asphyxiation without warning.
- Some may be toxic if inhaled at high concentrations.
- Contact with gas or liquefied gas may cause burns, severe injury and/or frostbite.
- Fire may produce irritating and/or toxic gases.

## PUBLIC SAFETY

- **CALL EMERGENCY RESPONSE Telephone Number on Shipping Paper first. If Shipping Paper not available or no answer, refer to appropriate telephone number listed on the inside back cover.**
- As an immediate precautionary measure, isolate spill or leak area for at least 100 meters (330 feet) in all directions.
- Keep unauthorized personnel away.
- Stay upwind, uphill and/or upstream.
- Many gases are heavier than air and will spread along ground and collect in low or confined areas (sewers, basements, tanks).

### PROTECTIVE CLOTHING

- Wear positive pressure self-contained breathing apparatus (SCBA).
- Structural firefighters' protective clothing will only provide limited protection.

### EVACUATION

**Large Spill**

- Consider initial downwind evacuation for at least 800 meters (1/2 mile).

**Fire**

- If tank, rail car or tank truck is involved in a fire, ISOLATE for 1600 meters (1 mile) in all directions; also, consider initial evacuation for 1600 meters (1 mile) in all directions.

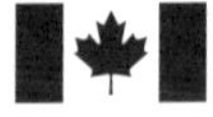

In Canada, an Emergency Response Assistance Plan (ERAP) may be required for this product. Please consult the shipping document and/or the ERAP Program Section (page 391).

## EMERGENCY RESPONSE

### FIRE

- **DO NOT EXTINGUISH A LEAKING GAS FIRE UNLESS LEAK CAN BE STOPPED.**

**Small Fire**

- Dry chemical or $CO_2$.

**Large Fire**

- Water spray or fog.
- Move containers from fire area if you can do it without risk.

**Fire involving Tanks**

- Fight fire from maximum distance or use unmanned hose holders or monitor nozzles.
- Cool containers with flooding quantities of water until well after fire is out.
- Do not direct water at source of leak or safety devices; icing may occur.
- Withdraw immediately in case of rising sound from venting safety devices or discoloration of tank.
- ALWAYS stay away from tanks engulfed in fire.
- For massive fire, use unmanned hose holders or monitor nozzles; if this is impossible, withdraw from area and let fire burn.

### SPILL OR LEAK

- ELIMINATE all ignition sources (no smoking, flares, sparks or flames in immediate area).
- All equipment used when handling the product must be grounded.
- Stop leak if you can do it without risk.
- Do not touch or walk through spilled material.
- Do not direct water at spill or source of leak.
- Use water spray to reduce vapors or divert vapor cloud drift. Avoid allowing water runoff to contact spilled material.
- If possible, turn leaking containers so that gas escapes rather than liquid.
- Prevent entry into waterways, sewers, basements or confined areas.
- Isolate area until gas has dispersed.

### FIRST AID

- Ensure that medical personnel are aware of the material(s) involved and take precautions to protect themselves.
- Move victim to fresh air.
- Call 911 or emergency medical service.
- Give artificial respiration if victim is not breathing.
- Administer oxygen if breathing is difficult.
- Remove and isolate contaminated clothing and shoes.
- In case of contact with liquefied gas, thaw frosted parts with lukewarm water.
- In case of burns, immediately cool affected skin for as long as possible with cold water. Do not remove clothing if adhering to skin.
- Keep victim calm and warm.

# GUIDE 117 GASES - TOXIC - FLAMMABLE (EXTREME HAZARD)

## POTENTIAL HAZARDS

### HEALTH

- **TOXIC; Extremely Hazardous.**
- May be fatal if inhaled or absorbed through skin.
- Initial odor may be irritating or foul and may deaden your sense of smell.
- Contact with gas or liquefied gas may cause burns, severe injury and/or frostbite.
- Fire will produce irritating, corrosive and/or toxic gases.
- Runoff from fire control may cause pollution.

### FIRE OR EXPLOSION

- These materials are extremely flammable.
- May form explosive mixtures with air.
- May be ignited by heat, sparks or flames.
- Vapors from liquefied gas are initially heavier than air and spread along ground.
- Vapors may travel to source of ignition and flash back.
- Runoff may create fire or explosion hazard.
- Cylinders exposed to fire may vent and release toxic and flammable gas through pressure relief devices.
- Containers may explode when heated.
- Ruptured cylinders may rocket.

## PUBLIC SAFETY

- **CALL EMERGENCY RESPONSE Telephone Number on Shipping Paper first. If Shipping Paper not available or no answer, refer to appropriate telephone number listed on the inside back cover.**
- As an immediate precautionary measure, isolate spill or leak area for at least 100 meters (330 feet) in all directions.
- Keep unauthorized personnel away.
- Stay upwind, uphill and/or upstream.
- Many gases are heavier than air and will spread along ground and collect in low or confined areas (sewers, basements, tanks).
- Ventilate closed spaces before entering.

### PROTECTIVE CLOTHING

- Wear positive pressure self-contained breathing apparatus (SCBA).
- Wear chemical protective clothing that is specifically recommended by the manufacturer. It may provide little or no thermal protection.
- Structural firefighters' protective clothing provides limited protection in fire situations ONLY; it is not effective in spill situations where direct contact with the substance is possible.

### EVACUATION

**Spill**

- See Table 1 - Initial Isolation and Protective Action Distances.

**Fire**

- If tank, rail car or tank truck is involved in a fire, ISOLATE for 1600 meters (1 mile) in all directions; also, consider initial evacuation for 1600 meters (1 mile) in all directions.

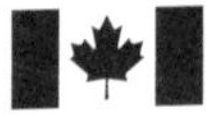

In Canada, an Emergency Response Assistance Plan (ERAP) may be required for this product. Please consult the shipping document and/or the ERAP Program Section (page 391).

## EMERGENCY RESPONSE

### FIRE

**DO NOT EXTINGUISH A LEAKING GAS FIRE UNLESS LEAK CAN BE STOPPED.**

**Small Fire**

- Dry chemical, $CO_2$, water spray or regular foam.

**Large Fire**

- Water spray, fog or regular foam.
- Move containers from fire area if you can do it without risk.
- Damaged cylinders should be handled only by specialists.

**Fire involving Tanks**

- Fight fire from maximum distance or use unmanned hose holders or monitor nozzles.
- Cool containers with flooding quantities of water until well after fire is out.
- Do not direct water at source of leak or safety devices; icing may occur.
- Withdraw immediately in case of rising sound from venting safety devices or discoloration of tank.
- ALWAYS stay away from tanks engulfed in fire.

### SPILL OR LEAK

- ELIMINATE all ignition sources (no smoking, flares, sparks or flames in immediate area).
- All equipment used when handling the product must be grounded.
- Fully encapsulating, vapor-protective clothing should be worn for spills and leaks with no fire.
- Do not touch or walk through spilled material.
- Stop leak if you can do it without risk.
- Use water spray to reduce vapors or divert vapor cloud drift. Avoid allowing water runoff to contact spilled material.
- Do not direct water at spill or source of leak.
- If possible, turn leaking containers so that gas escapes rather than liquid.
- Prevent entry into waterways, sewers, basements or confined areas.
- Isolate area until gas has dispersed.
- Consider igniting spill or leak to eliminate toxic gas concerns.

### FIRST AID

- Ensure that medical personnel are aware of the material(s) involved and take precautions to protect themselves.
- Move victim to fresh air.
- Call 911 or emergency medical service.
- Give artificial respiration if victim is not breathing.
- **Do not use mouth-to-mouth method if victim ingested or inhaled the substance; give artificial respiration with the aid of a pocket mask equipped with a one-way valve or other proper respiratory medical device.**
- Administer oxygen if breathing is difficult.
- Remove and isolate contaminated clothing and shoes.
- In case of contact with substance, immediately flush skin or eyes with running water for at least 20 minutes.
- In case of contact with liquefied gas, thaw frosted parts with lukewarm water.
- In case of burns, immediately cool affected skin for as long as possible with cold water. Do not remove clothing if adhering to skin.
- Keep victim calm and warm.
- Keep victim under observation.
- Effects of contact or inhalation may be delayed.

# GUIDE 118 GASES - FLAMMABLE - CORROSIVE

## POTENTIAL HAZARDS

### FIRE OR EXPLOSION

- **EXTREMELY FLAMMABLE.**
- May be ignited by heat, sparks or flames.
- May form explosive mixtures with air.
- Vapors from liquefied gas are initially heavier than air and spread along ground.
- Vapors may travel to source of ignition and flash back.
- Some of these materials may react violently with water.
- Cylinders exposed to fire may vent and release flammable gas through pressure relief devices.
- Containers may explode when heated.
- Ruptured cylinders may rocket.

### HEALTH

- May cause toxic effects if inhaled.
- Vapors are extremely irritating.
- Contact with gas or liquefied gas may cause burns, severe injury and/or frostbite.
- Fire will produce irritating, corrosive and/or toxic gases.
- Runoff from fire control may cause pollution.

## PUBLIC SAFETY

- **CALL EMERGENCY RESPONSE Telephone Number on Shipping Paper first. If Shipping Paper not available or no answer, refer to appropriate telephone number listed on the inside back cover.**
- As an immediate precautionary measure, isolate spill or leak area for at least 100 meters (330 feet) in all directions.
- Keep unauthorized personnel away.
- Stay upwind, uphill and/or upstream.
- Many gases are heavier than air and will spread along ground and collect in low or confined areas (sewers, basements, tanks).
- Ventilate closed spaces before entering.

### PROTECTIVE CLOTHING

- Wear positive pressure self-contained breathing apparatus (SCBA).
- Wear chemical protective clothing that is specifically recommended by the manufacturer. It may provide little or no thermal protection.
- Structural firefighters' protective clothing provides limited protection in fire situations ONLY; it is not effective in spill situations where direct contact with the substance is possible.

### EVACUATION

**Large Spill**

- Consider initial downwind evacuation for at least 800 meters (1/2 mile).

**Fire**

- If tank, rail car or tank truck is involved in a fire, ISOLATE for 1600 meters (1 mile) in all directions; also, consider initial evacuation for 1600 meters (1 mile) in all directions.

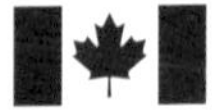

In Canada, an Emergency Response Assistance Plan (ERAP) may be required for this product. Please consult the shipping document and/or the ERAP Program Section (page 391).

## EMERGENCY RESPONSE

### FIRE

- **DO NOT EXTINGUISH A LEAKING GAS FIRE UNLESS LEAK CAN BE STOPPED.**

**Small Fire**

- Dry chemical or $CO_2$.

**Large Fire**

- Water spray, fog or regular foam.
- Move containers from fire area if you can do it without risk.
- Damaged cylinders should be handled only by specialists.

**Fire involving Tanks**

- Fight fire from maximum distance or use unmanned hose holders or monitor nozzles.
- Cool containers with flooding quantities of water until well after fire is out.
- Do not direct water at source of leak or safety devices; icing may occur.
- Withdraw immediately in case of rising sound from venting safety devices or discoloration of tank.
- ALWAYS stay away from tanks engulfed in fire.

### SPILL OR LEAK

- ELIMINATE all ignition sources (no smoking, flares, sparks or flames in immediate area).
- All equipment used when handling the product must be grounded.
- Fully encapsulating, vapor-protective clothing should be worn for spills and leaks with no fire.
- Do not touch or walk through spilled material.
- Stop leak if you can do it without risk.
- If possible, turn leaking containers so that gas escapes rather than liquid.
- Use water spray to reduce vapors or divert vapor cloud drift. Avoid allowing water runoff to contact spilled material.
- Do not direct water at spill or source of leak.
- Isolate area until gas has dispersed.

### FIRST AID

- Ensure that medical personnel are aware of the material(s) involved and take precautions to protect themselves.
- Move victim to fresh air.
- Call 911 or emergency medical service.
- Give artificial respiration if victim is not breathing.
- **Do not use mouth-to-mouth method if victim ingested or inhaled the substance; give artificial respiration with the aid of a pocket mask equipped with a one-way valve or other proper respiratory medical device.**
- Administer oxygen if breathing is difficult.
- Remove and isolate contaminated clothing and shoes.
- In case of contact with liquefied gas, thaw frosted parts with lukewarm water.
- In case of burns, immediately cool affected skin for as long as possible with cold water. Do not remove clothing if adhering to skin.
- Keep victim calm and warm.
- Keep victim under observation.
- Effects of contact or inhalation may be delayed.

# GUIDE 119 GASES - TOXIC - FLAMMABLE

## POTENTIAL HAZARDS

### HEALTH

- **TOXIC; may be fatal if inhaled or absorbed through skin.**
- Contact with gas or liquefied gas may cause burns, severe injury and/or frostbite.
- Fire will produce irritating, corrosive and/or toxic gases.
- Runoff from fire control may cause pollution.

### FIRE OR EXPLOSION

- Flammable; may be ignited by heat, sparks or flames.
- May form explosive mixtures with air.
- Those substances designated with a **(P)** may polymerize explosively when heated or involved in a fire.
- Vapors from liquefied gas are initially heavier than air and spread along ground.
- Vapors may travel to source of ignition and flash back.
- Some of these materials may react violently with water.
- Cylinders exposed to fire may vent and release toxic and flammable gas through pressure relief devices.
- Containers may explode when heated.
- Ruptured cylinders may rocket.
- Runoff may create fire or explosion hazard.

## PUBLIC SAFETY

- **CALL EMERGENCY RESPONSE Telephone Number on Shipping Paper first. If Shipping Paper not available or no answer, refer to appropriate telephone number listed on the inside back cover.**
- As an immediate precautionary measure, isolate spill or leak area for at least 100 meters (330 feet) in all directions.
- Keep unauthorized personnel away.
- Stay upwind, uphill and/or upstream.
- Many gases are heavier than air and will spread along ground and collect in low or confined areas (sewers, basements, tanks).
- Ventilate closed spaces before entering.

### PROTECTIVE CLOTHING

- Wear positive pressure self-contained breathing apparatus (SCBA).
- Wear chemical protective clothing that is specifically recommended by the manufacturer. It may provide little or no thermal protection.
- Structural firefighters' protective clothing provides limited protection in fire situations ONLY; it is not effective in spill situations where direct contact with the substance is possible.

### EVACUATION

**Spill**

- See Table 1 - Initial Isolation and Protective Action Distances for highlighted materials. For non-highlighted materials, increase, in the downwind direction, as necessary, the isolation distance shown under "PUBLIC SAFETY".

**Fire**

- If tank, rail car or tank truck is involved in a fire, ISOLATE for 1600 meters (1 mile) in all directions; also, consider initial evacuation for 1600 meters (1 mile) in all directions.

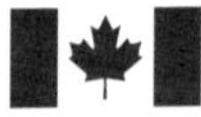

In Canada, an Emergency Response Assistance Plan (ERAP) may be required for this product. Please consult the shipping document and/or the ERAP Program Section (page 391).

## EMERGENCY RESPONSE

### FIRE

- **DO NOT EXTINGUISH A LEAKING GAS FIRE UNLESS LEAK CAN BE STOPPED.**

**Small Fire**

- Dry chemical, $CO_2$, water spray or alcohol-resistant foam.

**Large Fire**

- Water spray, fog or alcohol-resistant foam.
- **FOR CHLOROSILANES, DO NOT USE WATER;** use AFFF alcohol-resistant medium-expansion foam.
- Move containers from fire area if you can do it without risk.
- Damaged cylinders should be handled only by specialists.

**Fire involving Tanks**

- Fight fire from maximum distance or use unmanned hose holders or monitor nozzles.
- Cool containers with flooding quantities of water until well after fire is out.
- Do not direct water at source of leak or safety devices; icing may occur.
- Withdraw immediately in case of rising sound from venting safety devices or discoloration of tank.
- ALWAYS stay away from tanks engulfed in fire.

### SPILL OR LEAK

- ELIMINATE all ignition sources (no smoking, flares, sparks or flames in immediate area).
- All equipment used when handling the product must be grounded.
- Fully encapsulating, vapor-protective clothing should be worn for spills and leaks with no fire.
- Do not touch or walk through spilled material.
- Stop leak if you can do it without risk.
- Do not direct water at spill or source of leak.
- Use water spray to reduce vapors or divert vapor cloud drift. Avoid allowing water runoff to contact spilled material.
- **FOR CHLOROSILANES**, use AFFF alcohol-resistant medium-expansion foam to reduce vapors.
- If possible, turn leaking containers so that gas escapes rather than liquid.
- Prevent entry into waterways, sewers, basements or confined areas.
- Isolate area until gas has dispersed.

### FIRST AID

- Ensure that medical personnel are aware of the material(s) involved and take precautions to protect themselves.
- Move victim to fresh air.
- Call 911 or emergency medical service.
- Give artificial respiration if victim is not breathing.
- **Do not use mouth-to-mouth method if victim ingested or inhaled the substance; give artificial respiration with the aid of a pocket mask equipped with a one-way valve or other proper respiratory medical device.**
- Administer oxygen if breathing is difficult.
- Remove and isolate contaminated clothing and shoes.
- In case of contact with substance, immediately flush skin or eyes with running water for at least 20 minutes.
- In case of contact with liquefied gas, thaw frosted parts with lukewarm water.
- In case of burns, immediately cool affected skin for as long as possible with cold water. Do not remove clothing if adhering to skin.
- Keep victim calm and warm.
- Keep victim under observation.
- Effects of contact or inhalation may be delayed.

# GUIDE 120 GASES - INERT (INCLUDING REFRIGERATED LIQUIDS)

## POTENTIAL HAZARDS

### HEALTH

- Vapors may cause dizziness or asphyxiation without warning.
- Vapors from liquefied gas are initially heavier than air and spread along ground.
- Contact with gas or liquefied gas may cause burns, severe injury and/or frostbite.

### FIRE OR EXPLOSION

- **Non-flammable gases.**
- Containers may explode when heated.
- Ruptured cylinders may rocket.

## PUBLIC SAFETY

- **CALL EMERGENCY RESPONSE Telephone Number on Shipping Paper first. If Shipping Paper not available or no answer, refer to appropriate telephone number listed on the inside back cover.**
- As an immediate precautionary measure, isolate spill or leak area for at least 100 meters (330 feet) in all directions.
- Keep unauthorized personnel away.
- Stay upwind, uphill and/or upstream.
- Many gases are heavier than air and will spread along ground and collect in low or confined areas (sewers, basements, tanks).
- Ventilate closed spaces before entering.

### PROTECTIVE CLOTHING

- Wear positive pressure self-contained breathing apparatus (SCBA).
- Structural firefighters' protective clothing will only provide limited protection.
- Always wear thermal protective clothing when handling refrigerated/cryogenic liquids or solids.

### EVACUATION

**Large Spill**

- Consider initial downwind evacuation for at least 100 meters (330 feet).

**Fire**

- If tank, rail car or tank truck is involved in a fire, ISOLATE for 800 meters (1/2 mile) in all directions; also, consider initial evacuation for 800 meters (1/2 mile) in all directions.

## EMERGENCY RESPONSE

### FIRE

- Use extinguishing agent suitable for type of surrounding fire.
- Move containers from fire area if you can do it without risk.
- Damaged cylinders should be handled only by specialists.

**Fire involving Tanks**

- Fight fire from maximum distance or use unmanned hose holders or monitor nozzles.
- Cool containers with flooding quantities of water until well after fire is out.
- Do not direct water at source of leak or safety devices; icing may occur.
- Withdraw immediately in case of rising sound from venting safety devices or discoloration of tank.
- ALWAYS stay away from tanks engulfed in fire.

### SPILL OR LEAK

- Do not touch or walk through spilled material.
- Stop leak if you can do it without risk.
- Use water spray to reduce vapors or divert vapor cloud drift. Avoid allowing water runoff to contact spilled material.
- Do not direct water at spill or source of leak.
- If possible, turn leaking containers so that gas escapes rather than liquid.
- Prevent entry into waterways, sewers, basements or confined areas.
- Allow substance to evaporate.
- Ventilate the area.

**CAUTION: When in contact with refrigerated/cryogenic liquids, many materials become brittle and are likely to break without warning.**

### FIRST AID

- Ensure that medical personnel are aware of the material(s) involved and take precautions to protect themselves.
- Move victim to fresh air.
- Call 911 or emergency medical service.
- Give artificial respiration if victim is not breathing.
- Administer oxygen if breathing is difficult.
- Clothing frozen to the skin should be thawed before being removed.
- In case of contact with liquefied gas, thaw frosted parts with lukewarm water.
- Keep victim calm and warm.

# GUIDE 121 GASES - INERT

## POTENTIAL HAZARDS

### HEALTH

- Vapors may cause dizziness or asphyxiation without warning.
- Vapors from liquefied gas are initially heavier than air and spread along ground.

### FIRE OR EXPLOSION

- **Non-flammable gases.**
- Containers may explode when heated.
- Ruptured cylinders may rocket.

## PUBLIC SAFETY

- **CALL EMERGENCY RESPONSE Telephone Number on Shipping Paper first. If Shipping Paper not available or no answer, refer to appropriate telephone number listed on the inside back cover.**
- As an immediate precautionary measure, isolate spill or leak area for at least 100 meters (330 feet) in all directions.
- Keep unauthorized personnel away.
- Stay upwind, uphill and/or upstream.
- Many gases are heavier than air and will spread along ground and collect in low or confined areas (sewers, basements, tanks).
- Ventilate closed spaces before entering.

### PROTECTIVE CLOTHING

- Wear positive pressure self-contained breathing apparatus (SCBA).
- Structural firefighters' protective clothing will only provide limited protection.

### EVACUATION

**Large Spill**

- Consider initial downwind evacuation for at least 100 meters (330 feet).

**Fire**

- If tank, rail car or tank truck is involved in a fire, ISOLATE for 800 meters (1/2 mile) in all directions; also, consider initial evacuation for 800 meters (1/2 mile) in all directions.

## EMERGENCY RESPONSE

### FIRE

- Use extinguishing agent suitable for type of surrounding fire.
- Move containers from fire area if you can do it without risk.
- Damaged cylinders should be handled only by specialists.

**Fire involving Tanks**

- Fight fire from maximum distance or use unmanned hose holders or monitor nozzles.
- Cool containers with flooding quantities of water until well after fire is out.
- Do not direct water at source of leak or safety devices; icing may occur.
- Withdraw immediately in case of rising sound from venting safety devices or discoloration of tank.
- ALWAYS stay away from tanks engulfed in fire.

### SPILL OR LEAK

- Do not touch or walk through spilled material.
- Stop leak if you can do it without risk.
- Use water spray to reduce vapors or divert vapor cloud drift. Avoid allowing water runoff to contact spilled material.
- Do not direct water at spill or source of leak.
- If possible, turn leaking containers so that gas escapes rather than liquid.
- Prevent entry into waterways, sewers, basements or confined areas.
- Allow substance to evaporate.
- Ventilate the area.

### FIRST AID

- Ensure that medical personnel are aware of the material(s) involved and take precautions to protect themselves.
- Move victim to fresh air.
- Call 911 or emergency medical service.
- Give artificial respiration if victim is not breathing.
- Administer oxygen if breathing is difficult.
- Keep victim calm and warm.

# GUIDE 122 GASES - OXIDIZING (INCLUDING REFRIGERATED LIQUIDS)

## POTENTIAL HAZARDS

### FIRE OR EXPLOSION

- Substance does not burn but will support combustion.
- Some may react explosively with fuels.
- May ignite combustibles (wood, paper, oil, clothing, etc.).
- Vapors from liquefied gas are initially heavier than air and spread along ground.
- Runoff may create fire or explosion hazard.
- Containers may explode when heated.
- Ruptured cylinders may rocket.

### HEALTH

- Vapors may cause dizziness or asphyxiation without warning.
- Contact with gas or liquefied gas may cause burns, severe injury and/or frostbite.
- Fire may produce irritating and/or toxic gases.

## PUBLIC SAFETY

- **CALL EMERGENCY RESPONSE Telephone Number on Shipping Paper first. If Shipping Paper not available or no answer, refer to appropriate telephone number listed on the inside back cover.**
- As an immediate precautionary measure, isolate spill or leak area for at least 100 meters (330 feet) in all directions.
- Keep unauthorized personnel away.
- Stay upwind, uphill and/or upstream.
- Many gases are heavier than air and will spread along ground and collect in low or confined areas (sewers, basements, tanks).
- Ventilate closed spaces before entering.

### PROTECTIVE CLOTHING

- Wear positive pressure self-contained breathing apparatus (SCBA).
- Wear chemical protective clothing that is specifically recommended by the manufacturer. It may provide little or no thermal protection.
- Structural firefighters' protective clothing provides limited protection in fire situations ONLY; it is not effective in spill situations where direct contact with the substance is possible.
- Always wear thermal protective clothing when handling refrigerated/cryogenic liquids.

### EVACUATION

**Large Spill**

- Consider initial downwind evacuation for at least 500 meters (1/3 mile).

**Fire**

- If tank, rail car or tank truck is involved in a fire, ISOLATE for 800 meters (1/2 mile) in all directions; also, consider initial evacuation for 800 meters (1/2 mile) in all directions.

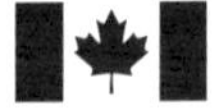

In Canada, an Emergency Response Assistance Plan (ERAP) may be required for this product. Please consult the shipping document and/or the ERAP Program Section (page 391).

## EMERGENCY RESPONSE

### FIRE

- Use extinguishing agent suitable for type of surrounding fire.

**Small Fire**

- Dry chemical or $CO_2$.

**Large Fire**

- Water spray, fog or regular foam.
- Move containers from fire area if you can do it without risk.
- Damaged cylinders should be handled only by specialists.

**Fire involving Tanks**

- Fight fire from maximum distance or use unmanned hose holders or monitor nozzles.
- Cool containers with flooding quantities of water until well after fire is out.
- Do not direct water at source of leak or safety devices; icing may occur.
- Withdraw immediately in case of rising sound from venting safety devices or discoloration of tank.
- ALWAYS stay away from tanks engulfed in fire.
- For massive fire, use unmanned hose holders or monitor nozzles; if this is impossible, withdraw from area and let fire burn.

### SPILL OR LEAK

- Keep combustibles (wood, paper, oil, etc.) away from spilled material.
- Do not touch or walk through spilled material.
- Stop leak if you can do it without risk.
- If possible, turn leaking containers so that gas escapes rather than liquid.
- Do not direct water at spill or source of leak.
- Use water spray to reduce vapors or divert vapor cloud drift. Avoid allowing water runoff to contact spilled material.
- Prevent entry into waterways, sewers, basements or confined areas.
- Allow substance to evaporate.
- Isolate area until gas has dispersed.

**CAUTION: When in contact with refrigerated/cryogenic liquids, many materials become brittle and are likely to break without warning.**

### FIRST AID

- Ensure that medical personnel are aware of the material(s) involved and take precautions to protect themselves.
- Move victim to fresh air.
- Call 911 or emergency medical service.
- Give artificial respiration if victim is not breathing.
- Administer oxygen if breathing is difficult.
- Remove and isolate contaminated clothing and shoes.
- Clothing frozen to the skin should be thawed before being removed.
- In case of contact with liquefied gas, thaw frosted parts with lukewarm water.
- Keep victim calm and warm.

# GUIDE 123 GASES - TOXIC AND/OR CORROSIVE

## POTENTIAL HAZARDS

### HEALTH

- **TOXIC; may be fatal if inhaled or absorbed through skin.**
- Vapors may be irritating.
- Contact with gas or liquefied gas may cause burns, severe injury and/or frostbite.
- Fire will produce irritating, corrosive and/or toxic gases.
- Runoff from fire control may cause pollution.

### FIRE OR EXPLOSION

- Some may burn but none ignite readily.
- Vapors from liquefied gas are initially heavier than air and spread along ground.
- Cylinders exposed to fire may vent and release toxic and/or corrosive gas through pressure relief devices.
- Containers may explode when heated.
- Ruptured cylinders may rocket.

## PUBLIC SAFETY

- **CALL EMERGENCY RESPONSE Telephone Number on Shipping Paper first. If Shipping Paper not available or no answer, refer to appropriate telephone number listed on the inside back cover.**
- As an immediate precautionary measure, isolate spill or leak area for at least 100 meters (330 feet) in all directions.
- Keep unauthorized personnel away.
- Stay upwind, uphill and/or upstream.
- Many gases are heavier than air and will spread along ground and collect in low or confined areas (sewers, basements, tanks).
- Ventilate closed spaces before entering.

### PROTECTIVE CLOTHING

- Wear positive pressure self-contained breathing apparatus (SCBA).
- Wear chemical protective clothing that is specifically recommended by the manufacturer. It may provide little or no thermal protection.
- Structural firefighters' protective clothing provides limited protection in fire situations ONLY; it is not effective in spill situations where direct contact with the substance is possible.

### EVACUATION

**Spill**

- See Table 1 - Initial Isolation and Protective Action Distances for highlighted materials. For non-highlighted materials, increase, in the downwind direction, as necessary, the isolation distance shown under "PUBLIC SAFETY".

**Fire**

- If tank, rail car or tank truck is involved in a fire, ISOLATE for 800 meters (1/2 mile) in all directions; also, consider initial evacuation for 800 meters (1/2 mile) in all directions.

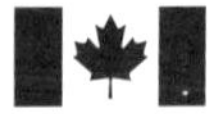

In Canada, an Emergency Response Assistance Plan (ERAP) may be required for this product. Please consult the shipping document and/or the ERAP Program Section (page 391).

## EMERGENCY RESPONSE

### FIRE

**Small Fire**

- Dry chemical or $CO_2$.

**Large Fire**

- Water spray, fog or regular foam.
- Do not get water inside containers.
- Move containers from fire area if you can do it without risk.
- Damaged cylinders should be handled only by specialists.

**Fire involving Tanks**

- Fight fire from maximum distance or use unmanned hose holders or monitor nozzles.
- Cool containers with flooding quantities of water until well after fire is out.
- Do not direct water at source of leak or safety devices; icing may occur.
- Withdraw immediately in case of rising sound from venting safety devices or discoloration of tank.
- ALWAYS stay away from tanks engulfed in fire.

### SPILL OR LEAK

- Fully encapsulating, vapor-protective clothing should be worn for spills and leaks with no fire.
- Do not touch or walk through spilled material.
- Stop leak if you can do it without risk.
- If possible, turn leaking containers so that gas escapes rather than liquid.
- Prevent entry into waterways, sewers, basements or confined areas.
- Use water spray to reduce vapors or divert vapor cloud drift. Avoid allowing water runoff to contact spilled material.
- Do not direct water at spill or source of leak.
- Isolate area until gas has dispersed.

### FIRST AID

- Ensure that medical personnel are aware of the material(s) involved and take precautions to protect themselves.
- Move victim to fresh air.
- Call 911 or emergency medical service.
- Give artificial respiration if victim is not breathing.
- **Do not use mouth-to-mouth method if victim ingested or inhaled the substance; give artificial respiration with the aid of a pocket mask equipped with a one-way valve or other proper respiratory medical device.**
- Administer oxygen if breathing is difficult.
- Remove and isolate contaminated clothing and shoes.
- In case of contact with liquefied gas, thaw frosted parts with lukewarm water.
- In case of contact with substance, immediately flush skin or eyes with running water for at least 20 minutes.
- Keep victim calm and warm.
- Keep victim under observation.
- Effects of contact or inhalation may be delayed.

# GUIDE 124 GASES - TOXIC AND/OR CORROSIVE - OXIDIZING

## POTENTIAL HAZARDS

### HEALTH

- **TOXIC; may be fatal if inhaled or absorbed through skin.**
- Fire will produce irritating, corrosive and/or toxic gases.
- Contact with gas or liquefied gas may cause burns, severe injury and/or frostbite.
- Runoff from fire control may cause pollution.

### FIRE OR EXPLOSION

- Substance does not burn but will support combustion.
- Vapors from liquefied gas are initially heavier than air and spread along ground.
- These are strong oxidizers and will react vigorously or explosively with many materials including fuels.
- May ignite combustibles (wood, paper, oil, clothing, etc.).
- Some will react violently with air, moist air and/or water.
- Cylinders exposed to fire may vent and release toxic and/or corrosive gas through pressure relief devices.
- Containers may explode when heated.
- Ruptured cylinders may rocket.

## PUBLIC SAFETY

- **CALL EMERGENCY RESPONSE Telephone Number on Shipping Paper first. If Shipping Paper not available or no answer, refer to appropriate telephone number listed on the inside back cover.**
- As an immediate precautionary measure, isolate spill or leak area for at least 100 meters (330 feet) in all directions.
- Keep unauthorized personnel away.
- Stay upwind, uphill and/or upstream.
- Many gases are heavier than air and will spread along ground and collect in low or confined areas (sewers, basements, tanks).
- Ventilate closed spaces before entering.

### PROTECTIVE CLOTHING

- Wear positive pressure self-contained breathing apparatus (SCBA).
- Wear chemical protective clothing that is specifically recommended by the manufacturer. It may provide little or no thermal protection.
- Structural firefighters' protective clothing provides limited protection in fire situations ONLY; it is not effective in spill situations where direct contact with the substance is possible.

### EVACUATION

**Spill**

- See Table 1 - Initial Isolation and Protective Action Distances.

**Fire**

- If tank, rail car or tank truck is involved in a fire, ISOLATE for 800 meters (1/2 mile) in all directions; also, consider initial evacuation for 800 meters (1/2 mile) in all directions.

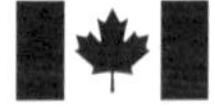

In Canada, an Emergency Response Assistance Plan (ERAP) may be required for this product. Please consult the shipping document and/or the ERAP Program Section (page 391).

## EMERGENCY RESPONSE

### FIRE

**Small Fire**

**CAUTION**: These materials do not burn but will support combustion. Some will react violently with water.

- Contain fire and let burn. If fire must be fought, water spray or fog is recommended.
- **Water only; no dry chemical, $CO_2$ or Halon®.**
- Do not get water inside containers.
- Move containers from fire area if you can do it without risk.
- Damaged cylinders should be handled only by specialists.

**Fire involving Tanks**

- Fight fire from maximum distance or use unmanned hose holders or monitor nozzles.
- Cool containers with flooding quantities of water until well after fire is out.
- Do not direct water at source of leak or safety devices; icing may occur.
- Withdraw immediately in case of rising sound from venting safety devices or discoloration of tank.
- ALWAYS stay away from tanks engulfed in fire.
- For massive fire, use unmanned hose holders or monitor nozzles; if this is impossible, withdraw from area and let fire burn.

### SPILL OR LEAK

- Fully encapsulating, vapor-protective clothing should be worn for spills and leaks with no fire.
- Do not touch or walk through spilled material.
- Keep combustibles (wood, paper, oil, etc.) away from spilled material.
- Stop leak if you can do it without risk.
- Use water spray to reduce vapors or divert vapor cloud drift. Avoid allowing water runoff to contact spilled material.
- Do not direct water at spill or source of leak.
- If possible, turn leaking containers so that gas escapes rather than liquid.
- Prevent entry into waterways, sewers, basements or confined areas.
- Isolate area until gas has dispersed.
- Ventilate the area.

### FIRST AID

- Ensure that medical personnel are aware of the material(s) involved and take precautions to protect themselves.
- Move victim to fresh air.
- Call 911 or emergency medical service.
- Give artificial respiration if victim is not breathing.
- **Do not use mouth-to-mouth method if victim ingested or inhaled the substance; give artificial respiration with the aid of a pocket mask equipped with a one-way valve or other proper respiratory medical device.**
- Administer oxygen if breathing is difficult.
- Clothing frozen to the skin should be thawed before being removed.
- Remove and isolate contaminated clothing and shoes.
- In case of contact with substance, immediately flush skin or eyes with running water for at least 20 minutes.
- Keep victim calm and warm.
- Keep victim under observation.
- Effects of contact or inhalation may be delayed.

# GUIDE 125 GASES - CORROSIVE

## POTENTIAL HAZARDS

### HEALTH

- **TOXIC; may be fatal if inhaled, ingested or absorbed through skin.**
- Vapors are extremely irritating and corrosive.
- Contact with gas or liquefied gas may cause burns, severe injury and/or frostbite.
- Fire will produce irritating, corrosive and/or toxic gases.
- Runoff from fire control may cause pollution.

### FIRE OR EXPLOSION

- Some may burn but none ignite readily.
- Vapors from liquefied gas are initially heavier than air and spread along ground.
- Some of these materials may react violently with water.
- Cylinders exposed to fire may vent and release toxic and/or corrosive gas through pressure relief devices.
- Containers may explode when heated.
- Ruptured cylinders may rocket.
- For UN1005: Anhydrous ammonia, at high concentrations in confined spaces, presents a flammability risk if a source of ignition is introduced.

## PUBLIC SAFETY

- **CALL EMERGENCY RESPONSE Telephone Number on Shipping Paper first. If Shipping Paper not available or no answer, refer to appropriate telephone number listed on the inside back cover.**
- As an immediate precautionary measure, isolate spill or leak area for at least 100 meters (330 feet) in all directions.
- Keep unauthorized personnel away.
- Stay upwind, uphill and/or upstream.
- Many gases are heavier than air and will spread along ground and collect in low or confined areas (sewers, basements, tanks).
- Ventilate closed spaces before entering.

### PROTECTIVE CLOTHING

- Wear positive pressure self-contained breathing apparatus (SCBA).
- Wear chemical protective clothing that is specifically recommended by the manufacturer. It may provide little or no thermal protection.
- Structural firefighters' protective clothing provides limited protection in fire situations ONLY; it is not effective in spill situations where direct contact with the substance is possible.

### EVACUATION

**Spill**

- See Table 1 - Initial Isolation and Protective Action Distances for highlighted materials. For non-highlighted materials, increase, in the downwind direction, as necessary, the isolation distance shown under "PUBLIC SAFETY".

**Fire**

- If tank, rail car or tank truck is involved in a fire, ISOLATE for 1600 meters (1 mile) in all directions; also, consider initial evacuation for 1600 meters (1 mile) in all directions.

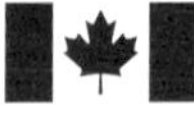

In Canada, an Emergency Response Assistance Plan (ERAP) may be required for this product. Please consult the shipping document and/or the ERAP Program Section (page 391).

## EMERGENCY RESPONSE

### FIRE

**Small Fire**

- Dry chemical or $CO_2$.

**Large Fire**

- Water spray, fog or regular foam.
- Move containers from fire area if you can do it without risk.
- Do not get water inside containers.
- Damaged cylinders should be handled only by specialists.

**Fire involving Tanks**

- Fight fire from maximum distance or use unmanned hose holders or monitor nozzles.
- Cool containers with flooding quantities of water until well after fire is out.
- Do not direct water at source of leak or safety devices; icing may occur.
- Withdraw immediately in case of rising sound from venting safety devices or discoloration of tank.
- ALWAYS stay away from tanks engulfed in fire.

### SPILL OR LEAK

- Fully encapsulating, vapor-protective clothing should be worn for spills and leaks with no fire.
- Do not touch or walk through spilled material.
- Stop leak if you can do it without risk.
- If possible, turn leaking containers so that gas escapes rather than liquid.
- Prevent entry into waterways, sewers, basements or confined areas.
- Do not direct water at spill or source of leak.
- Use water spray to reduce vapors or divert vapor cloud drift. Avoid allowing water runoff to contact spilled material.
- Isolate area until gas has dispersed.

### FIRST AID

- Ensure that medical personnel are aware of the material(s) involved and take precautions to protect themselves.
- Move victim to fresh air.
- Call 911 or emergency medical service.
- Give artificial respiration if victim is not breathing.
- **Do not use mouth-to-mouth method if victim ingested or inhaled the substance; give artificial respiration with the aid of a pocket mask equipped with a one-way valve or other proper respiratory medical device.**
- Administer oxygen if breathing is difficult.
- Remove and isolate contaminated clothing and shoes.
- In case of contact with liquefied gas, thaw frosted parts with lukewarm water.
- In case of contact with substance, immediately flush skin or eyes with running water for at least 20 minutes.
- **In case of contact with Hydrogen fluoride, anhydrous (UN1052),** flush with large amounts of water. For skin contact, if calcium gluconate gel is available, rinse 5 minutes, then apply gel. Otherwise, continue rinsing until medical treatment is available. For eyes, flush with water or a saline solution for 15 minutes.
- Keep victim calm and warm.
- Keep victim under observation.
- Effects of contact or inhalation may be delayed.

# GUIDE 126 GASES - COMPRESSED OR LIQUEFIED (INCLUDING REFRIGERANT GASES)

## POTENTIAL HAZARDS

### FIRE OR EXPLOSION

- Some may burn but none ignite readily.
- Containers may explode when heated.
- Ruptured cylinders may rocket.

### HEALTH

- Vapors may cause dizziness or asphyxiation without warning.
- Vapors from liquefied gas are initially heavier than air and spread along ground.
- Contact with gas or liquefied gas may cause burns, severe injury and/or frostbite.
- Fire may produce irritating, corrosive and/or toxic gases.

## PUBLIC SAFETY

- **CALL EMERGENCY RESPONSE Telephone Number on Shipping Paper first. If Shipping Paper not available or no answer, refer to appropriate telephone number listed on the inside back cover.**
- As an immediate precautionary measure, isolate spill or leak area for at least 100 meters (330 feet) in all directions.
- Keep unauthorized personnel away.
- Stay upwind, uphill and/or upstream.
- Many gases are heavier than air and will spread along ground and collect in low or confined areas (sewers, basements, tanks).
- Ventilate closed spaces before entering.

### PROTECTIVE CLOTHING

- Wear positive pressure self-contained breathing apparatus (SCBA).
- Wear chemical protective clothing that is specifically recommended by the manufacturer. It may provide little or no thermal protection.
- Structural firefighters' protective clothing will only provide limited protection.

### EVACUATION

**Large Spill**

- Consider initial downwind evacuation for at least 500 meters (1/3 mile).

**Fire**

- If tank, rail car or tank truck is involved in a fire, ISOLATE for 800 meters (1/2 mile) in all directions; also, consider initial evacuation for 800 meters (1/2 mile) in all directions.

## EMERGENCY RESPONSE

### FIRE

- Use extinguishing agent suitable for type of surrounding fire.

**Small Fire**

- Dry chemical or $CO_2$.

**Large Fire**

- Water spray, fog or regular foam.
- Move containers from fire area if you can do it without risk.
- Damaged cylinders should be handled only by specialists.

**Fire involving Tanks**

- Fight fire from maximum distance or use unmanned hose holders or monitor nozzles.
- Cool containers with flooding quantities of water until well after fire is out.
- Do not direct water at source of leak or safety devices; icing may occur.
- Withdraw immediately in case of rising sound from venting safety devices or discoloration of tank.
- ALWAYS stay away from tanks engulfed in fire.
- Some of these materials, if spilled, may evaporate leaving a flammable residue.

### SPILL OR LEAK

- Do not touch or walk through spilled material.
- Stop leak if you can do it without risk.
- Do not direct water at spill or source of leak.
- Use water spray to reduce vapors or divert vapor cloud drift. Avoid allowing water runoff to contact spilled material.
- If possible, turn leaking containers so that gas escapes rather than liquid.
- Prevent entry into waterways, sewers, basements or confined areas.
- Allow substance to evaporate.
- Ventilate the area.

### FIRST AID

- Ensure that medical personnel are aware of the material(s) involved and take precautions to protect themselves.
- Move victim to fresh air.
- Call 911 or emergency medical service.
- Give artificial respiration if victim is not breathing.
- Administer oxygen if breathing is difficult.
- Remove and isolate contaminated clothing and shoes.
- In case of contact with liquefied gas, thaw frosted parts with lukewarm water.
- Keep victim calm and warm.

# GUIDE 127 FLAMMABLE LIQUIDS (WATER-MISCIBLE)

## POTENTIAL HAZARDS

### FIRE OR EXPLOSION

- **HIGHLY FLAMMABLE: Will be easily ignited by heat, sparks or flames.**
- Vapors may form explosive mixtures with air.
- Vapors may travel to source of ignition and flash back.
- Most vapors are heavier than air. They will spread along ground and collect in low or confined areas (sewers, basements, tanks).
- Vapor explosion hazard indoors, outdoors or in sewers.
- Those substances designated with a **(P)** may polymerize explosively when heated or involved in a fire.
- Runoff to sewer may create fire or explosion hazard.
- Containers may explode when heated.
- Many liquids are lighter than water.

### HEALTH

- Inhalation or contact with material may irritate or burn skin and eyes.
- Fire may produce irritating, corrosive and/or toxic gases.
- Vapors may cause dizziness or suffocation.
- Runoff from fire control may cause pollution.

## PUBLIC SAFETY

- **CALL EMERGENCY RESPONSE Telephone Number on Shipping Paper first. If Shipping Paper not available or no answer, refer to appropriate telephone number listed on the inside back cover.**
- As an immediate precautionary measure, isolate spill or leak area for at least 50 meters (150 feet) in all directions.
- Keep unauthorized personnel away.
- Stay upwind, uphill and/or upstream.
- Ventilate closed spaces before entering.

### PROTECTIVE CLOTHING

- Wear positive pressure self-contained breathing apparatus (SCBA).
- Structural firefighters' protective clothing will only provide limited protection.

### EVACUATION

**Large Spill**

- Consider initial downwind evacuation for at least 300 meters (1000 feet).

**Fire**

- If tank, rail car or tank truck is involved in a fire, ISOLATE for 800 meters (1/2 mile) in all directions; also, consider initial evacuation for 800 meters (1/2 mile) in all directions.

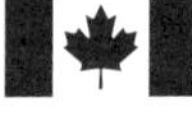

In Canada, an Emergency Response Assistance Plan (ERAP) may be required for this product. Please consult the shipping document and/or the ERAP Program Section (page 391).

## EMERGENCY RESPONSE

### FIRE

**CAUTION: All these products have a very low flash point: Use of water spray when fighting fire may be inefficient.**

**CAUTION: For fire involving UN1170, UN1987 or UN3475, alcohol-resistant foam should be used.**

**Small Fire**

- Dry chemical, $CO_2$, water spray or alcohol-resistant foam.

**Large Fire**

- Water spray, fog or alcohol-resistant foam.
- **Do not use straight streams**.
- Move containers from fire area if you can do it without risk.

**Fire involving Tanks or Car/Trailer Loads**

- Fight fire from maximum distance or use unmanned hose holders or monitor nozzles.
- Cool containers with flooding quantities of water until well after fire is out.
- Withdraw immediately in case of rising sound from venting safety devices or discoloration of tank.
- ALWAYS stay away from tanks engulfed in fire.
- For massive fire, use unmanned hose holders or monitor nozzles; if this is impossible, withdraw from area and let fire burn.

### SPILL OR LEAK

- ELIMINATE all ignition sources (no smoking, flares, sparks or flames in immediate area).
- All equipment used when handling the product must be grounded.
- Do not touch or walk through spilled material.
- Stop leak if you can do it without risk.
- Prevent entry into waterways, sewers, basements or confined areas.
- A vapor-suppressing foam may be used to reduce vapors.
- Absorb or cover with dry earth, sand or other non-combustible material and transfer to containers.
- Use clean, non-sparking tools to collect absorbed material.

**Large Spill**

- Dike far ahead of liquid spill for later disposal.
- Water spray may reduce vapor, but may not prevent ignition in closed spaces.

### FIRST AID

- Ensure that medical personnel are aware of the material(s) involved and take precautions to protect themselves.
- Move victim to fresh air.
- Call 911 or emergency medical service.
- Give artificial respiration if victim is not breathing.
- Administer oxygen if breathing is difficult.
- Remove and isolate contaminated clothing and shoes.
- In case of contact with substance, immediately flush skin or eyes with running water for at least 20 minutes.
- Wash skin with soap and water.
- In case of burns, immediately cool affected skin for as long as possible with cold water. Do not remove clothing if adhering to skin.
- Keep victim calm and warm.

# GUIDE 128 FLAMMABLE LIQUIDS (WATER-IMMISCIBLE)

## POTENTIAL HAZARDS

### FIRE OR EXPLOSION

- **HIGHLY FLAMMABLE: Will be easily ignited by heat, sparks or flames.**
- Vapors may form explosive mixtures with air.
- Vapors may travel to source of ignition and flash back.
- Most vapors are heavier than air. They will spread along ground and collect in low or confined areas (sewers, basements, tanks).
- Vapor explosion hazard indoors, outdoors or in sewers.
- Those substances designated with a **(P)** may polymerize explosively when heated or involved in a fire.
- Runoff to sewer may create fire or explosion hazard.
- Containers may explode when heated.
- Many liquids are lighter than water.
- Substance may be transported hot.
- For hybrid vehicles, GUIDE 147 (lithium ion batteries) or GUIDE 138 (sodium batteries) should also be consulted.
- **If molten aluminum is involved, refer to GUIDE 169.**

### HEALTH

- Inhalation or contact with material may irritate or burn skin and eyes.
- Fire may produce irritating, corrosive and/or toxic gases.
- Vapors may cause dizziness or suffocation.
- Runoff from fire control or dilution water may cause pollution.

## PUBLIC SAFETY

- **CALL EMERGENCY RESPONSE Telephone Number on Shipping Paper first. If Shipping Paper not available or no answer, refer to appropriate telephone number listed on the inside back cover.**
- As an immediate precautionary measure, isolate spill or leak area for at least 50 meters (150 feet) in all directions.
- Keep unauthorized personnel away.
- Stay upwind, uphill and/or upstream.
- Ventilate closed spaces before entering.

### PROTECTIVE CLOTHING

- Wear positive pressure self-contained breathing apparatus (SCBA).
- Structural firefighters' protective clothing will only provide limited protection.

### EVACUATION

**Large Spill**

- Consider initial downwind evacuation for at least 300 meters (1000 feet).

**Fire**

- If tank, rail car or tank truck is involved in a fire, ISOLATE for 800 meters (1/2 mile) in all directions; also, consider initial evacuation for 800 meters (1/2 mile) in all directions.

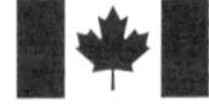

In Canada, an Emergency Response Assistance Plan (ERAP) may be required for this product. Please consult the shipping document and/or the ERAP Program Section (page 391).

## EMERGENCY RESPONSE

### FIRE

**CAUTION: All these products have a very low flash point: Use of water spray when fighting fire may be inefficient.**

**CAUTION: For mixtures containing alcohol or polar solvent, alcohol-resistant foam may be more effective.**

**Small Fire**
- Dry chemical, $CO_2$, water spray or regular foam.

**Large Fire**
- Water spray, fog or regular foam.
- **Do not use straight streams**.
- Move containers from fire area if you can do it without risk.

**Fire involving Tanks or Car/Trailer Loads**
- Fight fire from maximum distance or use unmanned hose holders or monitor nozzles.
- Cool containers with flooding quantities of water until well after fire is out.
- Withdraw immediately in case of rising sound from venting safety devices or discoloration of tank.
- ALWAYS stay away from tanks engulfed in fire.
- For massive fire, use unmanned hose holders or monitor nozzles; if this is impossible, withdraw from area and let fire burn.

### SPILL OR LEAK
- ELIMINATE all ignition sources (no smoking, flares, sparks or flames in immediate area).
- All equipment used when handling the product must be grounded.
- Do not touch or walk through spilled material.
- Stop leak if you can do it without risk.
- Prevent entry into waterways, sewers, basements or confined areas.
- A vapor-suppressing foam may be used to reduce vapors.
- Absorb or cover with dry earth, sand or other non-combustible material and transfer to containers.
- Use clean, non-sparking tools to collect absorbed material.

**Large Spill**
- Dike far ahead of liquid spill for later disposal.
- Water spray may reduce vapor, but may not prevent ignition in closed spaces.

### FIRST AID
- Ensure that medical personnel are aware of the material(s) involved and take precautions to protect themselves.
- Move victim to fresh air.
- Call 911 or emergency medical service.
- Give artificial respiration if victim is not breathing.
- Administer oxygen if breathing is difficult.
- Remove and isolate contaminated clothing and shoes.
- In case of contact with substance, immediately flush skin or eyes with running water for at least 20 minutes.
- Wash skin with soap and water.
- In case of burns, immediately cool affected skin for as long as possible with cold water. Do not remove clothing if adhering to skin.
- Keep victim calm and warm.

# GUIDE 129 FLAMMABLE LIQUIDS (WATER-MISCIBLE/NOXIOUS)

## POTENTIAL HAZARDS

### FIRE OR EXPLOSION

- **HIGHLY FLAMMABLE: Will be easily ignited by heat, sparks or flames.**
- Vapors may form explosive mixtures with air.
- Vapors may travel to source of ignition and flash back.
- Most vapors are heavier than air. They will spread along ground and collect in low or confined areas (sewers, basements, tanks).
- Vapor explosion hazard indoors, outdoors or in sewers.
- Those substances designated with a **(P)** may polymerize explosively when heated or involved in a fire.
- Runoff to sewer may create fire or explosion hazard.
- Containers may explode when heated.
- Many liquids are lighter than water.

### HEALTH

- May cause toxic effects if inhaled or absorbed through skin.
- Inhalation or contact with material may irritate or burn skin and eyes.
- Fire will produce irritating, corrosive and/or toxic gases.
- Vapors may cause dizziness or suffocation.
- Runoff from fire control or dilution water may cause pollution.

## PUBLIC SAFETY

- **CALL EMERGENCY RESPONSE Telephone Number on Shipping Paper first. If Shipping Paper not available or no answer, refer to appropriate telephone number listed on the inside back cover.**
- As an immediate precautionary measure, isolate spill or leak area for at least 50 meters (150 feet) in all directions.
- Keep unauthorized personnel away.
- Stay upwind, uphill and/or upstream.
- Ventilate closed spaces before entering.

### PROTECTIVE CLOTHING

- Wear positive pressure self-contained breathing apparatus (SCBA).
- Structural firefighters' protective clothing will only provide limited protection.

### EVACUATION

**Large Spill**

- Consider initial downwind evacuation for at least 300 meters (1000 feet).

**Fire**

- If tank, rail car or tank truck is involved in a fire, ISOLATE for 800 meters (1/2 mile) in all directions; also, consider initial evacuation for 800 meters (1/2 mile) in all directions.

In Canada, an Emergency Response Assistance Plan (ERAP) may be required for this product. Please consult the shipping document and/or the ERAP Program Section (page 391).

## EMERGENCY RESPONSE

### FIRE

**CAUTION: All these products have a very low flash point: Use of water spray when fighting fire may be inefficient.**

**Small Fire**

- Dry chemical, $CO_2$, water spray or alcohol-resistant foam.
- **Do not use dry chemical extinguishers to control fires involving nitromethane (UN1261) or nitroethane (UN2842).**

**Large Fire**

- Water spray, fog or alcohol-resistant foam.
- **Do not use straight streams.**
- Move containers from fire area if you can do it without risk.

**Fire involving Tanks or Car/Trailer Loads**

- Fight fire from maximum distance or use unmanned hose holders or monitor nozzles.
- Cool containers with flooding quantities of water until well after fire is out.
- Withdraw immediately in case of rising sound from venting safety devices or discoloration of tank.
- ALWAYS stay away from tanks engulfed in fire.
- For massive fire, use unmanned hose holders or monitor nozzles; if this is impossible, withdraw from area and let fire burn.

### SPILL OR LEAK

- ELIMINATE all ignition sources (no smoking, flares, sparks or flames in immediate area).
- All equipment used when handling the product must be grounded.
- Do not touch or walk through spilled material.
- Stop leak if you can do it without risk.
- Prevent entry into waterways, sewers, basements or confined areas.
- A vapor-suppressing foam may be used to reduce vapors.
- Absorb or cover with dry earth, sand or other non-combustible material and transfer to containers.
- Use clean, non-sparking tools to collect absorbed material.

**Large Spill**

- Dike far ahead of liquid spill for later disposal.
- Water spray may reduce vapor, but may not prevent ignition in closed spaces.

### FIRST AID

- Ensure that medical personnel are aware of the material(s) involved and take precautions to protect themselves.
- Move victim to fresh air.
- Call 911 or emergency medical service.
- Give artificial respiration if victim is not breathing.
- Administer oxygen if breathing is difficult.
- Remove and isolate contaminated clothing and shoes.
- In case of contact with substance, immediately flush skin or eyes with running water for at least 20 minutes.
- Wash skin with soap and water.
- In case of burns, immediately cool affected skin for as long as possible with cold water. Do not remove clothing if adhering to skin.
- Keep victim calm and warm.
- Effects of exposure (inhalation, ingestion or skin contact) to substance may be delayed.

# GUIDE 130 FLAMMABLE LIQUIDS (WATER-IMMISCIBLE/NOXIOUS)

## POTENTIAL HAZARDS

### FIRE OR EXPLOSION

- **HIGHLY FLAMMABLE: Will be easily ignited by heat, sparks or flames.**
- Vapors may form explosive mixtures with air.
- Vapors may travel to source of ignition and flash back.
- Most vapors are heavier than air. They will spread along ground and collect in low or confined areas (sewers, basements, tanks).
- Vapor explosion hazard indoors, outdoors or in sewers.
- Those substances designated with a **(P)** may polymerize explosively when heated or involved in a fire.
- Runoff to sewer may create fire or explosion hazard.
- Containers may explode when heated.
- Many liquids are lighter than water.

### HEALTH

- May cause toxic effects if inhaled or absorbed through skin.
- Inhalation or contact with material may irritate or burn skin and eyes.
- Fire will produce irritating, corrosive and/or toxic gases.
- Vapors may cause dizziness or suffocation.
- Runoff from fire control or dilution water may cause pollution.

## PUBLIC SAFETY

- **CALL EMERGENCY RESPONSE Telephone Number on Shipping Paper first. If Shipping Paper not available or no answer, refer to appropriate telephone number listed on the inside back cover.**
- As an immediate precautionary measure, isolate spill or leak area for at least 50 meters (150 feet) in all directions.
- Keep unauthorized personnel away.
- Stay upwind, uphill and/or upstream.
- Ventilate closed spaces before entering.

### PROTECTIVE CLOTHING

- Wear positive pressure self-contained breathing apparatus (SCBA).
- Structural firefighters' protective clothing will only provide limited protection.

### EVACUATION

**Large Spill**

- Consider initial downwind evacuation for at least 300 meters (1000 feet).

**Fire**

- If tank, rail car or tank truck is involved in a fire, ISOLATE for 800 meters (1/2 mile) in all directions; also, consider initial evacuation for 800 meters (1/2 mile) in all directions.

In Canada, an Emergency Response Assistance Plan (ERAP) may be required for this product. Please consult the shipping document and/or the ERAP Program Section (page 391).

## EMERGENCY RESPONSE

### FIRE

**CAUTION: All these products have a very low flash point: Use of water spray when fighting fire may be inefficient.**

**Small Fire**
- Dry chemical, $CO_2$, water spray or regular foam.

**Large Fire**
- Water spray, fog or regular foam.
- **Do not use straight streams.**
- Move containers from fire area if you can do it without risk.

**Fire involving Tanks or Car/Trailer Loads**
- Fight fire from maximum distance or use unmanned hose holders or monitor nozzles.
- Cool containers with flooding quantities of water until well after fire is out.
- Withdraw immediately in case of rising sound from venting safety devices or discoloration of tank.
- ALWAYS stay away from tanks engulfed in fire.
- For massive fire, use unmanned hose holders or monitor nozzles; if this is impossible, withdraw from area and let fire burn.

### SPILL OR LEAK
- ELIMINATE all ignition sources (no smoking, flares, sparks or flames in immediate area).
- All equipment used when handling the product must be grounded.
- Do not touch or walk through spilled material.
- Stop leak if you can do it without risk.
- Prevent entry into waterways, sewers, basements or confined areas.
- A vapor-suppressing foam may be used to reduce vapors.
- Absorb or cover with dry earth, sand or other non-combustible material and transfer to containers.
- Use clean, non-sparking tools to collect absorbed material.

**Large Spill**
- Dike far ahead of liquid spill for later disposal.
- Water spray may reduce vapor, but may not prevent ignition in closed spaces.

### FIRST AID
- Ensure that medical personnel are aware of the material(s) involved and take precautions to protect themselves.
- Move victim to fresh air.
- Call 911 or emergency medical service.
- Give artificial respiration if victim is not breathing.
- Administer oxygen if breathing is difficult.
- Remove and isolate contaminated clothing and shoes.
- In case of contact with substance, immediately flush skin or eyes with running water for at least 20 minutes.
- Wash skin with soap and water.
- In case of burns, immediately cool affected skin for as long as possible with cold water. Do not remove clothing if adhering to skin.
- Keep victim calm and warm.
- Effects of exposure (inhalation, ingestion or skin contact) to substance may be delayed.

# GUIDE 131 FLAMMABLE LIQUIDS - TOXIC

## POTENTIAL HAZARDS

### HEALTH

- **TOXIC; may be fatal if inhaled, ingested or absorbed through skin.**
- Inhalation or contact with some of these materials will irritate or burn skin and eyes.
- Fire will produce irritating, corrosive and/or toxic gases.
- Vapors may cause dizziness or suffocation.
- Runoff from fire control or dilution water may cause pollution.

### FIRE OR EXPLOSION

- **HIGHLY FLAMMABLE: Will be easily ignited by heat, sparks or flames.**
- Vapors may form explosive mixtures with air.
- Vapors may travel to source of ignition and flash back.
- Most vapors are heavier than air. They will spread along ground and collect in low or confined areas (sewers, basements, tanks).
- Vapor explosion and poison hazard indoors, outdoors or in sewers.
- Those substances designated with a **(P)** may polymerize explosively when heated or involved in a fire.
- Runoff to sewer may create fire or explosion hazard.
- Containers may explode when heated.
- Many liquids are lighter than water.

## PUBLIC SAFETY

- **CALL EMERGENCY RESPONSE Telephone Number on Shipping Paper first. If Shipping Paper not available or no answer, refer to appropriate telephone number listed on the inside back cover.**
- As an immediate precautionary measure, isolate spill or leak area for at least 50 meters (150 feet) in all directions.
- Keep unauthorized personnel away.
- Stay upwind, uphill and/or upstream.
- Ventilate closed spaces before entering.

### PROTECTIVE CLOTHING

- Wear positive pressure self-contained breathing apparatus (SCBA).
- Wear chemical protective clothing that is specifically recommended by the manufacturer. It may provide little or no thermal protection.
- Structural firefighters' protective clothing provides limited protection in fire situations ONLY; it is not effective in spill situations where direct contact with the substance is possible.

### EVACUATION

**Spill**

- See Table 1 - Initial Isolation and Protective Action Distances for highlighted materials. For non-highlighted materials, increase, in the downwind direction, as necessary, the isolation distance shown under "PUBLIC SAFETY".

**Fire**

- If tank, rail car or tank truck is involved in a fire, ISOLATE for 800 meters (1/2 mile) in all directions; also, consider initial evacuation for 800 meters (1/2 mile) in all directions.

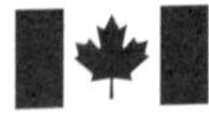

In Canada, an Emergency Response Assistance Plan (ERAP) may be required for this product. Please consult the shipping document and/or the ERAP Program Section (page 391).

## EMERGENCY RESPONSE

### FIRE

**CAUTION: All these products have a very low flash point: Use of water spray when fighting fire may be inefficient.**

**Small Fire**

- Dry chemical, $CO_2$, water spray or alcohol-resistant foam.

**Large Fire**

- Water spray, fog or alcohol-resistant foam.
- Move containers from fire area if you can do it without risk.
- Dike fire-control water for later disposal; do not scatter the material.
- Use water spray or fog; do not use straight streams.

**Fire involving Tanks or Car/Trailer Loads**

- Fight fire from maximum distance or use unmanned hose holders or monitor nozzles.
- Cool containers with flooding quantities of water until well after fire is out.
- Withdraw immediately in case of rising sound from venting safety devices or discoloration of tank.
- ALWAYS stay away from tanks engulfed in fire.
- For massive fire, use unmanned hose holders or monitor nozzles; if this is impossible, withdraw from area and let fire burn.

### SPILL OR LEAK

- Fully encapsulating, vapor-protective clothing should be worn for spills and leaks with no fire.
- ELIMINATE all ignition sources (no smoking, flares, sparks or flames in immediate area).
- All equipment used when handling the product must be grounded.
- Do not touch or walk through spilled material.
- Stop leak if you can do it without risk.
- Prevent entry into waterways, sewers, basements or confined areas.
- A vapor-suppressing foam may be used to reduce vapors.

**Small Spill**

- Absorb with earth, sand or other non-combustible material and transfer to containers for later disposal.
- Use clean, non-sparking tools to collect absorbed material.

**Large Spill**

- Dike far ahead of liquid spill for later disposal.
- Water spray may reduce vapor, but may not prevent ignition in closed spaces.

### FIRST AID

- Ensure that medical personnel are aware of the material(s) involved and take precautions to protect themselves.
- Move victim to fresh air.
- Call 911 or emergency medical service.
- Give artificial respiration if victim is not breathing.
- **Do not use mouth-to-mouth method if victim ingested or inhaled the substance; give artificial respiration with the aid of a pocket mask equipped with a one-way valve or other proper respiratory medical device.**
- Administer oxygen if breathing is difficult.
- Remove and isolate contaminated clothing and shoes.
- In case of contact with substance, immediately flush skin or eyes with running water for at least 20 minutes.
- Wash skin with soap and water.
- In case of burns, immediately cool affected skin for as long as possible with cold water. Do not remove clothing if adhering to skin.
- Keep victim calm and warm.
- Effects of exposure (inhalation, ingestion or skin contact) to substance may be delayed.

## POTENTIAL HAZARDS

### FIRE OR EXPLOSION

- Flammable/combustible material.
- May be ignited by heat, sparks or flames.
- Vapors may form explosive mixtures with air.
- Vapors may travel to source of ignition and flash back.
- Most vapors are heavier than air. They will spread along ground and collect in low or confined areas (sewers, basements, tanks).
- Vapor explosion hazard indoors, outdoors or in sewers.
- Those substances designated with a **(P)** may polymerize explosively when heated or involved in a fire.
- Runoff to sewer may create fire or explosion hazard.
- Containers may explode when heated.
- Many liquids are lighter than water.

### HEALTH

- May cause toxic effects if inhaled or ingested/swallowed.
- Contact with substance may cause severe burns to skin and eyes.
- Fire will produce irritating, corrosive and/or toxic gases.
- Vapors may cause dizziness or suffocation.
- Runoff from fire control or dilution water may cause pollution.

## PUBLIC SAFETY

- **CALL EMERGENCY RESPONSE Telephone Number on Shipping Paper first. If Shipping Paper not available or no answer, refer to appropriate telephone number listed on the inside back cover.**
- As an immediate precautionary measure, isolate spill or leak area for at least 50 meters (150 feet) in all directions.
- Keep unauthorized personnel away.
- Stay upwind, uphill and/or upstream.
- Ventilate closed spaces before entering.

### PROTECTIVE CLOTHING

- Wear positive pressure self-contained breathing apparatus (SCBA).
- Wear chemical protective clothing that is specifically recommended by the manufacturer. It may provide little or no thermal protection.
- Structural firefighters' protective clothing provides limited protection in fire situations ONLY; it is not effective in spill situations where direct contact with the substance is possible.

### EVACUATION

**Spill**

- See Table 1 - Initial Isolation and Protective Action Distances for highlighted materials. For non-highlighted materials, increase, in the downwind direction, as necessary, the isolation distance shown under "PUBLIC SAFETY".

**Fire**

- If tank, rail car or tank truck is involved in a fire, ISOLATE for 800 meters (1/2 mile) in all directions; also, consider initial evacuation for 800 meters (1/2 mile) in all directions.

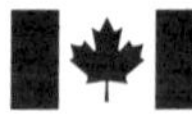

In Canada, an Emergency Response Assistance Plan (ERAP) may be required for this product. Please consult the shipping document and/or the ERAP Program Section (page 391).

## EMERGENCY RESPONSE

### FIRE

- **Some of these materials may react violently with water.**

**Small Fire**

- Dry chemical, $CO_2$, water spray or alcohol-resistant foam.

**Large Fire**

- Water spray, fog or alcohol-resistant foam.
- Move containers from fire area if you can do it without risk.
- Dike fire-control water for later disposal; do not scatter the material.
- Do not get water inside containers.

**Fire involving Tanks or Car/Trailer Loads**

- Fight fire from maximum distance or use unmanned hose holders or monitor nozzles.
- Cool containers with flooding quantities of water until well after fire is out.
- Withdraw immediately in case of rising sound from venting safety devices or discoloration of tank.
- ALWAYS stay away from tanks engulfed in fire.
- For massive fire, use unmanned hose holders or monitor nozzles; if this is impossible, withdraw from area and let fire burn.

### SPILL OR LEAK

- Fully encapsulating, vapor-protective clothing should be worn for spills and leaks with no fire.
- ELIMINATE all ignition sources (no smoking, flares, sparks or flames in immediate area).
- All equipment used when handling the product must be grounded.
- Do not touch or walk through spilled material.
- Stop leak if you can do it without risk.
- Prevent entry into waterways, sewers, basements or confined areas.
- A vapor-suppressing foam may be used to reduce vapors.
- Absorb with earth, sand or other non-combustible material and transfer to containers (except for Hydrazine).
- Use clean, non-sparking tools to collect absorbed material.

**Large Spill**

- Dike far ahead of liquid spill for later disposal.
- Water spray may reduce vapor, but may not prevent ignition in closed spaces.

### FIRST AID

- Ensure that medical personnel are aware of the material(s) involved and take precautions to protect themselves.
- Move victim to fresh air.
- Call 911 or emergency medical service.
- Give artificial respiration if victim is not breathing.
- **Do not use mouth-to-mouth method if victim ingested or inhaled the substance; give artificial respiration with the aid of a pocket mask equipped with a one-way valve or other proper respiratory medical device.**
- Administer oxygen if breathing is difficult.
- Remove and isolate contaminated clothing and shoes.
- In case of contact with substance, immediately flush skin or eyes with running water for at least 20 minutes.
- In case of burns, immediately cool affected skin for as long as possible with cold water. Do not remove clothing if adhering to skin.
- Keep victim calm and warm.
- Effects of exposure (inhalation, ingestion or skin contact) to substance may be delayed.

# GUIDE 133 FLAMMABLE SOLIDS

## POTENTIAL HAZARDS

### FIRE OR EXPLOSION

- Flammable/combustible material.
- May be ignited by friction, heat, sparks or flames.
- Some may burn rapidly with flare-burning effect.
- Powders, dusts, shavings, borings, turnings or cuttings may explode or burn with explosive violence.
- Substance may be transported in a molten form at a temperature that may be above its flash point.
- May re-ignite after fire is extinguished.

### HEALTH

- Fire may produce irritating and/or toxic gases.
- Contact may cause burns to skin and eyes.
- Contact with molten substance may cause severe burns to skin and eyes.
- Runoff from fire control may cause pollution.

## PUBLIC SAFETY

- **CALL EMERGENCY RESPONSE Telephone Number on Shipping Paper first. If Shipping Paper not available or no answer, refer to appropriate telephone number listed on the inside back cover.**
- As an immediate precautionary measure, isolate spill or leak area for at least 25 meters (75 feet) in all directions.
- Keep unauthorized personnel away.
- Stay upwind, uphill and/or upstream.

### PROTECTIVE CLOTHING

- Wear positive pressure self-contained breathing apparatus (SCBA).
- Structural firefighters' protective clothing will only provide limited protection.

### EVACUATION

**Large Spill**

- Consider initial downwind evacuation for at least 100 meters (330 feet).

**Fire**

- If tank, rail car or tank truck is involved in a fire, ISOLATE for 800 meters (1/2 mile) in all directions; also, consider initial evacuation for 800 meters (1/2 mile) in all directions.

In Canada, an Emergency Response Assistance Plan (ERAP) may be required for this product. Please consult the shipping document and/or the ERAP Program Section (page 391).

## EMERGENCY RESPONSE

### FIRE

**Small Fire**

- Dry chemical, $CO_2$, sand, earth, water spray or regular foam.

**Large Fire**

- Water spray, fog or regular foam.
- Move containers from fire area if you can do it without risk.

**Fire Involving Metal Pigments or Pastes (e.g. "Aluminum Paste")**

- Aluminum Paste fires should be treated as a combustible metal fire. Use DRY sand, graphite powder, dry sodium chloride-based extinguishers, G-1® or Met-L-X® powder.
  Also, see GUIDE 170.

**Fire involving Tanks or Car/Trailer Loads**

- Cool containers with flooding quantities of water until well after fire is out.
- For massive fire, use unmanned hose holders or monitor nozzles; if this is impossible, withdraw from area and let fire burn.
- Withdraw immediately in case of rising sound from venting safety devices or discoloration of tank.
- ALWAYS stay away from tanks engulfed in fire.

### SPILL OR LEAK

- ELIMINATE all ignition sources (no smoking, flares, sparks or flames in immediate area).
- Do not touch or walk through spilled material.

**Small Dry Spill**

- With clean shovel, place material into clean, dry container and cover loosely; move containers from spill area.

**Large Spill**

- Wet down with water and dike for later disposal.
- Prevent entry into waterways, sewers, basements or confined areas.

### FIRST AID

- Ensure that medical personnel are aware of the material(s) involved and take precautions to protect themselves.
- Move victim to fresh air.
- Call 911 or emergency medical service.
- Give artificial respiration if victim is not breathing.
- Administer oxygen if breathing is difficult.
- Remove and isolate contaminated clothing and shoes.
- In case of contact with substance, immediately flush skin or eyes with running water for at least 20 minutes.
- Removal of solidified molten material from skin requires medical assistance.
- Keep victim calm and warm.

# GUIDE 134 FLAMMABLE SOLIDS - TOXIC AND/OR CORROSIVE

## POTENTIAL HAZARDS

### FIRE OR EXPLOSION

- Flammable/combustible material.
- May be ignited by heat, sparks or flames.
- When heated, vapors may form explosive mixtures with air: indoors, outdoors and sewers explosion hazards.
- Contact with metals may evolve flammable hydrogen gas.
- Containers may explode when heated.

### HEALTH

- **TOXIC;** inhalation, ingestion or skin contact with material may cause severe injury or death.
- Fire will produce irritating, corrosive and/or toxic gases.
- Runoff from fire control or dilution water may be corrosive and/or toxic and cause pollution.

## PUBLIC SAFETY

- **CALL EMERGENCY RESPONSE Telephone Number on Shipping Paper first. If Shipping Paper not available or no answer, refer to appropriate telephone number listed on the inside back cover.**
- As an immediate precautionary measure, isolate spill or leak area for at least 25 meters (75 feet) in all directions.
- Stay upwind, uphill and/or upstream.
- Keep unauthorized personnel away.
- Ventilate enclosed areas.

### PROTECTIVE CLOTHING

- Wear positive pressure self-contained breathing apparatus (SCBA).
- Wear chemical protective clothing that is specifically recommended by the manufacturer. It may provide little or no thermal protection.
- Structural firefighters' protective clothing provides limited protection in fire situations ONLY; it is not effective in spill situations where direct contact with the substance is possible.

### EVACUATION

**Large Spill**

- Consider initial downwind evacuation for at least 100 meters (330 feet).

**Fire**

- If tank, rail car or tank truck is involved in a fire, ISOLATE for 800 meters (1/2 mile) in all directions; also, consider initial evacuation for 800 meters (1/2 mile) in all directions.

In Canada, an Emergency Response Assistance Plan (ERAP) may be required for this product. Please consult the shipping document and/or the ERAP Program Section (page 391).

## EMERGENCY RESPONSE

### FIRE

**Small Fire**

- Dry chemical, $CO_2$, water spray or alcohol-resistant foam.

**Large Fire**

- Water spray, fog or alcohol-resistant foam.
- Move containers from fire area if you can do it without risk.
- Use water spray or fog; do not use straight streams.
- Do not get water inside containers.
- Dike fire-control water for later disposal; do not scatter the material.

**Fire involving Tanks or Car/Trailer Loads**

- Fight fire from maximum distance or use unmanned hose holders or monitor nozzles.
- Cool containers with flooding quantities of water until well after fire is out.
- Withdraw immediately in case of rising sound from venting safety devices or discoloration of tank.
- ALWAYS stay away from tanks engulfed in fire.

### SPILL OR LEAK

- Fully encapsulating, vapor-protective clothing should be worn for spills and leaks with no fire.
- ELIMINATE all ignition sources (no smoking, flares, sparks or flames in immediate area).
- Stop leak if you can do it without risk.
- Do not touch damaged containers or spilled material unless wearing appropriate protective clothing.
- Prevent entry into waterways, sewers, basements or confined areas.
- Use clean, non-sparking tools to collect material and place it into loosely covered plastic containers for later disposal.

### FIRST AID

- Ensure that medical personnel are aware of the material(s) involved and take precautions to protect themselves.
- Move victim to fresh air.
- Call 911 or emergency medical service.
- Give artificial respiration if victim is not breathing.
- **Do not use mouth-to-mouth method if victim ingested or inhaled the substance; give artificial respiration with the aid of a pocket mask equipped with a one-way valve or other proper respiratory medical device.**
- Administer oxygen if breathing is difficult.
- Remove and isolate contaminated clothing and shoes.
- In case of contact with substance, immediately flush skin or eyes with running water for at least 20 minutes.
- For minor skin contact, avoid spreading material on unaffected skin.
- Keep victim calm and warm.
- Effects of exposure (inhalation, ingestion or skin contact) to substance may be delayed.

# GUIDE 135 SUBSTANCES - SPONTANEOUSLY COMBUSTIBLE

## POTENTIAL HAZARDS

### FIRE OR EXPLOSION

- Flammable/combustible material.
- May ignite on contact with moist air or moisture.
- May burn rapidly with flare-burning effect.
- Some react vigorously or explosively on contact with water.
- Some may decompose explosively when heated or involved in a fire.
- May re-ignite after fire is extinguished.
- Runoff may create fire or explosion hazard.
- Containers may explode when heated.

### HEALTH

- Fire will produce irritating, corrosive and/or toxic gases.
- Inhalation of decomposition products may cause severe injury or death.
- Contact with substance may cause severe burns to skin and eyes.
- Runoff from fire control may cause pollution.

## PUBLIC SAFETY

- **CALL EMERGENCY RESPONSE Telephone Number on Shipping Paper first. If Shipping Paper not available or no answer, refer to appropriate telephone number listed on the inside back cover.**
- As an immediate precautionary measure, isolate spill or leak area in all directions for at least 50 meters (150 feet) for liquids and at least 25 meters (75 feet) for solids.
- Stay upwind, uphill and/or upstream.
- Keep unauthorized personnel away.

### PROTECTIVE CLOTHING

- Wear positive pressure self-contained breathing apparatus (SCBA).
- Wear chemical protective clothing that is specifically recommended by the manufacturer. It may provide little or no thermal protection.
- Structural firefighters' protective clothing will only provide limited protection.

### EVACUATION

**Spill**

- See Table 1 - Initial Isolation and Protective Action Distances for highlighted materials. For non-highlighted materials, increase, in the downwind direction, as necessary, the isolation distance shown under "PUBLIC SAFETY".

**Fire**

- If tank, rail car or tank truck is involved in a fire, ISOLATE for 800 meters (1/2 mile) in all directions; also, consider initial evacuation for 800 meters (1/2 mile) in all directions.

In Canada, an Emergency Response Assistance Plan (ERAP) may be required for this product. Please consult the shipping document and/or the ERAP Program Section (page 391).

## EMERGENCY RESPONSE

### FIRE

- **DO NOT USE WATER, $CO_2$ OR FOAM ON MATERIAL ITSELF.**
- Some of these materials may react violently with water.

**EXCEPTION: For Xanthates, UN3342 and for Dithionite (Hydrosulfite/Hydrosulphite) UN1384, UN1923 and UN1929, USE FLOODING AMOUNTS OF WATER for SMALL AND LARGE fires to stop the reaction. Smothering will not work for these materials, they do not need air to burn.**

**Small Fire**

- Dry chemical, soda ash, lime or DRY sand, **EXCEPT for UN1384, UN1923, UN1929 and UN3342**.

**Large Fire**

- DRY sand, dry chemical, soda ash or lime **EXCEPT for UN1384, UN1923, UN1929 and UN3342**, or withdraw from area and let fire burn.
- **CAUTION**: **UN3342** when flooded with water will continue to evolve flammable Carbon disulfide/Carbon disulphide vapors.
- Move containers from fire area if you can do it without risk.

**Fire involving Tanks or Car/Trailer Loads**

- Fight fire from maximum distance or use unmanned hose holders or monitor nozzles.
- Do not get water inside containers or in contact with substance.
- Cool containers with flooding quantities of water until well after fire is out.
- Withdraw immediately in case of rising sound from venting safety devices or discoloration of tank.
- ALWAYS stay away from tanks engulfed in fire.

### SPILL OR LEAK

- Fully encapsulating, vapor-protective clothing should be worn for spills and leaks with no fire.
- ELIMINATE all ignition sources (no smoking, flares, sparks or flames in immediate area).
- Do not touch or walk through spilled material.
- Stop leak if you can do it without risk.

**Small Spill**

**EXCEPTION: For spills of Xanthates, UN3342 and for Dithionite (Hydrosulfite/Hydrosulphite), UN1384, UN1923 and UN1929, dissolve in 5 parts water and collect for proper disposal.**

- **CAUTION**: **UN3342** when flooded with water will continue to evolve flammable Carbon disulfide/Carbon disulphide vapors.
- Cover with DRY earth, DRY sand or other non-combustible material followed with plastic sheet to minimize spreading or contact with rain.
- Use clean, non-sparking tools to collect material and place it into loosely covered plastic containers for later disposal.
- Prevent entry into waterways, sewers, basements or confined areas.

### FIRST AID

- Ensure that medical personnel are aware of the material(s) involved and take precautions to protect themselves.
- Move victim to fresh air.
- Call 911 or emergency medical service.
- Give artificial respiration if victim is not breathing.
- Administer oxygen if breathing is difficult.
- Remove and isolate contaminated clothing and shoes.
- In case of contact with substance, immediately flush skin or eyes with running water for at least 20 minutes.
- Keep victim calm and warm.

# GUIDE 136 SUBSTANCES - SPONTANEOUSLY COMBUSTIBLE - TOXIC AND/OR CORROSIVE (AIR-REACTIVE)

## POTENTIAL HAZARDS

### FIRE OR EXPLOSION

- Extremely flammable; will ignite itself if exposed to air.
- Burns rapidly, releasing dense, white, irritating fumes.
- Substance may be transported in a molten form.
- May re-ignite after fire is extinguished.
- Corrosive substances in contact with metals may produce flammable hydrogen gas.
- Containers may explode when heated.

### HEALTH

- Fire will produce irritating, corrosive and/or toxic gases.
- **TOXIC**; ingestion of substance or inhalation of decomposition products will cause severe injury or death.
- Contact with substance may cause severe burns to skin and eyes.
- Some effects may be experienced due to skin absorption.
- Runoff from fire control may be corrosive and/or toxic and cause pollution.

## PUBLIC SAFETY

- **CALL EMERGENCY RESPONSE Telephone Number on Shipping Paper first. If Shipping Paper not available or no answer, refer to appropriate telephone number listed on the inside back cover.**
- As an immediate precautionary measure, isolate spill or leak area in all directions for at least 50 meters (150 feet) for liquids and at least 25 meters (75 feet) for solids.
- Stay upwind, uphill and/or upstream.
- Keep unauthorized personnel away.

### PROTECTIVE CLOTHING

- Wear positive pressure self-contained breathing apparatus (SCBA).
- Wear chemical protective clothing that is specifically recommended by the manufacturer. It may provide little or no thermal protection.
- Structural firefighters' protective clothing provides limited protection in fire situations ONLY; it is not effective in spill situations where direct contact with the substance is possible.
- **For Phosphorus (UN1381): Special aluminized protective clothing should be worn when direct contact with the substance is possible.**

### EVACUATION

**Spill**

- Consider initial downwind evacuation for at least 300 meters (1000 feet).

**Fire**

- If tank, rail car or tank truck is involved in a fire, ISOLATE for 800 meters (1/2 mile) in all directions; also, consider initial evacuation for 800 meters (1/2 mile) in all directions.

In Canada, an Emergency Response Assistance Plan (ERAP) may be required for this product. Please consult the shipping document and/or the ERAP Program Section (page 391).

## EMERGENCY RESPONSE

### FIRE

**Small Fire**

- Water spray, wet sand or wet earth.

**Large Fire**

- Water spray or fog.
- **Do not scatter spilled material with high-pressure water streams.**
- Move containers from fire area if you can do it without risk.

**Fire involving Tanks or Car/Trailer Loads**

- Fight fire from maximum distance or use unmanned hose holders or monitor nozzles.
- Cool containers with flooding quantities of water until well after fire is out.
- Withdraw immediately in case of rising sound from venting safety devices or discoloration of tank.
- ALWAYS stay away from tanks engulfed in fire.

### SPILL OR LEAK

- Fully encapsulating, vapor-protective clothing should be worn for spills and leaks with no fire.
- ELIMINATE all ignition sources (no smoking, flares, sparks or flames in immediate area).
- Do not touch or walk through spilled material.
- Do not touch damaged containers or spilled material unless wearing appropriate protective clothing.
- Stop leak if you can do it without risk.

**Small Spill**

- Cover with water, sand or earth. Shovel into metal container and keep material under water.

**Large Spill**

- Dike for later disposal and cover with wet sand or earth.
- Prevent entry into waterways, sewers, basements or confined areas.

### FIRST AID

- Ensure that medical personnel are aware of the material(s) involved and take precautions to protect themselves.
- Move victim to fresh air.
- Call 911 or emergency medical service.
- Give artificial respiration if victim is not breathing.
- Administer oxygen if breathing is difficult.
- In case of contact with substance, keep exposed skin areas immersed in water or covered with wet bandages until medical attention is received.
- Removal of solidified molten material from skin requires medical assistance.
- Remove and isolate contaminated clothing and shoes at the site and place in metal container filled with water. Fire hazard if allowed to dry.
- Effects of exposure (inhalation, ingestion or skin contact) to substance may be delayed.
- Keep victim calm and warm.

# GUIDE 137 SUBSTANCES - WATER-REACTIVE - CORROSIVE

## POTENTIAL HAZARDS

### HEALTH

- CORROSIVE and/or TOXIC; inhalation, ingestion or contact (skin, eyes) with vapors, dusts or substance may cause severe injury, burns or death.
- Fire will produce irritating, corrosive and/or toxic gases.
- Reaction with water may generate much heat that will increase the concentration of fumes in the air.
- Contact with molten substance may cause severe burns to skin and eyes.
- Runoff from fire control or dilution water may cause pollution.

### FIRE OR EXPLOSION

- **EXCEPT FOR ACETIC ANHYDRIDE (UN1715), THAT IS FLAMMABLE,** some of these materials may burn, but none ignite readily.
- May ignite combustibles (wood, paper, oil, clothing, etc.).
- Substance will react with water (some violently), releasing corrosive and/or toxic gases and runoff.
- Flammable/toxic gases may accumulate in confined areas (basement, tanks, hopper/tank cars, etc.).
- Contact with metals may evolve flammable hydrogen gas.
- Containers may explode when heated or if contaminated with water.
- Substance may be transported in a molten form.

## PUBLIC SAFETY

- **CALL EMERGENCY RESPONSE Telephone Number on Shipping Paper first. If Shipping Paper not available or no answer, refer to appropriate telephone number listed on the inside back cover.**
- As an immediate precautionary measure, isolate spill or leak area in all directions for at least 50 meters (150 feet) for liquids and at least 25 meters (75 feet) for solids.
- Keep unauthorized personnel away.
- Stay upwind, uphill and/or upstream.
- Ventilate enclosed areas.

### PROTECTIVE CLOTHING

- Wear positive pressure self-contained breathing apparatus (SCBA).
- Wear chemical protective clothing that is specifically recommended by the manufacturer. It may provide little or no thermal protection.
- Structural firefighters' protective clothing provides limited protection in fire situations ONLY; it is not effective in spill situations where direct contact with the substance is possible.

### EVACUATION

**Spill**

- See Table 1 - Initial Isolation and Protective Action Distances for highlighted materials. For non-highlighted materials, increase, in the downwind direction, as necessary, the isolation distance shown under "PUBLIC SAFETY".

**Fire**

- If tank, rail car or tank truck is involved in a fire, ISOLATE for 800 meters (1/2 mile) in all directions; also, consider initial evacuation for 800 meters (1/2 mile) in all directions.

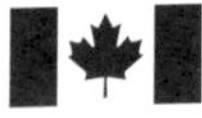

In Canada, an Emergency Response Assistance Plan (ERAP) may be required for this product. Please consult the shipping document and/or the ERAP Program Section (page 391).

## EMERGENCY RESPONSE

### FIRE

- **When material is not involved in fire, do not use water on material itself.**

**Small Fire**

- Dry chemical or $CO_2$.
- Move containers from fire area if you can do it without risk.

**Large Fire**

- Flood fire area with large quantities of water, while knocking down vapors with water fog. If insufficient water supply: knock down vapors only.

**Fire involving Tanks or Car/Trailer Loads**

- Cool containers with flooding quantities of water until well after fire is out.
- Do not get water inside containers.
- Withdraw immediately in case of rising sound from venting safety devices or discoloration of tank.
- ALWAYS stay away from tanks engulfed in fire.

### SPILL OR LEAK

- Fully encapsulating, vapor-protective clothing should be worn for spills and leaks with no fire.
- Do not touch damaged containers or spilled material unless wearing appropriate protective clothing.
- Stop leak if you can do it without risk.
- Use water spray to reduce vapors; do not put water directly on leak, spill area or inside container.
- Keep combustibles (wood, paper, oil, etc.) away from spilled material.

**Small Spill**

- Cover with DRY earth, DRY sand or other non-combustible material followed with plastic sheet to minimize spreading or contact with rain.
- Use clean, non-sparking tools to collect material and place it into loosely covered plastic containers for later disposal.
- Prevent entry into waterways, sewers, basements or confined areas.

### FIRST AID

- Ensure that medical personnel are aware of the material(s) involved and take precautions to protect themselves.
- Move victim to fresh air.
- Call 911 or emergency medical service.
- Give artificial respiration if victim is not breathing.
- **Do not use mouth-to-mouth method if victim ingested or inhaled the substance; give artificial respiration with the aid of a pocket mask equipped with a one-way valve or other proper respiratory medical device.**
- Administer oxygen if breathing is difficult.
- Remove and isolate contaminated clothing and shoes.
- In case of contact with substance, immediately flush skin or eyes with running water for at least 20 minutes.
- For minor skin contact, avoid spreading material on unaffected skin.
- Removal of solidified molten material from skin requires medical assistance.
- Keep victim calm and warm.
- Effects of exposure (inhalation, ingestion or skin contact) to substance may be delayed.

# GUIDE 138 SUBSTANCES - WATER-REACTIVE (EMITTING FLAMMABLE GASES)

## POTENTIAL HAZARDS

### FIRE OR EXPLOSION

- Produce flammable gases on contact with water.
- May ignite on contact with water or moist air.
- Some react vigorously or explosively on contact with water.
- May be ignited by heat, sparks or flames.
- May re-ignite after fire is extinguished.
- Some are transported in highly flammable liquids.
- Runoff may create fire or explosion hazard.

### HEALTH

- Inhalation or contact with vapors, substance or decomposition products may cause severe injury or death.
- May produce corrosive solutions on contact with water.
- Fire will produce irritating, corrosive and/or toxic gases.
- Runoff from fire control may cause pollution.

## PUBLIC SAFETY

- **CALL EMERGENCY RESPONSE Telephone Number on Shipping Paper first. If Shipping Paper not available or no answer, refer to appropriate telephone number listed on the inside back cover.**
- As an immediate precautionary measure, isolate spill or leak area in all directions for at least 50 meters (150 feet) for liquids and at least 25 meters (75 feet) for solids.
- Keep unauthorized personnel away.
- Stay upwind, uphill and/or upstream.
- Ventilate the area before entry.

### PROTECTIVE CLOTHING

- Wear positive pressure self-contained breathing apparatus (SCBA).
- Wear chemical protective clothing that is specifically recommended by the manufacturer. It may provide little or no thermal protection.
- Structural firefighters' protective clothing provides limited protection in fire situations ONLY; it is not effective in spill situations where direct contact with the substance is possible.

### EVACUATION

**Spill**

- See Table 1 - Initial Isolation and Protective Action Distances for highlighted materials. For non-highlighted materials, increase, in the downwind direction, as necessary, the isolation distance shown under "PUBLIC SAFETY".

**Fire**

- If tank, rail car or tank truck is involved in a fire, ISOLATE for 800 meters (1/2 mile) in all directions; also, consider initial evacuation for 800 meters (1/2 mile) in all directions.

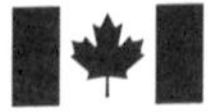

In Canada, an Emergency Response Assistance Plan (ERAP) may be required for this product. Please consult the shipping document and/or the ERAP Program Section (page 391).

## EMERGENCY RESPONSE

### FIRE

- **DO NOT USE WATER OR FOAM.**

**Small Fire**

- Dry chemical, soda ash, lime or sand.

**Large Fire**

- DRY sand, dry chemical, soda ash or lime or withdraw from area and let fire burn.
- Move containers from fire area if you can do it without risk.

**Fire Involving Metals or Powders (Aluminum, Lithium, Magnesium, etc.)**

- Use dry chemical, DRY sand, sodium chloride powder, graphite powder or Met-L-X® powder; in addition, for Lithium you may use Lith-X® powder or copper powder.
  Also, see GUIDE 170.

**Fire involving Tanks or Car/Trailer Loads**

- Fight fire from maximum distance or use unmanned hose holders or monitor nozzles.
- Do not get water inside containers.
- Cool containers with flooding quantities of water until well after fire is out.
- Withdraw immediately in case of rising sound from venting safety devices or discoloration of tank.
- ALWAYS stay away from tanks engulfed in fire.

### SPILL OR LEAK

- ELIMINATE all ignition sources (no smoking, flares, sparks or flames in immediate area).
- Do not touch or walk through spilled material.
- Stop leak if you can do it without risk.
- Use water spray to reduce vapors or divert vapor cloud drift. Avoid allowing water runoff to contact spilled material.
- **DO NOT GET WATER on spilled substance or inside containers.**

**Small Spill**

- Cover with DRY earth, DRY sand or other non-combustible material followed with plastic sheet to minimize spreading or contact with rain.
- Dike for later disposal; do not apply water unless directed to do so.

**Powder Spill**

- Cover powder spill with plastic sheet or tarp to minimize spreading and keep powder dry.
- **DO NOT CLEAN-UP OR DISPOSE OF, EXCEPT UNDER SUPERVISION OF A SPECIALIST.**

### FIRST AID

- Ensure that medical personnel are aware of the material(s) involved and take precautions to protect themselves.
- Move victim to fresh air.
- Call 911 or emergency medical service.
- Give artificial respiration if victim is not breathing.
- Administer oxygen if breathing is difficult.
- Remove and isolate contaminated clothing and shoes.
- In case of contact with substance, wipe from skin immediately; flush skin or eyes with running water for at least 20 minutes.
- Keep victim calm and warm.

## POTENTIAL HAZARDS

### FIRE OR EXPLOSION

- Produce flammable and toxic gases on contact with water.
- May ignite on contact with water or moist air.
- Some react vigorously or explosively on contact with water.
- May be ignited by heat, sparks or flames.
- May re-ignite after fire is extinguished.
- Some are transported in highly flammable liquids.
- Containers may explode when heated.
- Runoff may create fire or explosion hazard.

### HEALTH

- Highly toxic: contact with water produces toxic gas, may be fatal if inhaled.
- Inhalation or contact with vapors, substance or decomposition products may cause severe injury or death.
- May produce corrosive solutions on contact with water.
- Fire will produce irritating, corrosive and/or toxic gases.
- Runoff from fire control may cause pollution.

## PUBLIC SAFETY

- **CALL EMERGENCY RESPONSE Telephone Number on Shipping Paper first. If Shipping Paper not available or no answer, refer to appropriate telephone number listed on the inside back cover.**
- As an immediate precautionary measure, isolate spill or leak area in all directions for at least 50 meters (150 feet) for liquids and at least 25 meters (75 feet) for solids.
- Keep unauthorized personnel away.
- Stay upwind, uphill and/or upstream.
- Ventilate the area before entry.

### PROTECTIVE CLOTHING

- Wear positive pressure self-contained breathing apparatus (SCBA).
- Wear chemical protective clothing that is specifically recommended by the manufacturer. It may provide little or no thermal protection.
- Structural firefighters' protective clothing provides limited protection in fire situations ONLY; it is not effective in spill situations where direct contact with the substance is possible.

### EVACUATION

**Spill**

- See Table 1 - Initial Isolation and Protective Action Distances for highlighted materials. For non-highlighted materials, increase, in the downwind direction, as necessary, the isolation distance shown under "PUBLIC SAFETY".

**Fire**

- If tank, rail car or tank truck is involved in a fire, ISOLATE for 800 meters (1/2 mile) in all directions; also, consider initial evacuation for 800 meters (1/2 mile) in all directions.

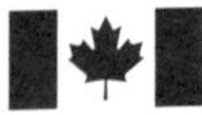

In Canada, an Emergency Response Assistance Plan (ERAP) may be required for this product. Please consult the shipping document and/or the ERAP Program Section (page 391).

## EMERGENCY RESPONSE

### FIRE

- **DO NOT USE WATER OR FOAM. (FOAM MAY BE USED FOR CHLOROSILANES, SEE BELOW)**

**Small Fire**

- Dry chemical, soda ash, lime or sand.

**Large Fire**

- DRY sand, dry chemical, soda ash or lime or withdraw from area and let fire burn.
- **FOR CHLOROSILANES, DO NOT USE WATER**; use AFFF alcohol-resistant medium-expansion foam; **DO NOT USE** dry chemicals, soda ash or lime on chlorosilane fires (large or small) as they may release large quantities of hydrogen gas that may explode.
- Move containers from fire area if you can do it without risk.

**Fire involving Tanks or Car/Trailer Loads**

- Fight fire from maximum distance or use unmanned hose holders or monitor nozzles.
- Cool containers with flooding quantities of water until well after fire is out.
- Do not get water inside containers.
- Withdraw immediately in case of rising sound from venting safety devices or discoloration of tank.
- ALWAYS stay away from tanks engulfed in fire.

### SPILL OR LEAK

- Fully encapsulating, vapor-protective clothing should be worn for spills and leaks with no fire.
- ELIMINATE all ignition sources (no smoking, flares, sparks or flames in immediate area).
- Do not touch or walk through spilled material.
- Stop leak if you can do it without risk.
- **DO NOT GET WATER on spilled substance or inside containers.**
- Use water spray to reduce vapors or divert vapor cloud drift. Avoid allowing water runoff to contact spilled material.
- **FOR CHLOROSILANES**, use AFFF alcohol-resistant medium-expansion foam to reduce vapors.

**Small Spill**

- Cover with DRY earth, DRY sand or other non-combustible material followed with plastic sheet to minimize spreading or contact with rain.
- Dike for later disposal; do not apply water unless directed to do so.

**Powder Spill**

- Cover powder spill with plastic sheet or tarp to minimize spreading and keep powder dry.
- **DO NOT CLEAN-UP OR DISPOSE OF, EXCEPT UNDER SUPERVISION OF A SPECIALIST.**

### FIRST AID

- Ensure that medical personnel are aware of the material(s) involved and take precautions to protect themselves.
- Move victim to fresh air.
- Call 911 or emergency medical service.
- Give artificial respiration if victim is not breathing.
- **Do not use mouth-to-mouth method if victim ingested or inhaled the substance; give artificial respiration with the aid of a pocket mask equipped with a one-way valve or other proper respiratory medical device.**
- Administer oxygen if breathing is difficult.
- Remove and isolate contaminated clothing and shoes.
- In case of contact with substance, wipe from skin immediately; flush skin or eyes with running water for at least 20 minutes.
- Keep victim calm and warm.

# GUIDE 140 OXIDIZERS

## POTENTIAL HAZARDS

### FIRE OR EXPLOSION

- These substances will accelerate burning when involved in a fire.
- Some may decompose explosively when heated or involved in a fire.
- May explode from heat or contamination.
- Some will react explosively with hydrocarbons (fuels).
- May ignite combustibles (wood, paper, oil, clothing, etc.).
- Containers may explode when heated.
- Runoff may create fire or explosion hazard.

### HEALTH

- Inhalation, ingestion or contact (skin, eyes) with vapors or substance may cause severe injury, burns or death.
- Fire may produce irritating, corrosive and/or toxic gases.
- Runoff from fire control or dilution water may cause pollution.

## PUBLIC SAFETY

- **CALL EMERGENCY RESPONSE Telephone Number on Shipping Paper first. If Shipping Paper not available or no answer, refer to appropriate telephone number listed on the inside back cover.**
- As an immediate precautionary measure, isolate spill or leak area in all directions for at least 50 meters (150 feet) for liquids and at least 25 meters (75 feet) for solids.
- Keep unauthorized personnel away.
- Stay upwind, uphill and/or upstream.
- Ventilate closed spaces before entering.

### PROTECTIVE CLOTHING

- Wear positive pressure self-contained breathing apparatus (SCBA).
- Wear chemical protective clothing that is specifically recommended by the manufacturer. It may provide little or no thermal protection.
- Structural firefighters' protective clothing will only provide limited protection.

### EVACUATION

**Large Spill**

- Consider initial downwind evacuation for at least 100 meters (330 feet).

**Fire**

- If tank, rail car or tank truck is involved in a fire, ISOLATE for 800 meters (1/2 mile) in all directions; also, consider initial evacuation for 800 meters (1/2 mile) in all directions.

In Canada, an Emergency Response Assistance Plan (ERAP) may be required for this product. Please consult the shipping document and/or the ERAP Program Section (page 391).

## EMERGENCY RESPONSE

### FIRE

**Small Fire**

- Use water. Do not use dry chemicals or foams. $CO_2$ or Halon® may provide limited control.

**Large Fire**

- Flood fire area with water from a distance.
- Do not move cargo or vehicle if cargo has been exposed to heat.
- Move containers from fire area if you can do it without risk.

**Fire involving Tanks or Car/Trailer Loads**

- Fight fire from maximum distance or use unmanned hose holders or monitor nozzles.
- Cool containers with flooding quantities of water until well after fire is out.
- ALWAYS stay away from tanks engulfed in fire.
- For massive fire, use unmanned hose holders or monitor nozzles; if this is impossible, withdraw from area and let fire burn.

### SPILL OR LEAK

- Keep combustibles (wood, paper, oil, etc.) away from spilled material.
- Do not touch damaged containers or spilled material unless wearing appropriate protective clothing.
- Stop leak if you can do it without risk.
- Do not get water inside containers.

**Small Dry Spill**

- With clean shovel, place material into clean, dry container and cover loosely; move containers from spill area.

**Small Liquid Spill**

- Use a non-combustible material like vermiculite or sand to soak up the product and place into a container for later disposal.

**Large Spill**

- Dike far ahead of liquid spill for later disposal.
- **Following product recovery, flush area with water.**

### FIRST AID

- Ensure that medical personnel are aware of the material(s) involved and take precautions to protect themselves.
- Move victim to fresh air.
- Call 911 or emergency medical service.
- Give artificial respiration if victim is not breathing.
- Administer oxygen if breathing is difficult.
- Remove and isolate contaminated clothing and shoes.
- Contaminated clothing may be a fire risk when dry.
- In case of contact with substance, immediately flush skin or eyes with running water for at least 20 minutes.
- Keep victim calm and warm.

# GUIDE 141 OXIDIZERS - TOXIC

## POTENTIAL HAZARDS

### FIRE OR EXPLOSION

- These substances will accelerate burning when involved in a fire.
- May explode from heat or contamination.
- Some may burn rapidly.
- Some will react explosively with hydrocarbons (fuels).
- May ignite combustibles (wood, paper, oil, clothing, etc.).
- Containers may explode when heated.
- Runoff may create fire or explosion hazard.

### HEALTH

- Toxic by ingestion.
- Inhalation of dust is toxic.
- Fire may produce irritating, corrosive and/or toxic gases.
- Contact with substance may cause severe burns to skin and eyes.
- Runoff from fire control or dilution water may cause pollution.

## PUBLIC SAFETY

- **CALL EMERGENCY RESPONSE Telephone Number on Shipping Paper first. If Shipping Paper not available or no answer, refer to appropriate telephone number listed on the inside back cover.**
- As an immediate precautionary measure, isolate spill or leak area in all directions for at least 50 meters (150 feet) for liquids and at least 25 meters (75 feet) for solids.
- Keep unauthorized personnel away.
- Stay upwind, uphill and/or upstream.
- Ventilate closed spaces before entering.

### PROTECTIVE CLOTHING

- Wear positive pressure self-contained breathing apparatus (SCBA).
- Wear chemical protective clothing that is specifically recommended by the manufacturer. It may provide little or no thermal protection.
- Structural firefighters' protective clothing will only provide limited protection.

### EVACUATION

**Large Spill**

- Consider initial downwind evacuation for at least 100 meters (330 feet).

**Fire**

- If tank, rail car or tank truck is involved in a fire, ISOLATE for 800 meters (1/2 mile) in all directions; also, consider initial evacuation for 800 meters (1/2 mile) in all directions.

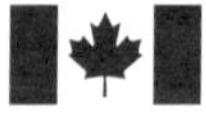

In Canada, an Emergency Response Assistance Plan (ERAP) may be required for this product. Please consult the shipping document and/or the ERAP Program Section (page 391).

## EMERGENCY RESPONSE

### FIRE

**Small Fire**

- Use water. Do not use dry chemicals or foams. $CO_2$ or Halon® may provide limited control.

**Large Fire**

- Flood fire area with water from a distance.
- Do not move cargo or vehicle if cargo has been exposed to heat.
- Move containers from fire area if you can do it without risk.

**Fire involving Tanks or Car/Trailer Loads**

- Fight fire from maximum distance or use unmanned hose holders or monitor nozzles.
- Cool containers with flooding quantities of water until well after fire is out.
- ALWAYS stay away from tanks engulfed in fire.
- For massive fire, use unmanned hose holders or monitor nozzles; if this is impossible, withdraw from area and let fire burn.

### SPILL OR LEAK

- Keep combustibles (wood, paper, oil, etc.) away from spilled material.
- Do not touch damaged containers or spilled material unless wearing appropriate protective clothing.
- Stop leak if you can do it without risk.

**Small Dry Spill**

- With clean shovel, place material into clean, dry container and cover loosely; move containers from spill area.

**Large Spill**

- Dike far ahead of spill for later disposal.

### FIRST AID

- Ensure that medical personnel are aware of the material(s) involved and take precautions to protect themselves.
- Move victim to fresh air.
- Call 911 or emergency medical service.
- Give artificial respiration if victim is not breathing.
- Administer oxygen if breathing is difficult.
- Remove and isolate contaminated clothing and shoes.
- Contaminated clothing may be a fire risk when dry.
- In case of contact with substance, immediately flush skin or eyes with running water for at least 20 minutes.
- Keep victim calm and warm.

# GUIDE 142 Oxidizers - Toxic (Liquid)

## POTENTIAL HAZARDS

### FIRE OR EXPLOSION

- These substances will accelerate burning when involved in a fire.
- May explode from heat or contamination.
- Some will react explosively with hydrocarbons (fuels).
- May ignite combustibles (wood, paper, oil, clothing, etc.).
- Containers may explode when heated.
- Runoff may create fire or explosion hazard.

### HEALTH

- **TOXIC;** inhalation, ingestion or contact (skin, eyes) with vapors or substance may cause severe injury, burns or death.
- Fire may produce irritating, corrosive and/or toxic gases.
- Toxic/flammable fumes may accumulate in confined areas (basement, tanks, tank cars, etc.).
- Runoff from fire control or dilution water may cause pollution.

## PUBLIC SAFETY

- **CALL EMERGENCY RESPONSE Telephone Number on Shipping Paper first. If Shipping Paper not available or no answer, refer to appropriate telephone number listed on the inside back cover.**
- As an immediate precautionary measure, isolate spill or leak area for at least 50 meters (150 feet) in all directions.
- Keep unauthorized personnel away.
- Stay upwind, uphill and/or upstream.
- Ventilate closed spaces before entering.

### PROTECTIVE CLOTHING

- Wear positive pressure self-contained breathing apparatus (SCBA).
- Wear chemical protective clothing that is specifically recommended by the manufacturer. It may provide little or no thermal protection.
- Structural firefighters' protective clothing provides limited protection in fire situations ONLY; it is not effective in spill situations where direct contact with the substance is possible.

### EVACUATION

**Spill**

- See Table 1 - Initial Isolation and Protective Action Distances for highlighted materials. For non-highlighted materials, increase, in the downwind direction, as necessary, the isolation distance shown under "PUBLIC SAFETY".

**Fire**

- If tank, rail car or tank truck is involved in a fire, ISOLATE for 800 meters (1/2 mile) in all directions; also, consider initial evacuation for 800 meters (1/2 mile) in all directions.

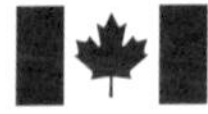

In Canada, an Emergency Response Assistance Plan (ERAP) may be required for this product. Please consult the shipping document and/or the ERAP Program Section (page 391).

## EMERGENCY RESPONSE

### FIRE

**Small Fire**

- Use water. Do not use dry chemicals or foams. $CO_2$ or Halon® may provide limited control.

**Large Fire**

- Flood fire area with water from a distance.
- Do not move cargo or vehicle if cargo has been exposed to heat.
- Move containers from fire area if you can do it without risk.

**Fire involving Tanks or Car/Trailer Loads**

- Fight fire from maximum distance or use unmanned hose holders or monitor nozzles.
- Cool containers with flooding quantities of water until well after fire is out.
- ALWAYS stay away from tanks engulfed in fire.
- For massive fire, use unmanned hose holders or monitor nozzles; if this is impossible, withdraw from area and let fire burn.

### SPILL OR LEAK

- Keep combustibles (wood, paper, oil, etc.) away from spilled material.
- Fully encapsulating, vapor-protective clothing should be worn for spills and leaks with no fire.
- Do not touch damaged containers or spilled material unless wearing appropriate protective clothing.
- Stop leak if you can do it without risk.
- Use water spray to reduce vapors or divert vapor cloud drift.
- Do not get water inside containers.

**Small Liquid Spill**

- Use a non-combustible material like vermiculite or sand to soak up the product and place into a container for later disposal.

**Large Spill**

- Dike far ahead of liquid spill for later disposal.

### FIRST AID

- Ensure that medical personnel are aware of the material(s) involved and take precautions to protect themselves.
- Move victim to fresh air.
- Call 911 or emergency medical service.
- Give artificial respiration if victim is not breathing.
- **Do not use mouth-to-mouth method if victim ingested or inhaled the substance; give artificial respiration with the aid of a pocket mask equipped with a one-way valve or other proper respiratory medical device.**
- Administer oxygen if breathing is difficult.
- Remove and isolate contaminated clothing and shoes.
- Contaminated clothing may be a fire risk when dry.
- In case of contact with substance, immediately flush skin or eyes with running water for at least 20 minutes.
- Keep victim calm and warm.

# GUIDE 143 OXIDIZERS (UNSTABLE)

## POTENTIAL HAZARDS

### FIRE OR EXPLOSION

- May explode from friction, heat or contamination.
- These substances will accelerate burning when involved in a fire.
- May ignite combustibles (wood, paper, oil, clothing, etc.).
- Some will react explosively with hydrocarbons (fuels).
- Containers may explode when heated.
- Runoff may create fire or explosion hazard.

### HEALTH

- **TOXIC;** inhalation, ingestion or contact (skin, eyes) with vapors, dusts or substance may cause severe injury, burns or death.
- Fire may produce irritating and/or toxic gases.
- Toxic fumes or dust may accumulate in confined areas (basement, tanks, hopper/tank cars, etc.).
- Runoff from fire control or dilution water may cause pollution.

## PUBLIC SAFETY

- **CALL EMERGENCY RESPONSE Telephone Number on Shipping Paper first. If Shipping Paper not available or no answer, refer to appropriate telephone number listed on the inside back cover.**
- As an immediate precautionary measure, isolate spill or leak area in all directions for at least 50 meters (150 feet) for liquids and at least 25 meters (75 feet) for solids.
- Keep unauthorized personnel away.
- Stay upwind, uphill and/or upstream.
- Ventilate closed spaces before entering.

### PROTECTIVE CLOTHING

- Wear positive pressure self-contained breathing apparatus (SCBA).
- Wear chemical protective clothing that is specifically recommended by the manufacturer. It may provide little or no thermal protection.
- Structural firefighters' protective clothing provides limited protection in fire situations ONLY; it is not effective in spill situations where direct contact with the substance is possible.

### EVACUATION

**Spill**

- See Table 1 - Initial Isolation and Protective Action Distances for highlighted materials. For non-highlighted materials, increase, in the downwind direction, as necessary, the isolation distance shown under "PUBLIC SAFETY".

**Fire**

- If tank, rail car or tank truck is involved in a fire, ISOLATE for 800 meters (1/2 mile) in all directions; also, consider initial evacuation for 800 meters (1/2 mile) in all directions.

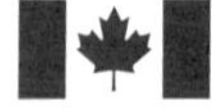

In Canada, an Emergency Response Assistance Plan (ERAP) may be required for this product. Please consult the shipping document and/or the ERAP Program Section (page 391).

## EMERGENCY RESPONSE

### FIRE

**Small Fire**

- Use water. Do not use dry chemicals or foams. $CO_2$ or Halon® may provide limited control.

**Large Fire**

- Flood fire area with water from a distance.
- Do not move cargo or vehicle if cargo has been exposed to heat.
- Move containers from fire area if you can do it without risk.
- Do not get water inside containers: a violent reaction may occur.

**Fire involving Tanks or Car/Trailer Loads**

- Cool containers with flooding quantities of water until well after fire is out.
- Dike fire-control water for later disposal.
- ALWAYS stay away from tanks engulfed in fire.
- For massive fire, use unmanned hose holders or monitor nozzles; if this is impossible, withdraw from area and let fire burn.

### SPILL OR LEAK

- Keep combustibles (wood, paper, oil, etc.) away from spilled material.
- Do not touch damaged containers or spilled material unless wearing appropriate protective clothing.
- Use water spray to reduce vapors or divert vapor cloud drift.
- Prevent entry into waterways, sewers, basements or confined areas.

**Small Spill**

- Flush area with flooding quantities of water.

**Large Spill**

- **DO NOT CLEAN-UP OR DISPOSE OF, EXCEPT UNDER SUPERVISION OF A SPECIALIST.**

### FIRST AID

- Ensure that medical personnel are aware of the material(s) involved and take precautions to protect themselves.
- Move victim to fresh air.
- Call 911 or emergency medical service.
- Give artificial respiration if victim is not breathing.
- Administer oxygen if breathing is difficult.
- Remove and isolate contaminated clothing and shoes.
- Contaminated clothing may be a fire risk when dry.
- In case of contact with substance, immediately flush skin or eyes with running water for at least 20 minutes.
- Keep victim calm and warm.

# GUIDE 144 OXIDIZERS (WATER-REACTIVE)

## POTENTIAL HAZARDS

### FIRE OR EXPLOSION

- May ignite combustibles (wood, paper, oil, clothing, etc.).
- React vigorously and/or explosively with water.
- Produce toxic and/or corrosive substances on contact with water.
- Flammable/toxic gases may accumulate in tanks and hopper cars.
- Some may produce flammable hydrogen gas upon contact with metals.
- Containers may explode when heated.
- Runoff may create fire or explosion hazard.

### HEALTH

- **TOXIC;** inhalation or contact with vapor, substance, or decomposition products may cause severe injury or death.
- Fire will produce irritating, corrosive and/or toxic gases.
- Runoff from fire control or dilution water may cause pollution.

## PUBLIC SAFETY

- **CALL EMERGENCY RESPONSE Telephone Number on Shipping Paper first. If Shipping Paper not available or no answer, refer to appropriate telephone number listed on the inside back cover.**
- As an immediate precautionary measure, isolate spill or leak area in all directions for at least 50 meters (150 feet) for liquids and at least 25 meters (75 feet) for solids.
- Keep unauthorized personnel away.
- Stay upwind, uphill and/or upstream.
- Ventilate closed spaces before entering.

### PROTECTIVE CLOTHING

- Wear positive pressure self-contained breathing apparatus (SCBA).
- Wear chemical protective clothing that is specifically recommended by the manufacturer. It may provide little or no thermal protection.
- Structural firefighters' protective clothing provides limited protection in fire situations ONLY; it is not effective in spill situations where direct contact with the substance is possible.

### EVACUATION

**Spill**

- See Table 1 - Initial Isolation and Protective Action Distances for highlighted materials. For non-highlighted materials, increase, in the downwind direction, as necessary, the isolation distance shown under "PUBLIC SAFETY".

**Fire**

- If tank, rail car or tank truck is involved in a fire, ISOLATE for 800 meters (1/2 mile) in all directions; also, consider initial evacuation for 800 meters (1/2 mile) in all directions.

In Canada, an Emergency Response Assistance Plan (ERAP) may be required for this product. Please consult the shipping document and/or the ERAP Program Section (page 391).

## EMERGENCY RESPONSE

### FIRE

- **DO NOT USE WATER OR FOAM.**

**Small Fire**

- Dry chemical, soda ash or lime.

**Large Fire**

- DRY sand, dry chemical, soda ash or lime or withdraw from area and let fire burn.
- Do not move cargo or vehicle if cargo has been exposed to heat.
- Move containers from fire area if you can do it without risk.

**Fire involving Tanks or Car/Trailer Loads**

- Fight fire from maximum distance or use unmanned hose holders or monitor nozzles.
- Cool containers with flooding quantities of water until well after fire is out.
- Withdraw immediately in case of rising sound from venting safety devices or discoloration of tank.
- ALWAYS stay away from tanks engulfed in fire.

### SPILL OR LEAK

- ELIMINATE all ignition sources (no smoking, flares, sparks or flames in immediate area).
- Do not touch damaged containers or spilled material unless wearing appropriate protective clothing.
- Stop leak if you can do it without risk.
- Use water spray to reduce vapors or divert vapor cloud drift. Avoid allowing water runoff to contact spilled material.
- **DO NOT GET WATER on spilled substance or inside containers.**

**Small Spill**

- Cover with DRY earth, DRY sand or other non-combustible material followed with plastic sheet to minimize spreading or contact with rain.

**Large Spill**

- **DO NOT CLEAN-UP OR DISPOSE OF, EXCEPT UNDER SUPERVISION OF A SPECIALIST.**

### FIRST AID

- Ensure that medical personnel are aware of the material(s) involved and take precautions to protect themselves.
- Move victim to fresh air.
- Call 911 or emergency medical service.
- Give artificial respiration if victim is not breathing.
- **Do not use mouth-to-mouth method if victim ingested or inhaled the substance; give artificial respiration with the aid of a pocket mask equipped with a one-way valve or other proper respiratory medical device.**
- Administer oxygen if breathing is difficult.
- Remove and isolate contaminated clothing and shoes.
- Contaminated clothing may be a fire risk when dry.
- In case of contact with substance, immediately flush skin or eyes with running water for at least 20 minutes.
- Keep victim calm and warm.
- Keep victim under observation.
- Effects of contact or inhalation may be delayed.

# GUIDE 145 ORGANIC PEROXIDES (HEAT AND CONTAMINATION SENSITIVE)

## POTENTIAL HAZARDS

### FIRE OR EXPLOSION

- May explode from heat or contamination.
- May ignite combustibles (wood, paper, oil, clothing, etc.).
- May be ignited by heat, sparks or flames.
- May burn rapidly with flare-burning effect.
- Containers may explode when heated.
- Runoff may create fire or explosion hazard.

### HEALTH

- Fire may produce irritating, corrosive and/or toxic gases.
- Ingestion or contact (skin, eyes) with substance may cause severe injury or burns.
- Runoff from fire control or dilution water may cause pollution.

## PUBLIC SAFETY

- **CALL EMERGENCY RESPONSE Telephone Number on Shipping Paper first. If Shipping Paper not available or no answer, refer to appropriate telephone number listed on the inside back cover.**
- As an immediate precautionary measure, isolate spill or leak area in all directions for at least 50 meters (150 feet) for liquids and at least 25 meters (75 feet) for solids.
- Keep unauthorized personnel away.
- Stay upwind, uphill and/or upstream.

### PROTECTIVE CLOTHING

- Wear positive pressure self-contained breathing apparatus (SCBA).
- Wear chemical protective clothing that is specifically recommended by the manufacturer. It may provide little or no thermal protection.
- Structural firefighters' protective clothing will only provide limited protection.

### EVACUATION

**Large Spill**

- Consider initial evacuation for at least 250 meters (800 feet) in all directions.

**Fire**

- If tank, rail car or tank truck is involved in a fire, ISOLATE for 800 meters (1/2 mile) in all directions; also, consider initial evacuation for 800 meters (1/2 mile) in all directions.

## EMERGENCY RESPONSE

### FIRE

**Small Fire**

- Water spray or fog is preferred; if water not available use dry chemical, $CO_2$ or regular foam.

**Large Fire**

- Flood fire area with water from a distance.
- Use water spray or fog; do not use straight streams.
- Do not move cargo or vehicle if cargo has been exposed to heat.
- Move containers from fire area if you can do it without risk.

**Fire involving Tanks or Car/Trailer Loads**

- Fight fire from maximum distance or use unmanned hose holders or monitor nozzles.
- Cool containers with flooding quantities of water until well after fire is out.
- ALWAYS stay away from tanks engulfed in fire.
- For massive fire, use unmanned hose holders or monitor nozzles; if this is impossible, withdraw from area and let fire burn.

### SPILL OR LEAK

- ELIMINATE all ignition sources (no smoking, flares, sparks or flames in immediate area).
- Keep combustibles (wood, paper, oil, etc.) away from spilled material.
- Do not touch damaged containers or spilled material unless wearing appropriate protective clothing.
- Keep substance wet using water spray.
- Stop leak if you can do it without risk.

**Small Spill**

- Pick up with inert, damp, non-combustible material using clean, non-sparking tools and place into loosely covered plastic containers for later disposal.

**Large Spill**

- Wet down with water and dike for later disposal.
- Prevent entry into waterways, sewers, basements or confined areas.
- **DO NOT CLEAN-UP OR DISPOSE OF, EXCEPT UNDER SUPERVISION OF A SPECIALIST.**

### FIRST AID

- Ensure that medical personnel are aware of the material(s) involved and take precautions to protect themselves.
- Move victim to fresh air.
- Call 911 or emergency medical service.
- Give artificial respiration if victim is not breathing.
- Administer oxygen if breathing is difficult.
- Remove and isolate contaminated clothing and shoes.
- Contaminated clothing may be a fire risk when dry.
- Remove material from skin immediately.
- In case of contact with substance, immediately flush skin or eyes with running water for at least 20 minutes.
- Keep victim calm and warm.

# GUIDE 146 ORGANIC PEROXIDES (HEAT, CONTAMINATION AND FRICTION SENSITIVE)

## POTENTIAL HAZARDS

### FIRE OR EXPLOSION

- May explode from heat, shock, friction or contamination.
- May ignite combustibles (wood, paper, oil, clothing, etc.).
- May be ignited by heat, sparks or flames.
- May burn rapidly with flare-burning effect.
- Containers may explode when heated.
- Runoff may create fire or explosion hazard.

### HEALTH

- Fire may produce irritating, corrosive and/or toxic gases.
- Ingestion or contact (skin, eyes) with substance may cause severe injury or burns.
- Runoff from fire control or dilution water may cause pollution.

## PUBLIC SAFETY

- **CALL EMERGENCY RESPONSE Telephone Number on Shipping Paper first. If Shipping Paper not available or no answer, refer to appropriate telephone number listed on the inside back cover.**
- As an immediate precautionary measure, isolate spill or leak area in all directions for at least 50 meters (150 feet) for liquids and at least 25 meters (75 feet) for solids.
- Keep unauthorized personnel away.
- Stay upwind, uphill and/or upstream.

### PROTECTIVE CLOTHING

- Wear positive pressure self-contained breathing apparatus (SCBA).
- Wear chemical protective clothing that is specifically recommended by the manufacturer. It may provide little or no thermal protection.
- Structural firefighters' protective clothing will only provide limited protection.

### EVACUATION

**Large Spill**

- Consider initial evacuation for at least 250 meters (800 feet) in all directions.

**Fire**

- If tank, rail car or tank truck is involved in a fire, ISOLATE for 800 meters (1/2 mile) in all directions; also, consider initial evacuation for 800 meters (1/2 mile) in all directions.

In Canada, an Emergency Response Assistance Plan (ERAP) may be required for this product. Please consult the shipping document and/or the ERAP Program Section (page 391).

## EMERGENCY RESPONSE

### FIRE

**Small Fire**

- Water spray or fog is preferred; if water not available use dry chemical, $CO_2$ or regular foam.

**Large Fire**

- Flood fire area with water from a distance.
- Use water spray or fog; do not use straight streams.
- Do not move cargo or vehicle if cargo has been exposed to heat.
- Move containers from fire area if you can do it without risk.

**Fire involving Tanks or Car/Trailer Loads**

- Fight fire from maximum distance or use unmanned hose holders or monitor nozzles.
- Cool containers with flooding quantities of water until well after fire is out.
- ALWAYS stay away from tanks engulfed in fire.
- For massive fire, use unmanned hose holders or monitor nozzles; if this is impossible, withdraw from area and let fire burn.

### SPILL OR LEAK

- ELIMINATE all ignition sources (no smoking, flares, sparks or flames in immediate area).
- Keep combustibles (wood, paper, oil, etc.) away from spilled material.
- Do not touch damaged containers or spilled material unless wearing appropriate protective clothing.
- Keep substance wet using water spray.
- Stop leak if you can do it without risk.

**Small Spill**

- Pick up with inert, damp, non-combustible material using clean, non-sparking tools and place into loosely covered plastic containers for later disposal.

**Large Spill**

- Wet down with water and dike for later disposal.
- Prevent entry into waterways, sewers, basements or confined areas.
- **DO NOT CLEAN-UP OR DISPOSE OF, EXCEPT UNDER SUPERVISION OF A SPECIALIST.**

### FIRST AID

- Ensure that medical personnel are aware of the material(s) involved and take precautions to protect themselves.
- Move victim to fresh air.
- Call 911 or emergency medical service.
- Give artificial respiration if victim is not breathing.
- Administer oxygen if breathing is difficult.
- Remove and isolate contaminated clothing and shoes.
- Contaminated clothing may be a fire risk when dry.
- Remove material from skin immediately.
- In case of contact with substance, immediately flush skin or eyes with running water for at least 20 minutes.
- Keep victim calm and warm.

# GUIDE 147 LITHIUM ION BATTERIES

## POTENTIAL HAZARDS

### FIRE OR EXPLOSION

- Lithium ion batteries contain flammable liquid electrolyte that may vent, ignite and produce sparks when subjected to high temperatures (> 150 °C (302 °F)), when damaged or abused (e.g., mechanical damage or electrical overcharging).
- May burn rapidly with flare-burning effect.
- May ignite other batteries in close proximity.

### HEALTH

- Contact with battery electrolyte may be irritating to skin, eyes and mucous membranes.
- Fire will produce irritating, corrosive and/or toxic gases.
- Burning batteries may produce toxic hydrogen fluoride gas (see GUIDE 125).
- Fumes may cause dizziness or suffocation.

## PUBLIC SAFETY

- **CALL Emergency Response Telephone Number on Shipping Paper first. If Shipping Paper not available or no answer, refer to appropriate telephone number listed on the inside back cover.**
- As an immediate precautionary measure, isolate spill or leak area for at least 25 meters (75 feet) in all directions.
- Keep unauthorized personnel away.
- Stay upwind, uphill and/or upstream.
- Ventilate closed spaces before entering.

### PROTECTIVE CLOTHING

- Wear positive pressure self-contained breathing apparatus (SCBA).
- Structural firefighters' protective clothing will only provide limited protection.

### EVACUATION

**Large Spill**

- Consider initial downwind evacuation for at least 100 meters (330 feet).

**Fire**

- If rail car or trailer is involved in a fire, ISOLATE for 500 meters (1/3 mile) in all directions; also initiate evacuation including emergency responders for 500 meters (1/3 mile) in all directions.

## EMERGENCY RESPONSE

### FIRE

**Small Fire**

- Dry chemical, $CO_2$, water spray or regular foam.

**Large Fire**

- Water spray, fog or regular foam.
- Move containers from fire area if you can do it without risk.

### SPILL OR LEAK

- ELIMINATE all ignition sources (no smoking, flares, sparks or flames in immediate area).
- Do not touch or walk through spilled material.
- Absorb with earth, sand or other non-combustible material.
- Leaking batteries and contaminated absorbent material should be placed in metal containers.

### FIRST AID

- Ensure that medical personnel are aware of the material(s) involved and take precautions to protect themselves.
- Move victim to fresh air.
- Call 911 or emergency medical service.
- Give artificial respiration if victim is not breathing.
- Administer oxygen if breathing is difficult.
- Remove and isolate contaminated clothing and shoes.
- In case of contact with substance, immediately flush skin or eyes with running water for at least 20 minutes.

# GUIDE 148 ORGANIC PEROXIDES (HEAT AND CONTAMINATION SENSITIVE/TEMPERATURE CONTROLLED)

## POTENTIAL HAZARDS

### FIRE OR EXPLOSION

- May explode from heat, contamination or loss of temperature control.
- These materials are particularly sensitive to temperature rises. Above a given "Control Temperature" they decompose violently and catch fire.
- May ignite combustibles (wood, paper, oil, clothing, etc.).
- May ignite spontaneously if exposed to air.
- May be ignited by heat, sparks or flames.
- May burn rapidly with flare-burning effect.
- Containers may explode when heated.
- Runoff may create fire or explosion hazard.

### HEALTH

- Fire may produce irritating, corrosive and/or toxic gases.
- Ingestion or contact (skin, eyes) with substance may cause severe injury or burns.
- Runoff from fire control or dilution water may cause pollution.

## PUBLIC SAFETY

- **CALL EMERGENCY RESPONSE Telephone Number on Shipping Paper first. If Shipping Paper not available or no answer, refer to appropriate telephone number listed on the inside back cover.**
- As an immediate precautionary measure, isolate spill or leak area in all directions for at least 50 meters (150 feet) for liquids and at least 25 meters (75 feet) for solids.
- Keep unauthorized personnel away.
- Stay upwind, uphill and/or upstream.
- **DO NOT allow the substance to warm up. Obtain liquid nitrogen (wear thermal protective clothing, see GUIDE 120), dry ice or ice for cooling. If this is not possible or none can be obtained, evacuate the area immediately.**

### PROTECTIVE CLOTHING

- Wear positive pressure self-contained breathing apparatus (SCBA).
- Wear chemical protective clothing that is specifically recommended by the manufacturer. It may provide little or no thermal protection.
- Structural firefighters' protective clothing will only provide limited protection.

### EVACUATION

**Large Spill**

- Consider initial evacuation for at least 250 meters (800 feet) in all directions.

**Fire**

- If tank, rail car or tank truck is involved in a fire, ISOLATE for 800 meters (1/2 mile) in all directions; also, consider initial evacuation for 800 meters (1/2 mile) in all directions.

In Canada, an Emergency Response Assistance Plan (ERAP) may be required for this product. Please consult the shipping document and/or the ERAP Program Section (page 391).

## EMERGENCY RESPONSE

### FIRE

- **The temperature of the substance must be maintained at or below the "Control Temperature" at all times.**

**Small Fire**

- Water spray or fog is preferred; if water not available use dry chemical, $CO_2$ or regular foam.

**Large Fire**

- Flood fire area with water from a distance.
- Use water spray or fog; do not use straight streams.
- Do not move cargo or vehicle if cargo has been exposed to heat.
- Move containers from fire area if you can do it without risk.

**Fire involving Tanks or Car/Trailer Loads**

- Fight fire from maximum distance or use unmanned hose holders or monitor nozzles.
- Cool containers with flooding quantities of water until well after fire is out.
- **BEWARE OF POSSIBLE CONTAINER EXPLOSION.**
- ALWAYS stay away from tanks engulfed in fire.
- For massive fire, use unmanned hose holders or monitor nozzles; if this is impossible, withdraw from area and let fire burn.

### SPILL OR LEAK

- ELIMINATE all ignition sources (no smoking, flares, sparks or flames in immediate area).
- Keep combustibles (wood, paper, oil, etc.) away from spilled material.
- Do not touch or walk through spilled material.
- Stop leak if you can do it without risk.

**Small Spill**

- Pick up with inert, damp, non-combustible material using clean, non-sparking tools and place into loosely covered plastic containers for later disposal.

**Large Spill**

- Dike far ahead of liquid spill for later disposal.
- Prevent entry into waterways, sewers, basements or confined areas.
- **DO NOT CLEAN-UP OR DISPOSE OF, EXCEPT UNDER SUPERVISION OF A SPECIALIST.**

### FIRST AID

- Ensure that medical personnel are aware of the material(s) involved and take precautions to protect themselves.
- Move victim to fresh air.
- Call 911 or emergency medical service.
- Give artificial respiration if victim is not breathing.
- Administer oxygen if breathing is difficult.
- Remove and isolate contaminated clothing and shoes.
- Contaminated clothing may be a fire risk when dry.
- Remove material from skin immediately.
- In case of contact with substance, immediately flush skin or eyes with running water for at least 20 minutes.
- Keep victim calm and warm.

# GUIDE 149 SUBSTANCES (SELF-REACTIVE)

## POTENTIAL HAZARDS

### FIRE OR EXPLOSION

- **Self-decomposition, self-polymerization, or self-ignition may be triggered by heat, chemical reaction, friction or impact.**
- May be ignited by heat, sparks or flames.
- Some may decompose explosively when heated or involved in a fire.
- Those substances designated with a **(P)** may polymerize explosively when heated or involved in a fire.
- May burn violently. Decomposition or polymerization may be self-accelerating and produce large amounts of gases.
- Vapors or dust may form explosive mixtures with air.

### HEALTH

- Inhalation or contact with vapors, substance or decomposition products may cause severe injury or death.
- May produce irritating, toxic and/or corrosive gases.
- Runoff from fire control may cause pollution.

## PUBLIC SAFETY

- **CALL EMERGENCY RESPONSE Telephone Number on Shipping Paper first. If Shipping Paper not available or no answer, refer to appropriate telephone number listed on the inside back cover.**
- As an immediate precautionary measure, isolate spill or leak area in all directions for at least 50 meters (150 feet) for liquids and at least 25 meters (75 feet) for solids.
- Keep unauthorized personnel away.
- Stay upwind, uphill and/or upstream.

### PROTECTIVE CLOTHING

- Wear positive pressure self-contained breathing apparatus (SCBA).
- Wear chemical protective clothing that is specifically recommended by the manufacturer. It may provide little or no thermal protection.
- Structural firefighters' protective clothing will only provide limited protection.

### EVACUATION

**Large Spill**

- Consider initial evacuation for at least 250 meters (800 feet) in all directions.

**Fire**

- If tank, rail car or tank truck is involved in a fire, ISOLATE for 800 meters (1/2 mile) in all directions; also, consider initial evacuation for 800 meters (1/2 mile) in all directions.

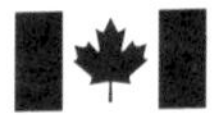

In Canada, an Emergency Response Assistance Plan (ERAP) may be required for this product. Please consult the shipping document and/or the ERAP Program Section (page 391).

## EMERGENCY RESPONSE

### FIRE

**Small Fire**

- Dry chemical, $CO_2$, water spray or regular foam.

**Large Fire**

- Flood fire area with water from a distance.
- Move containers from fire area if you can do it without risk.

**Fire involving Tanks or Car/Trailer Loads**

- **BEWARE OF POSSIBLE CONTAINER EXPLOSION.**
- Fight fire from maximum distance or use unmanned hose holders or monitor nozzles.
- Cool containers with flooding quantities of water until well after fire is out.
- Withdraw immediately in case of rising sound from venting safety devices or discoloration of tank.
- ALWAYS stay away from tanks engulfed in fire.

### SPILL OR LEAK

- ELIMINATE all ignition sources (no smoking, flares, sparks or flames in immediate area).
- Do not touch or walk through spilled material.
- Stop leak if you can do it without risk.

**Small Spill**

- Pick up with inert, damp, non-combustible material using clean, non-sparking tools and place into loosely covered plastic containers for later disposal.
- Prevent entry into waterways, sewers, basements or confined areas.

### FIRST AID

- Ensure that medical personnel are aware of the material(s) involved and take precautions to protect themselves.
- Move victim to fresh air.
- Call 911 or emergency medical service.
- Give artificial respiration if victim is not breathing.
- Administer oxygen if breathing is difficult.
- Remove and isolate contaminated clothing and shoes.
- In case of contact with substance, immediately flush skin or eyes with running water for at least 20 minutes.
- Keep victim calm and warm.

## POTENTIAL HAZARDS

### FIRE OR EXPLOSION

- **Self-decomposition, self-polymerization, or self-ignition may be triggered by heat, chemical reaction, friction or impact.**
- Self-accelerating decomposition may occur if the specific control temperature is not maintained.
- These materials are particularly sensitive to temperature rises. Above a given "Control Temperature" they decompose or polymerize violently and may catch fire.
- May be ignited by heat, sparks or flames.
- Those substances designated with a **(P)** may polymerize explosively when heated or involved in a fire.
- Some may decompose explosively when heated or involved in a fire.
- May burn violently. Decomposition or polymerization may be self-accelerating and produce large amounts of gases.
- Vapors or dust may form explosive mixtures with air.

### HEALTH

- Inhalation or contact with vapors, substance or decomposition products may cause severe injury or death.
- May produce irritating, toxic and/or corrosive gases.
- Runoff from fire control may cause pollution.

## PUBLIC SAFETY

- **CALL EMERGENCY RESPONSE Telephone Number on Shipping Paper first. If Shipping Paper not available or no answer, refer to appropriate telephone number listed on the inside back cover.**
- As an immediate precautionary measure, isolate spill or leak area in all directions for at least 50 meters (150 feet) for liquids and at least 25 meters (75 feet) for solids.
- Keep unauthorized personnel away.
- Stay upwind, uphill and/or upstream.
- **DO NOT allow the substance to warm up. Obtain liquid nitrogen (wear thermal protective clothing, see GUIDE 120), dry ice or ice for cooling. If this is not possible or none can be obtained, evacuate the area immediately.**

### PROTECTIVE CLOTHING

- Wear positive pressure self-contained breathing apparatus (SCBA).
- Wear chemical protective clothing that is specifically recommended by the manufacturer. It may provide little or no thermal protection.
- Structural firefighters' protective clothing will only provide limited protection.

### EVACUATION

**Large Spill**

- Consider initial evacuation for at least 250 meters (800 feet) in all directions.

**Fire**

- If tank, rail car or tank truck is involved in a fire, ISOLATE for 800 meters (1/2 mile) in all directions; also, consider initial evacuation for 800 meters (1/2 mile) in all directions.

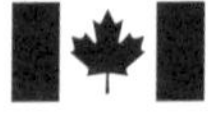

In Canada, an Emergency Response Assistance Plan (ERAP) may be required for this product. Please consult the shipping document and/or the ERAP Program Section (page 391).

## EMERGENCY RESPONSE

### FIRE

- **The temperature of the substance must be maintained at or below the "Control Temperature" at all times.**

**Small Fire**

- Dry chemical, $CO_2$, water spray or regular foam.

**Large Fire**

- Flood fire area with water from a distance.
- Move containers from fire area if you can do it without risk.

**Fire involving Tanks or Car/Trailer Loads**

- **BEWARE OF POSSIBLE CONTAINER EXPLOSION.**
- Fight fire from maximum distance or use unmanned hose holders or monitor nozzles.
- Cool containers with flooding quantities of water until well after fire is out.
- Withdraw immediately in case of rising sound from venting safety devices or discoloration of tank.
- ALWAYS stay away from tanks engulfed in fire.

### SPILL OR LEAK

- ELIMINATE all ignition sources (no smoking, flares, sparks or flames in immediate area).
- Do not touch or walk through spilled material.
- Stop leak if you can do it without risk.

**Small Spill**

- Pick up with inert, damp, non-combustible material using clean, non-sparking tools and place into loosely covered plastic containers for later disposal.
- Prevent entry into waterways, sewers, basements or confined areas.
- **DO NOT CLEAN-UP OR DISPOSE OF, EXCEPT UNDER SUPERVISION OF A SPECIALIST.**

### FIRST AID

- Ensure that medical personnel are aware of the material(s) involved and take precautions to protect themselves.
- Move victim to fresh air.
- Call 911 or emergency medical service.
- Give artificial respiration if victim is not breathing.
- Administer oxygen if breathing is difficult.
- Remove and isolate contaminated clothing and shoes.
- In case of contact with substance, immediately flush skin or eyes with running water for at least 20 minutes.
- Keep victim calm and warm.

# GUIDE 151 SUBSTANCES - TOXIC (NON-COMBUSTIBLE)

## POTENTIAL HAZARDS

### HEALTH

- **Highly toxic**, may be fatal if inhaled, swallowed or absorbed through skin.
- Avoid any skin contact.
- Effects of contact or inhalation may be delayed.
- Fire may produce irritating, corrosive and/or toxic gases.
- Runoff from fire control or dilution water may be corrosive and/or toxic and cause pollution.

### FIRE OR EXPLOSION

- Non-combustible, substance itself does not burn but may decompose upon heating to produce corrosive and/or toxic fumes.
- Containers may explode when heated.
- Runoff may pollute waterways.

## PUBLIC SAFETY

- **CALL EMERGENCY RESPONSE Telephone Number on Shipping Paper first. If Shipping Paper not available or no answer, refer to appropriate telephone number listed on the inside back cover.**
- As an immediate precautionary measure, isolate spill or leak area in all directions for at least 50 meters (150 feet) for liquids and at least 25 meters (75 feet) for solids.
- Keep unauthorized personnel away.
- Stay upwind, uphill and/or upstream.

### PROTECTIVE CLOTHING

- Wear positive pressure self-contained breathing apparatus (SCBA).
- Wear chemical protective clothing that is specifically recommended by the manufacturer. It may provide little or no thermal protection.
- Structural firefighters' protective clothing provides limited protection in fire situations ONLY; it is not effective in spill situations where direct contact with the substance is possible.

### EVACUATION

**Spill**

- See Table 1 - Initial Isolation and Protective Action Distances for highlighted materials. For non-highlighted materials, increase, in the downwind direction, as necessary, the isolation distance shown under "PUBLIC SAFETY".

**Fire**

- If tank, rail car or tank truck is involved in a fire, ISOLATE for 800 meters (1/2 mile) in all directions; also, consider initial evacuation for 800 meters (1/2 mile) in all directions.

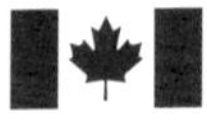

In Canada, an Emergency Response Assistance Plan (ERAP) may be required for this product. Please consult the shipping document and/or the ERAP Program Section (page 391).

## EMERGENCY RESPONSE

### FIRE

**Small Fire**

- Dry chemical, $CO_2$ or water spray.

**Large Fire**

- Water spray, fog or regular foam.
- Move containers from fire area if you can do it without risk.
- Dike fire-control water for later disposal; do not scatter the material.
- Use water spray or fog; do not use straight streams.

**Fire involving Tanks or Car/Trailer Loads**

- Fight fire from maximum distance or use unmanned hose holders or monitor nozzles.
- Do not get water inside containers.
- Cool containers with flooding quantities of water until well after fire is out.
- Withdraw immediately in case of rising sound from venting safety devices or discoloration of tank.
- ALWAYS stay away from tanks engulfed in fire.
- For massive fire, use unmanned hose holders or monitor nozzles; if this is impossible, withdraw from area and let fire burn.

### SPILL OR LEAK

- Do not touch damaged containers or spilled material unless wearing appropriate protective clothing.
- Stop leak if you can do it without risk.
- Prevent entry into waterways, sewers, basements or confined areas.
- Cover with plastic sheet to prevent spreading.
- Absorb or cover with dry earth, sand or other non-combustible material and transfer to containers.
- DO NOT GET WATER INSIDE CONTAINERS.

### FIRST AID

- Ensure that medical personnel are aware of the material(s) involved and take precautions to protect themselves.
- Move victim to fresh air.
- Call 911 or emergency medical service.
- Give artificial respiration if victim is not breathing.
- **Do not use mouth-to-mouth method if victim ingested or inhaled the substance; give artificial respiration with the aid of a pocket mask equipped with a one-way valve or other proper respiratory medical device.**
- Administer oxygen if breathing is difficult.
- Remove and isolate contaminated clothing and shoes.
- In case of contact with substance, immediately flush skin or eyes with running water for at least 20 minutes.
- For minor skin contact, avoid spreading material on unaffected skin.
- Keep victim calm and warm.
- Effects of exposure (inhalation, ingestion or skin contact) to substance may be delayed.

# GUIDE 152 SUBSTANCES - TOXIC (COMBUSTIBLE)

## POTENTIAL HAZARDS

### HEALTH

- **Highly toxic,** may be fatal if inhaled, swallowed or absorbed through skin.
- Contact with molten substance may cause severe burns to skin and eyes.
- Avoid any skin contact.
- Effects of contact or inhalation may be delayed.
- Fire may produce irritating, corrosive and/or toxic gases.
- Runoff from fire control or dilution water may be corrosive and/or toxic and cause pollution.

### FIRE OR EXPLOSION

- Combustible material: may burn but does not ignite readily.
- Containers may explode when heated.
- Runoff may pollute waterways.
- Substance may be transported in a molten form.

## PUBLIC SAFETY

- **CALL EMERGENCY RESPONSE Telephone Number on Shipping Paper first. If Shipping Paper not available or no answer, refer to appropriate telephone number listed on the inside back cover.**
- As an immediate precautionary measure, isolate spill or leak area in all directions for at least 50 meters (150 feet) for liquids and at least 25 meters (75 feet) for solids.
- Keep unauthorized personnel away.
- Stay upwind, uphill and/or upstream.

### PROTECTIVE CLOTHING

- Wear positive pressure self-contained breathing apparatus (SCBA).
- Wear chemical protective clothing that is specifically recommended by the manufacturer. It may provide little or no thermal protection.
- Structural firefighters' protective clothing provides limited protection in fire situations ONLY; it is not effective in spill situations where direct contact with the substance is possible.

### EVACUATION

**Spill**

- See Table 1 - Initial Isolation and Protective Action Distances for highlighted materials. For non-highlighted materials, increase, in the downwind direction, as necessary, the isolation distance shown under "PUBLIC SAFETY".

**Fire**

- If tank, rail car or tank truck is involved in a fire, ISOLATE for 800 meters (1/2 mile) in all directions; also, consider initial evacuation for 800 meters (1/2 mile) in all directions.

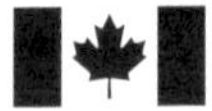

In Canada, an Emergency Response Assistance Plan (ERAP) may be required for this product. Please consult the shipping document and/or the ERAP Program Section (page 391).

## EMERGENCY RESPONSE

### FIRE

**Small Fire**

- Dry chemical, $CO_2$ or water spray.

**Large Fire**

- Water spray, fog or regular foam.
- Move containers from fire area if you can do it without risk.
- Dike fire-control water for later disposal; do not scatter the material.
- Use water spray or fog; do not use straight streams.

**Fire involving Tanks or Car/Trailer Loads**

- Fight fire from maximum distance or use unmanned hose holders or monitor nozzles.
- Do not get water inside containers.
- Cool containers with flooding quantities of water until well after fire is out.
- Withdraw immediately in case of rising sound from venting safety devices or discoloration of tank.
- ALWAYS stay away from tanks engulfed in fire.
- For massive fire, use unmanned hose holders or monitor nozzles; if this is impossible, withdraw from area and let fire burn.

### SPILL OR LEAK

- ELIMINATE all ignition sources (no smoking, flares, sparks or flames in immediate area).
- Do not touch damaged containers or spilled material unless wearing appropriate protective clothing.
- Stop leak if you can do it without risk.
- Prevent entry into waterways, sewers, basements or confined areas.
- Cover with plastic sheet to prevent spreading.
- Absorb or cover with dry earth, sand or other non-combustible material and transfer to containers.
- DO NOT GET WATER INSIDE CONTAINERS.

### FIRST AID

- Ensure that medical personnel are aware of the material(s) involved and take precautions to protect themselves.
- Move victim to fresh air.
- Call 911 or emergency medical service.
- Give artificial respiration if victim is not breathing.
- **Do not use mouth-to-mouth method if victim ingested or inhaled the substance; give artificial respiration with the aid of a pocket mask equipped with a one-way valve or other proper respiratory medical device.**
- Administer oxygen if breathing is difficult.
- Remove and isolate contaminated clothing and shoes.
- In case of contact with substance, immediately flush skin or eyes with running water for at least 20 minutes.
- For minor skin contact, avoid spreading material on unaffected skin.
- Keep victim calm and warm.
- Effects of exposure (inhalation, ingestion or skin contact) to substance may be delayed.

# GUIDE 153 SUBSTANCES - TOXIC AND/OR CORROSIVE (COMBUSTIBLE)

## POTENTIAL HAZARDS

### HEALTH

- **TOXIC**; inhalation, ingestion or skin contact with material may cause severe injury or death.
- Contact with molten substance may cause severe burns to skin and eyes.
- Avoid any skin contact.
- Effects of contact or inhalation may be delayed.
- Fire may produce irritating, corrosive and/or toxic gases.
- Runoff from fire control or dilution water may be corrosive and/or toxic and cause pollution.

### FIRE OR EXPLOSION

- Combustible material: may burn but does not ignite readily.
- When heated, vapors may form explosive mixtures with air: indoors, outdoors and sewers explosion hazards.
- Those substances designated with a **(P)** may polymerize explosively when heated or involved in a fire.
- Contact with metals may evolve flammable hydrogen gas.
- Containers may explode when heated.
- Runoff may pollute waterways.
- Substance may be transported in a molten form.

## PUBLIC SAFETY

- **CALL EMERGENCY RESPONSE Telephone Number on Shipping Paper first. If Shipping Paper not available or no answer, refer to appropriate telephone number listed on the inside back cover.**
- As an immediate precautionary measure, isolate spill or leak area in all directions for at least 50 meters (150 feet) for liquids and at least 25 meters (75 feet) for solids.
- Keep unauthorized personnel away.
- Stay upwind, uphill and/or upstream.
- Ventilate enclosed areas.

### PROTECTIVE CLOTHING

- Wear positive pressure self-contained breathing apparatus (SCBA).
- Wear chemical protective clothing that is specifically recommended by the manufacturer. It may provide little or no thermal protection.
- Structural firefighters' protective clothing provides limited protection in fire situations ONLY; it is not effective in spill situations where direct contact with the substance is possible.

### EVACUATION

**Spill**

- See Table 1 - Initial Isolation and Protective Action Distances for highlighted materials. For non-highlighted materials, increase, in the downwind direction, as necessary, the isolation distance shown under "PUBLIC SAFETY".

**Fire**

- If tank, rail car or tank truck is involved in a fire, ISOLATE for 800 meters (1/2 mile) in all directions; also, consider initial evacuation for 800 meters (1/2 mile) in all directions.

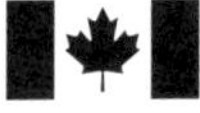

In Canada, an Emergency Response Assistance Plan (ERAP) may be required for this product. Please consult the shipping document and/or the ERAP Program Section (page 391).

## EMERGENCY RESPONSE

### FIRE

**Small Fire**
- Dry chemical, $CO_2$ or water spray.

**Large Fire**
- Dry chemical, $CO_2$, alcohol-resistant foam or water spray.
- Move containers from fire area if you can do it without risk.
- Dike fire-control water for later disposal; do not scatter the material.

**Fire involving Tanks or Car/Trailer Loads**
- Fight fire from maximum distance or use unmanned hose holders or monitor nozzles.
- Do not get water inside containers.
- Cool containers with flooding quantities of water until well after fire is out.
- Withdraw immediately in case of rising sound from venting safety devices or discoloration of tank.
- ALWAYS stay away from tanks engulfed in fire.

### SPILL OR LEAK

- ELIMINATE all ignition sources (no smoking, flares, sparks or flames in immediate area).
- Do not touch damaged containers or spilled material unless wearing appropriate protective clothing.
- Stop leak if you can do it without risk.
- Prevent entry into waterways, sewers, basements or confined areas.
- Absorb or cover with dry earth, sand or other non-combustible material and transfer to containers.
- DO NOT GET WATER INSIDE CONTAINERS.

### FIRST AID

- Ensure that medical personnel are aware of the material(s) involved and take precautions to protect themselves.
- Move victim to fresh air.
- Call 911 or emergency medical service.
- Give artificial respiration if victim is not breathing.
- **Do not use mouth-to-mouth method if victim ingested or inhaled the substance; give artificial respiration with the aid of a pocket mask equipped with a one-way valve or other proper respiratory medical device.**
- Administer oxygen if breathing is difficult.
- Remove and isolate contaminated clothing and shoes.
- In case of contact with substance, immediately flush skin or eyes with running water for at least 20 minutes.
- For minor skin contact, avoid spreading material on unaffected skin.
- Keep victim calm and warm.
- Effects of exposure (inhalation, ingestion or skin contact) to substance may be delayed.

## POTENTIAL HAZARDS

### HEALTH

- **TOXIC**; inhalation, ingestion or skin contact with material may cause severe injury or death.
- Contact with molten substance may cause severe burns to skin and eyes.
- Avoid any skin contact.
- Effects of contact or inhalation may be delayed.
- Fire may produce irritating, corrosive and/or toxic gases.
- Runoff from fire control or dilution water may be corrosive and/or toxic and cause pollution.

### FIRE OR EXPLOSION

- Non-combustible, substance itself does not burn but may decompose upon heating to produce corrosive and/or toxic fumes.
- Some are oxidizers and may ignite combustibles (wood, paper, oil, clothing, etc.).
- Contact with metals may evolve flammable hydrogen gas.
- Containers may explode when heated.
- For electric vehicles or equipment, GUIDE 147 (lithium ion batteries) or GUIDE 138 (sodium batteries) should also be consulted.

## PUBLIC SAFETY

- **CALL EMERGENCY RESPONSE Telephone Number on Shipping Paper first. If Shipping Paper not available or no answer, refer to appropriate telephone number listed on the inside back cover.**
- As an immediate precautionary measure, isolate spill or leak area in all directions for at least 50 meters (150 feet) for liquids and at least 25 meters (75 feet) for solids.
- Keep unauthorized personnel away.
- Stay upwind, uphill and/or upstream.
- Ventilate enclosed areas.

### PROTECTIVE CLOTHING

- Wear positive pressure self-contained breathing apparatus (SCBA).
- Wear chemical protective clothing that is specifically recommended by the manufacturer. It may provide little or no thermal protection.
- Structural firefighters' protective clothing provides limited protection in fire situations ONLY; it is not effective in spill situations where direct contact with the substance is possible.

### EVACUATION

**Spill**

- See Table 1 - Initial Isolation and Protective Action Distances for highlighted materials. For non-highlighted materials, increase, in the downwind direction, as necessary, the isolation distance shown under "PUBLIC SAFETY".

**Fire**

- If tank, rail car or tank truck is involved in a fire, ISOLATE for 800 meters (1/2 mile) in all directions; also, consider initial evacuation for 800 meters (1/2 mile) in all directions.

In Canada, an Emergency Response Assistance Plan (ERAP) may be required for this product. Please consult the shipping document and/or the ERAP Program Section (page 391).

## EMERGENCY RESPONSE

### FIRE

**Small Fire**

- Dry chemical, $CO_2$ or water spray.

**Large Fire**

- Dry chemical, $CO_2$, alcohol-resistant foam or water spray.
- Move containers from fire area if you can do it without risk.
- Dike fire-control water for later disposal; do not scatter the material.

**Fire involving Tanks or Car/Trailer Loads**

- Fight fire from maximum distance or use unmanned hose holders or monitor nozzles.
- Do not get water inside containers.
- Cool containers with flooding quantities of water until well after fire is out.
- Withdraw immediately in case of rising sound from venting safety devices or discoloration of tank.
- ALWAYS stay away from tanks engulfed in fire.

### SPILL OR LEAK

- ELIMINATE all ignition sources (no smoking, flares, sparks or flames in immediate area).
- Do not touch damaged containers or spilled material unless wearing appropriate protective clothing.
- Stop leak if you can do it without risk.
- Prevent entry into waterways, sewers, basements or confined areas.
- Absorb or cover with dry earth, sand or other non-combustible material and transfer to containers.
- DO NOT GET WATER INSIDE CONTAINERS.

### FIRST AID

- Ensure that medical personnel are aware of the material(s) involved and take precautions to protect themselves.
- Move victim to fresh air.
- Call 911 or emergency medical service.
- Give artificial respiration if victim is not breathing.
- **Do not use mouth-to-mouth method if victim ingested or inhaled the substance; give artificial respiration with the aid of a pocket mask equipped with a one-way valve or other proper respiratory medical device.**
- Administer oxygen if breathing is difficult.
- Remove and isolate contaminated clothing and shoes.
- In case of contact with substance, immediately flush skin or eyes with running water for at least 20 minutes.
- For minor skin contact, avoid spreading material on unaffected skin.
- Keep victim calm and warm.
- Effects of exposure (inhalation, ingestion or skin contact) to substance may be delayed.

# GUIDE 155 SUBSTANCES - TOXIC AND/OR CORROSIVE (FLAMMABLE/WATER-SENSITIVE)

## POTENTIAL HAZARDS

### FIRE OR EXPLOSION

- **HIGHLY FLAMMABLE: Will be easily ignited by heat, sparks or flames.**
- Vapors form explosive mixtures with air: indoors, outdoors and sewers explosion hazards.
- Most vapors are heavier than air. They will spread along ground and collect in low or confined areas (sewers, basements, tanks).
- Vapors may travel to source of ignition and flash back.
- Those substances designated with a **(P)** may polymerize explosively when heated or involved in a fire.
- Substance will react with water (some violently) releasing flammable, toxic or corrosive gases and runoff.
- Contact with metals may evolve flammable hydrogen gas.
- Containers may explode when heated or if contaminated with water.

### HEALTH

- **TOXIC**; inhalation, ingestion or contact (skin, eyes) with vapors, dusts or substance may cause severe injury, burns or death.
- **Bromoacetates and chloroacetates are extremely irritating/lachrymators.**
- Reaction with water or moist air will release toxic, corrosive or flammable gases.
- Reaction with water may generate much heat that will increase the concentration of fumes in the air.
- Fire will produce irritating, corrosive and/or toxic gases.
- Runoff from fire control or dilution water may be corrosive and/or toxic and cause pollution.

## PUBLIC SAFETY

- **CALL EMERGENCY RESPONSE Telephone Number on Shipping Paper first. If Shipping Paper not available or no answer, refer to appropriate telephone number listed on the inside back cover.**
- As an immediate precautionary measure, isolate spill or leak area in all directions for at least 50 meters (150 feet) for liquids and at least 25 meters (75 feet) for solids.
- Keep unauthorized personnel away.
- Stay upwind, uphill and/or upstream.
- Ventilate enclosed areas.

### PROTECTIVE CLOTHING

- Wear positive pressure self-contained breathing apparatus (SCBA).
- Wear chemical protective clothing that is specifically recommended by the manufacturer. It may provide little or no thermal protection.
- Structural firefighters' protective clothing provides limited protection in fire situations ONLY; it is not effective in spill situations where direct contact with the substance is possible.

### EVACUATION

**Spill**

- See Table 1 - Initial Isolation and Protective Action Distances for highlighted materials. For non-highlighted materials, increase, in the downwind direction, as necessary, the isolation distance shown under "PUBLIC SAFETY".

**Fire**

- If tank, rail car or tank truck is involved in a fire, ISOLATE for 800 meters (1/2 mile) in all directions; also, consider initial evacuation for 800 meters (1/2 mile) in all directions.

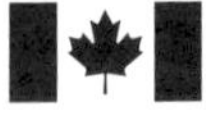

In Canada, an Emergency Response Assistance Plan (ERAP) may be required for this product. Please consult the shipping document and/or the ERAP Program Section (page 391).

## EMERGENCY RESPONSE

### FIRE

- Note: Most foams will react with the material and release corrosive/toxic gases.

**CAUTION: For Acetyl chloride (UN1717), use $CO_2$ or dry chemical only.**

**Small Fire**

- $CO_2$, dry chemical, dry sand, alcohol-resistant foam.

**Large Fire**

- Water spray, fog or alcohol-resistant foam.
- **FOR CHLOROSILANES, DO NOT USE WATER**; use AFFF alcohol-resistant medium-expansion foam.
- Move containers from fire area if you can do it without risk.
- Use water spray or fog; do not use straight streams.

**Fire involving Tanks or Car/Trailer Loads**

- Fight fire from maximum distance or use unmanned hose holders or monitor nozzles.
- Do not get water inside containers.
- Cool containers with flooding quantities of water until well after fire is out.
- Withdraw immediately in case of rising sound from venting safety devices or discoloration of tank.
- ALWAYS stay away from tanks engulfed in fire.

### SPILL OR LEAK

- ELIMINATE all ignition sources (no smoking, flares, sparks or flames in immediate area).
- All equipment used when handling the product must be grounded.
- Do not touch damaged containers or spilled material unless wearing appropriate protective clothing.
- Stop leak if you can do it without risk.
- A vapor-suppressing foam may be used to reduce vapors.
- **FOR CHLOROSILANES**, use AFFF alcohol-resistant medium-expansion foam to reduce vapors.
- **DO NOT GET WATER on spilled substance or inside containers.**
- Use water spray to reduce vapors or divert vapor cloud drift. Avoid allowing water runoff to contact spilled material.
- Prevent entry into waterways, sewers, basements or confined areas.

**Small Spill**

- Cover with DRY earth, DRY sand or other non-combustible material followed with plastic sheet to minimize spreading or contact with rain.
- Use clean, non-sparking tools to collect material and place it into loosely covered plastic containers for later disposal.

### FIRST AID

- Ensure that medical personnel are aware of the material(s) involved and take precautions to protect themselves.
- Move victim to fresh air.
- Call 911 or emergency medical service.
- Give artificial respiration if victim is not breathing.
- **Do not use mouth-to-mouth method if victim ingested or inhaled the substance; give artificial respiration with the aid of a pocket mask equipped with a one-way valve or other proper respiratory medical device.**
- Administer oxygen if breathing is difficult.
- Remove and isolate contaminated clothing and shoes.
- In case of contact with substance, immediately flush skin or eyes with running water for at least 20 minutes.
- For minor skin contact, avoid spreading material on unaffected skin.
- Keep victim calm and warm.
- Effects of exposure (inhalation, ingestion or skin contact) to substance may be delayed.

# GUIDE 156 SUBSTANCES - TOXIC AND/OR CORROSIVE (COMBUSTIBLE/WATER-SENSITIVE)

## POTENTIAL HAZARDS

### FIRE OR EXPLOSION

- Combustible material: may burn but does not ignite readily.
- Substance will react with water (some violently) releasing flammable, toxic or corrosive gases and runoff.
- When heated, vapors may form explosive mixtures with air: indoors, outdoors and sewers explosion hazards.
- Most vapors are heavier than air. They will spread along ground and collect in low or confined areas (sewers, basements, tanks).
- Vapors may travel to source of ignition and flash back.
- Contact with metals may evolve flammable hydrogen gas.
- Containers may explode when heated or if contaminated with water.

### HEALTH

- **TOXIC;** inhalation, ingestion or contact (skin, eyes) with vapors, dusts or substance may cause severe injury, burns or death.
- Contact with molten substance may cause severe burns to skin and eyes.
- Reaction with water or moist air will release toxic, corrosive or flammable gases.
- Reaction with water may generate much heat that will increase the concentration of fumes in the air.
- Fire will produce irritating, corrosive and/or toxic gases.
- Runoff from fire control or dilution water may be corrosive and/or toxic and cause pollution.

## PUBLIC SAFETY

- **CALL EMERGENCY RESPONSE Telephone Number on Shipping Paper first. If Shipping Paper not available or no answer, refer to appropriate telephone number listed on the inside back cover.**
- As an immediate precautionary measure, isolate spill or leak area in all directions for at least 50 meters (150 feet) for liquids and at least 25 meters (75 feet) for solids.
- Keep unauthorized personnel away.
- Stay upwind, uphill and/or upstream.
- Ventilate enclosed areas.

### PROTECTIVE CLOTHING

- Wear positive pressure self-contained breathing apparatus (SCBA).
- Wear chemical protective clothing that is specifically recommended by the manufacturer. It may provide little or no thermal protection.
- Structural firefighters' protective clothing provides limited protection in fire situations ONLY; it is not effective in spill situations where direct contact with the substance is possible.

### EVACUATION

**Spill**

- See Table 1 - Initial Isolation and Protective Action Distances for highlighted materials. For non-highlighted materials, increase, in the downwind direction, as necessary, the isolation distance shown under "PUBLIC SAFETY".

**Fire**

- If tank, rail car or tank truck is involved in a fire, ISOLATE for 800 meters (1/2 mile) in all directions; also, consider initial evacuation for 800 meters (1/2 mile) in all directions.

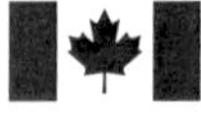

In Canada, an Emergency Response Assistance Plan (ERAP) may be required for this product. Please consult the shipping document and/or the ERAP Program Section (page 391).

## EMERGENCY RESPONSE

### FIRE

- Note: Most foams will react with the material and release corrosive/toxic gases.

**Small Fire**

- $CO_2$, dry chemical, dry sand, alcohol-resistant foam.

**Large Fire**

- Water spray, fog or alcohol-resistant foam.
- **FOR CHLOROSILANES, DO NOT USE WATER**; use AFFF alcohol-resistant medium-expansion foam.
- Move containers from fire area if you can do it without risk.
- Use water spray or fog; do not use straight streams.

**Fire involving Tanks or Car/Trailer Loads**

- Fight fire from maximum distance or use unmanned hose holders or monitor nozzles.
- Do not get water inside containers.
- Cool containers with flooding quantities of water until well after fire is out.
- Withdraw immediately in case of rising sound from venting safety devices or discoloration of tank.
- ALWAYS stay away from tanks engulfed in fire.

### SPILL OR LEAK

- ELIMINATE all ignition sources (no smoking, flares, sparks or flames in immediate area).
- All equipment used when handling the product must be grounded.
- Do not touch damaged containers or spilled material unless wearing appropriate protective clothing.
- Stop leak if you can do it without risk.
- A vapor-suppressing foam may be used to reduce vapors.
- **FOR CHLOROSILANES**, use AFFF alcohol-resistant medium-expansion foam to reduce vapors.
- **DO NOT GET WATER on spilled substance or inside containers.**
- Use water spray to reduce vapors or divert vapor cloud drift. Avoid allowing water runoff to contact spilled material.
- Prevent entry into waterways, sewers, basements or confined areas.

**Small Spill**

- Cover with DRY earth, DRY sand or other non-combustible material followed with plastic sheet to minimize spreading or contact with rain.
- Use clean, non-sparking tools to collect material and place it into loosely covered plastic containers for later disposal.

### FIRST AID

- Ensure that medical personnel are aware of the material(s) involved and take precautions to protect themselves.
- Move victim to fresh air.
- Call 911 or emergency medical service.
- Give artificial respiration if victim is not breathing.
- **Do not use mouth-to-mouth method if victim ingested or inhaled the substance; give artificial respiration with the aid of a pocket mask equipped with a one-way valve or other proper respiratory medical device.**
- Administer oxygen if breathing is difficult.
- Remove and isolate contaminated clothing and shoes.
- In case of contact with substance, immediately flush skin or eyes with running water for at least 20 minutes.
- For minor skin contact, avoid spreading material on unaffected skin.
- Keep victim calm and warm.
- Effects of exposure (inhalation, ingestion or skin contact) to substance may be delayed.

# GUIDE 157 SUBSTANCES - TOXIC AND/OR CORROSIVE (NON-COMBUSTIBLE/WATER-SENSITIVE)

## POTENTIAL HAZARDS

### HEALTH

- **TOXIC**; inhalation, ingestion or contact (skin, eyes) with vapors, dusts or substance may cause severe injury, burns or death.
- Reaction with water or moist air may release toxic, corrosive or flammable gases.
- Reaction with water may generate much heat that will increase the concentration of fumes in the air.
- Fire will produce irritating, corrosive and/or toxic gases.
- Runoff from fire control or dilution water may be corrosive and/or toxic and cause pollution.

### FIRE OR EXPLOSION

- Non-combustible, substance itself does not burn but may decompose upon heating to produce corrosive and/or toxic fumes.
- For UN1796, UN1826, UN2031 at high concentrations and for UN2032, these may act as oxidizers, also consult GUIDE 140.
- Vapors may accumulate in confined areas (basement, tanks, hopper/tank cars, etc.).
- Substance may react with water (some violently), releasing corrosive and/or toxic gases and runoff.
- Contact with metals may evolve flammable hydrogen gas.
- Containers may explode when heated or if contaminated with water.

## PUBLIC SAFETY

- **CALL EMERGENCY RESPONSE Telephone Number on Shipping Paper first. If Shipping Paper not available or no answer, refer to appropriate telephone number listed on the inside back cover.**
- As an immediate precautionary measure, isolate spill or leak area in all directions for at least 50 meters (150 feet) for liquids and at least 25 meters (75 feet) for solids.
- Keep unauthorized personnel away.
- Stay upwind, uphill and/or upstream.
- Ventilate enclosed areas.

### PROTECTIVE CLOTHING

- Wear positive pressure self-contained breathing apparatus (SCBA).
- Wear chemical protective clothing that is specifically recommended by the manufacturer. It may provide little or no thermal protection.
- Structural firefighters' protective clothing provides limited protection in fire situations ONLY; it is not effective in spill situations where direct contact with the substance is possible.

### EVACUATION

**Spill**

- See Table 1 - Initial Isolation and Protective Action Distances for highlighted materials. For non-highlighted materials, increase, in the downwind direction, as necessary, the isolation distance shown under "PUBLIC SAFETY".

**Fire**

- If tank, rail car or tank truck is involved in a fire, ISOLATE for 800 meters (1/2 mile) in all directions; also, consider initial evacuation for 800 meters (1/2 mile) in all directions.

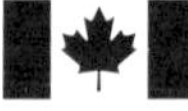

In Canada, an Emergency Response Assistance Plan (ERAP) may be required for this product. Please consult the shipping document and/or the ERAP Program Section (page 391).

## EMERGENCY RESPONSE

### FIRE

- Note: Some foams will react with the material and release corrosive/toxic gases.

**Small Fire**

- $CO_2$ (except for Cyanides), dry chemical, dry sand, alcohol-resistant foam.

**Large Fire**

- Water spray, fog or alcohol-resistant foam.
- Move containers from fire area if you can do it without risk.
- Use water spray or fog; do not use straight streams.
- Dike fire-control water for later disposal; do not scatter the material.

**Fire involving Tanks or Car/Trailer Loads**

- Fight fire from maximum distance or use unmanned hose holders or monitor nozzles.
- Do not get water inside containers.
- Cool containers with flooding quantities of water until well after fire is out.
- Withdraw immediately in case of rising sound from venting safety devices or discoloration of tank.
- ALWAYS stay away from tanks engulfed in fire.

### SPILL OR LEAK

- ELIMINATE all ignition sources (no smoking, flares, sparks or flames in immediate area).
- All equipment used when handling the product must be grounded.
- Do not touch damaged containers or spilled material unless wearing appropriate protective clothing.
- Stop leak if you can do it without risk.
- A vapor-suppressing foam may be used to reduce vapors.
- DO NOT GET WATER INSIDE CONTAINERS.
- Use water spray to reduce vapors or divert vapor cloud drift. Avoid allowing water runoff to contact spilled material.
- Prevent entry into waterways, sewers, basements or confined areas.

**Small Spill**

- Cover with DRY earth, DRY sand or other non-combustible material followed with plastic sheet to minimize spreading or contact with rain.
- Use clean, non-sparking tools to collect material and place it into loosely covered plastic containers for later disposal.

### FIRST AID

- Ensure that medical personnel are aware of the material(s) involved and take precautions to protect themselves.
- Move victim to fresh air.
- Call 911 or emergency medical service.
- Give artificial respiration if victim is not breathing.
- **Do not use mouth-to-mouth method if victim ingested or inhaled the substance; give artificial respiration with the aid of a pocket mask equipped with a one-way valve or other proper respiratory medical device.**
- Administer oxygen if breathing is difficult.
- Remove and isolate contaminated clothing and shoes.
- In case of contact with substance, immediately flush skin or eyes with running water for at least 20 minutes.
- **In case of contact with Hydrofluoric acid (UN1790)**, flush with large amounts of water. For skin contact, if calcium gluconate gel is available, rinse 5 minutes, then apply gel. Otherwise, continue rinsing until medical treatment is available. For eyes, flush with water or a saline solution for 15 minutes.
- For minor skin contact, avoid spreading material on unaffected skin.
- Keep victim calm and warm.
- Effects of exposure (inhalation, ingestion or skin contact) to substance may be delayed.

## POTENTIAL HAZARDS

### HEALTH

- Inhalation or contact with substance may cause infection, disease or death.
- Category A Infections Substances (UN2814 or UN2900) are more hazardous, or are in a more hazardous form, than infectious substances shipped as Category B Biological Substances (UN3373) or clinical waste / medical waste (UN3291).
- Runoff from fire control may cause environmental contamination.
- **Note: Damaged packages containing solid $CO_2$ as a refrigerant may produce water or frost from condensation of air. Do not touch this solid or liquid as it could be contaminated by the contents of the parcel.**
- Contact with solid $CO_2$ may cause burns, severe injury and/or frostbite.

### FIRE OR EXPLOSION

- Some of these materials may burn, but none ignite readily.
- Some may be transported in flammable liquids.

## PUBLIC SAFETY

- **CALL EMERGENCY RESPONSE Telephone Number on Shipping Paper first. If Shipping Paper not available or no answer, refer to appropriate telephone number listed on the inside back cover.**
- As an immediate precautionary measure, isolate spill or leak area for at least 25 meters (75 feet) in all directions.
- Keep unauthorized personnel away.
- Stay upwind, uphill and/or upstream.
- Identify the substance involved.

### PROTECTIVE CLOTHING

- Wear respiratory protection, such as fit-tested N95 respirator (at minimum), powered air purifying respirator (PAPR), or positive pressure self-contained breathing apparatus (SCBA).
- Wear full coverage body protection (e.g., Tyvek suit), faceshield, and disposable fluid-resistant gloves (e.g., latex or nitrile).
- Wear appropriate footwear; disposable shoe covers can be worn to protect against contamination.
- Puncture- and cut-resistant gloves should be worn over fluid-resistant gloves if sharp objects (e.g., broken glass, needles) are present.
- Wear insulated gloves (e.g. cryo gloves) over fluid-resistant gloves when handling dry ice (UN1845).
- Decontaminate protective clothing and personal protective equipment after use and before cleaning or disposal with an appropriate chemical disinfectant (e.g., 10% solution of bleach, equivalent to 0.5% sodium hypochlorite) or through a validated decontamination technology (e.g., autoclave) or process.
- Structural firefighters' protective clothing will only provide limited protection.

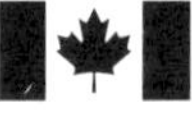

In Canada, an Emergency Response Assistance Plan (ERAP) may be required for this product. Please consult the shipping document and/or the ERAP Program Section (page 391).

## EMERGENCY RESPONSE

### FIRE

**Small Fire**

- Dry chemical, soda ash, lime or sand.

**Large Fire**

- Use extinguishing agent suitable for type of surrounding fire.
- Do not scatter spilled material with high-pressure water streams.
- Move containers from fire area if you can do it without risk.

### SPILL OR LEAK

- Do not touch or walk through spilled material.
- Do not touch damaged containers or spilled material unless wearing appropriate protective clothing.
- Absorb with earth, sand or other non-combustible material.
- Cover damaged package or spilled material with absorbent material such as paper towel, towel or rag to absorb any liquids, and, beginning from outside edge, pour liquid bleach or other chemical disinfectant to saturate. Keep wet with liquid bleach or other disinfectant.
- **DO NOT CLEAN-UP OR DISPOSE OF, EXCEPT UNDER SUPERVISION OF A SPECIALIST.**

### FIRST AID

- Ensure that medical personnel are aware of the material(s) involved and take precautions to protect themselves.
- Move victim to a safe isolated area.

**CAUTION: Victim may be a source of contamination.**

- Call 911 or emergency medical service.
- Remove and isolate contaminated clothing and shoes.
- In case of contact with substance, immediately flush skin or eyes with running water for at least 20 minutes.
- Effects of exposure (inhalation, ingestion, injection/inoculation or skin contact) to substance may be delayed. Victim should consult medical professional for information regarding symptoms and treatment.
- **For further assistance, contact your local Poison Control Center.**

# GUIDE 159 SUBSTANCES (IRRITATING)

## POTENTIAL HAZARDS

### HEALTH

- Inhalation of vapors or dust is extremely irritating.
- May cause burning of eyes and flow of tears.
- May cause coughing, difficult breathing and nausea.
- Brief exposure effects last only a few minutes.
- Exposure in an enclosed area may be very harmful.
- Fire will produce irritating, corrosive and/or toxic gases.
- Runoff from fire control or dilution water may cause pollution.

### FIRE OR EXPLOSION

- Some of these materials may burn, but none ignite readily.
- Containers may explode when heated.

## PUBLIC SAFETY

- **CALL EMERGENCY RESPONSE Telephone Number on Shipping Paper first. If Shipping Paper not available or no answer, refer to appropriate telephone number listed on the inside back cover.**
- As an immediate precautionary measure, isolate spill or leak area in all directions for at least 50 meters (150 feet) for liquids and at least 25 meters (75 feet) for solids.
- Keep unauthorized personnel away.
- Stay upwind, uphill and/or upstream.
- Ventilate closed spaces before entering.

### PROTECTIVE CLOTHING

- Wear positive pressure self-contained breathing apparatus (SCBA).
- Wear chemical protective clothing that is specifically recommended by the manufacturer. It may provide little or no thermal protection.
- Structural firefighters' protective clothing provides limited protection in fire situations ONLY; it is not effective in spill situations where direct contact with the substance is possible.

### EVACUATION

**Spill**

- See Table 1 - Initial Isolation and Protective Action Distances for highlighted materials. For non-highlighted materials, increase, in the downwind direction, as necessary, the isolation distance shown under “PUBLIC SAFETY”.

**Fire**

- If tank, rail car or tank truck is involved in a fire, ISOLATE for 800 meters (1/2 mile) in all directions; also, consider initial evacuation for 800 meters (1/2 mile) in all directions.

In Canada, an Emergency Response Assistance Plan (ERAP) may be required for this product. Please consult the shipping document and/or the ERAP Program Section (page 391).

## EMERGENCY RESPONSE

### FIRE

**Small Fire**

- Dry chemical, $CO_2$, water spray or regular foam.

**Large Fire**

- Water spray, fog or regular foam.
- Move containers from fire area if you can do it without risk.
- Dike fire-control water for later disposal; do not scatter the material.

**Fire involving Tanks or Car/Trailer Loads**

- Fight fire from maximum distance or use unmanned hose holders or monitor nozzles.
- Do not get water inside containers.
- Cool containers with flooding quantities of water until well after fire is out.
- Withdraw immediately in case of rising sound from venting safety devices or discoloration of tank.
- ALWAYS stay away from tanks engulfed in fire.
- For massive fire, use unmanned hose holders or monitor nozzles; if this is impossible, withdraw from area and let fire burn.

### SPILL OR LEAK

- Do not touch or walk through spilled material.
- Stop leak if you can do it without risk.
- Fully encapsulating, vapor-protective clothing should be worn for spills and leaks with no fire.

**Small Spill**

- Pick up with sand or other non-combustible absorbent material and place into containers for later disposal.

**Large Spill**

- Dike far ahead of liquid spill for later disposal.
- Prevent entry into waterways, sewers, basements or confined areas.

### FIRST AID

- Ensure that medical personnel are aware of the material(s) involved and take precautions to protect themselves.
- Move victim to fresh air.
- Call 911 or emergency medical service.
- Give artificial respiration if victim is not breathing.
- **Do not use mouth-to-mouth method if victim ingested or inhaled the substance; give artificial respiration with the aid of a pocket mask equipped with a one-way valve or other proper respiratory medical device.**
- Administer oxygen if breathing is difficult.
- Remove and isolate contaminated clothing and shoes.
- In case of contact with substance, immediately flush skin or eyes with running water for at least 20 minutes.
- For minor skin contact, avoid spreading material on unaffected skin.
- Keep victim calm and warm.
- Effects should disappear after individual has been exposed to fresh air for approximately 10 minutes.

# GUIDE 160 HALOGENATED SOLVENTS

## POTENTIAL HAZARDS

### HEALTH

- Toxic by ingestion.
- Vapors may cause dizziness or suffocation.
- Exposure in an enclosed area may be very harmful.
- Contact may irritate or burn skin and eyes.
- Fire may produce irritating and/or toxic gases.
- Runoff from fire control or dilution water may cause pollution.

### FIRE OR EXPLOSION

- Some of these materials may burn, but none ignite readily.
- Most vapors are heavier than air.
- Air/vapor mixtures may explode when ignited.
- Container may explode in heat of fire.

## PUBLIC SAFETY

- **CALL EMERGENCY RESPONSE Telephone Number on Shipping Paper first. If Shipping Paper not available or no answer, refer to appropriate telephone number listed on the inside back cover.**
- As an immediate precautionary measure, isolate spill or leak area for at least 50 meters (150 feet) in all directions.
- Keep unauthorized personnel away.
- Stay upwind, uphill and/or upstream.
- Many gases are heavier than air and will spread along ground and collect in low or confined areas (sewers, basements, tanks).
- Ventilate closed spaces before entering.

### PROTECTIVE CLOTHING

- Wear positive pressure self-contained breathing apparatus (SCBA).
- Wear chemical protective clothing that is specifically recommended by the manufacturer.
- Structural firefighters' protective clothing will only provide limited protection.

### EVACUATION

**Large Spill**

- Consider initial downwind evacuation for at least 100 meters (330 feet).

**Fire**

- If tank, rail car or tank truck is involved in a fire, ISOLATE for 800 meters (1/2 mile) in all directions; also, consider initial evacuation for 800 meters (1/2 mile) in all directions.

## EMERGENCY RESPONSE

### FIRE

**Small Fire**

- Dry chemical, $CO_2$ or water spray.

**Large Fire**

- Dry chemical, $CO_2$, alcohol-resistant foam or water spray.
- Move containers from fire area if you can do it without risk.
- Dike fire-control water for later disposal; do not scatter the material.

**Fire involving Tanks or Car/Trailer Loads**

- Fight fire from maximum distance or use unmanned hose holders or monitor nozzles.
- Cool containers with flooding quantities of water until well after fire is out.
- Withdraw immediately in case of rising sound from venting safety devices or discoloration of tank.
- ALWAYS stay away from tanks engulfed in fire.

### SPILL OR LEAK

- ELIMINATE all ignition sources (no smoking, flares, sparks or flames in immediate area).
- Stop leak if you can do it without risk.

**Small Liquid Spill**

- Pick up with sand, earth or other non-combustible absorbent material.

**Large Spill**

- Dike far ahead of liquid spill for later disposal.
- Prevent entry into waterways, sewers, basements or confined areas.

### FIRST AID

- Ensure that medical personnel are aware of the material(s) involved and take precautions to protect themselves.
- Move victim to fresh air.
- Call 911 or emergency medical service.
- Give artificial respiration if victim is not breathing.
- Administer oxygen if breathing is difficult.
- Remove and isolate contaminated clothing and shoes.
- In case of contact with substance, immediately flush skin or eyes with running water for at least 20 minutes.
- For minor skin contact, avoid spreading material on unaffected skin.
- Wash skin with soap and water.
- Keep victim calm and warm.

# GUIDE 161 RADIOACTIVE MATERIALS (LOW LEVEL RADIATION)

## POTENTIAL HAZARDS

### HEALTH

- Radiation presents minimal risk to transport workers, emergency response personnel and the public during transportation accidents. Packaging durability increases as potential hazard of radioactive content increases.
- Very low levels of contained radioactive materials and low radiation levels outside packages result in low risks to people. Damaged packages may release measurable amounts of radioactive material, but the resulting risks are expected to be low.
- Some radioactive materials cannot be detected by commonly available instruments.
- Packages do not have RADIOACTIVE I, II, or III labels. Some may have EMPTY labels or may have the word "Radioactive" in the package marking.

### FIRE OR EXPLOSION

- Some of these materials may burn, but most do not ignite readily.
- Many have cardboard outer packaging; content (physically large or small) can be of many different physical forms.
- Radioactivity does not change flammability or other properties of materials.

## PUBLIC SAFETY

- **CALL EMERGENCY RESPONSE Telephone Number on Shipping Paper first. If Shipping Paper not available or no answer, refer to appropriate telephone number listed on the inside back cover.**
- **Priorities for rescue, life-saving, first aid, fire control and other hazards are higher than the priority for measuring radiation levels.**
- Radiation Authority must be notified of accident conditions. Radiation Authority is usually responsible for decisions about radiological consequences and closure of emergencies.
- As an immediate precautionary measure, isolate spill or leak area for at least 25 meters (75 feet) in all directions.
- Stay upwind, uphill and/or upstream.
- Keep unauthorized personnel away.
- Detain or isolate uninjured persons or equipment suspected to be contaminated; delay decontamination and cleanup until instructions are received from Radiation Authority.

### PROTECTIVE CLOTHING

- Positive pressure self-contained breathing apparatus (SCBA) and structural firefighters' protective clothing will provide adequate protection.

### EVACUATION

**Large Spill**

- Consider initial downwind evacuation for at least 100 meters (330 feet).

**Fire**

- When a large quantity of this material is involved in a major fire, consider an initial evacuation distance of 300 meters (1000 feet) in all directions.

## EMERGENCY RESPONSE

### FIRE

- Presence of radioactive material will not influence the fire control processes and should not influence selection of techniques.
- Move containers from fire area if you can do it without risk.
- Do not move damaged packages; move undamaged packages out of fire zone.

**Small Fire**

- Dry chemical, $CO_2$, water spray or regular foam.

**Large Fire**

- Water spray, fog (flooding amounts).

### SPILL OR LEAK

- Do not touch damaged packages or spilled material.
- Cover liquid spill with sand, earth or other non-combustible absorbent material.
- Cover powder spill with plastic sheet or tarp to minimize spreading.

### FIRST AID

- Ensure that medical personnel are aware of the material(s) involved, take precautions to protect themselves and prevent spread of contamination.
- Call 911 or emergency medical service.
- Medical problems take priority over radiological concerns.
- Use first aid treatment according to the nature of the injury.
- Do not delay care and transport of a seriously injured person.
- Give artificial respiration if victim is not breathing.
- Administer oxygen if breathing is difficult.
- In case of contact with substance, immediately flush skin or eyes with running water for at least 20 minutes.
- Injured persons contaminated by contact with released material are not a serious hazard to health care personnel, equipment or facilities.

# GUIDE 162 RADIOACTIVE MATERIALS (LOW TO MODERATE LEVEL RADIATION)

## POTENTIAL HAZARDS

### HEALTH

- Radiation presents minimal risk to transport workers, emergency response personnel and the public during transportation accidents. Packaging durability increases as potential hazard of radioactive content increases.
- Undamaged packages are safe. Contents of damaged packages may cause higher external radiation exposure, or both external and internal radiation exposure if contents are released.
- Low radiation hazard when material is inside container. If material is released from package or bulk container, hazard will vary from low to moderate. Level of hazard will depend on the type and amount of radioactivity, the kind of material it is in, and/or the surfaces it is on.
- Some material may be released from packages during accidents of moderate severity but risks to people are not great.
- Released radioactive materials or contaminated objects usually will be visible if packaging fails.
- Some exclusive use shipments of bulk and packaged materials will not have "RADIOACTIVE" labels. Placards, markings and shipping papers provide identification.
- Some packages may have a "RADIOACTIVE" label and a second hazard label. The second hazard is usually greater than the radiation hazard; so follow this GUIDE as well as the response GUIDE for the second hazard class label.
- Some radioactive materials cannot be detected by commonly available instruments.
- Runoff from control of cargo fire may cause low-level pollution.

### FIRE OR EXPLOSION

- Some of these materials may burn, but most do not ignite readily.
- Uranium and Thorium metal cuttings may ignite spontaneously if exposed to air (see GUIDE 136).
- Nitrates are oxidizers and may ignite other combustibles (see GUIDE 141).

## PUBLIC SAFETY

- **CALL EMERGENCY RESPONSE Telephone Number on Shipping Paper first. If Shipping Paper not available or no answer, refer to appropriate telephone number listed on the inside back cover.**
- **Priorities for rescue, life-saving, first aid, fire control and other hazards are higher than the priority for measuring radiation levels.**
- Radiation Authority must be notified of accident conditions. Radiation Authority is usually responsible for decisions about radiological consequences and closure of emergencies.
- As an immediate precautionary measure, isolate spill or leak area for at least 25 meters (75 feet) in all directions.
- Stay upwind, uphill and/or upstream.
- Keep unauthorized personnel away.
- Detain or isolate uninjured persons or equipment suspected to be contaminated; delay decontamination and cleanup until instructions are received from Radiation Authority.

### PROTECTIVE CLOTHING

- Positive pressure self-contained breathing apparatus (SCBA) and structural firefighters' protective clothing will provide adequate protection.

### EVACUATION

**Large Spill**

- Consider initial downwind evacuation for at least 100 meters (330 feet).

**Fire**

- When a large quantity of this material is involved in a major fire, consider an initial evacuation distance of 300 meters (1000 feet) in all directions.

In Canada, an Emergency Response Assistance Plan (ERAP) may be required for this product. Please consult the shipping document and/or the ERAP Program Section (page 391).

## EMERGENCY RESPONSE

### FIRE

- Presence of radioactive material will not influence the fire control processes and should not influence selection of techniques.
- Move containers from fire area if you can do it without risk.
- Do not move damaged packages; move undamaged packages out of fire zone.

**Small Fire**

- Dry chemical, $CO_2$, water spray or regular foam.

**Large Fire**

- Water spray, fog (flooding amounts).
- Dike fire-control water for later disposal.

### SPILL OR LEAK

- Do not touch damaged packages or spilled material.
- Cover liquid spill with sand, earth or other non-combustible absorbent material.
- Dike to collect large liquid spills.
- Cover powder spill with plastic sheet or tarp to minimize spreading.

### FIRST AID

- Ensure that medical personnel are aware of the material(s) involved, take precautions to protect themselves.
- Call 911 or emergency medical service.
- Medical problems take priority over radiological concerns.
- Use first aid treatment according to the nature of the injury.
- Do not delay care and transport of a seriously injured person.
- Give artificial respiration if victim is not breathing.
- Administer oxygen if breathing is difficult.
- In case of contact with substance, wipe from skin immediately; flush skin or eyes with running water for at least 20 minutes.
- Injured persons contaminated by contact with released material are not a serious hazard to health care personnel, equipment or facilities.

# GUIDE 163 RADIOACTIVE MATERIALS (LOW TO HIGH LEVEL RADIATION)

## POTENTIAL HAZARDS

### HEALTH

- Radiation presents minimal risk to transport workers, emergency response personnel and the public during transportation accidents. Packaging durability increases as potential hazard of radioactive content increases.
- Undamaged packages are safe. Contents of damaged packages may cause higher external radiation exposure, or both external and internal radiation exposure if contents are released.
- Type A packages (cartons, boxes, drums, articles, etc.) identified as "Type A" by marking on packages or by shipping papers contain non-life-endangering amounts. Partial releases might be expected if "Type A" packages are damaged in moderately severe accidents.
- Type B packages, and the rarely occurring Type C packages (large and small, usually metal), contain the most hazardous amounts. They can be identified by package markings or by shipping papers. Life-threatening conditions may exist only if contents are released or package shielding fails. Because of design, evaluation and testing of packages, these conditions would be expected only for accidents of utmost severity.
- The rarely occurring "Special Arrangement" shipments may be of Type A, Type B or Type C packages. Package type will be marked on packages, and shipment details will be on shipping papers.
- Radioactive White-I labels indicate radiation levels outside single, isolated, undamaged packages are very low (less than 0.005 mSv/h (0.5 mrem/h)).
- Radioactive Yellow-II and Yellow-III labeled packages have higher radiation levels. The transport index (TI) on the label identifies the maximum radiation level in mrem/h one meter from a single, isolated, undamaged package.
- Some radioactive materials cannot be detected by commonly available instruments.
- Water from cargo fire control may cause pollution.

### FIRE OR EXPLOSION

- Some of these materials may burn, but most do not ignite readily.
- Radioactivity does not change flammability or other properties of materials.
- Type B packages are designed and evaluated to withstand total engulfment in flames at temperatures of 800°C (1475°F) for a period of 30 minutes.

## PUBLIC SAFETY

- **CALL EMERGENCY RESPONSE Telephone Number on Shipping Paper first. If Shipping Paper not available or no answer, refer to appropriate telephone number listed on the inside back cover.**
- **Priorities for rescue, life-saving, first aid, fire control and other hazards are higher than the priority for measuring radiation levels.**
- Radiation Authority must be notified of accident conditions. Radiation Authority is usually responsible for decisions about radiological consequences and closure of emergencies.
- As an immediate precautionary measure, isolate spill or leak area for at least 25 meters (75 feet) in all directions.
- Stay upwind, uphill and/or upstream.
- Keep unauthorized personnel away.
- Detain or isolate uninjured persons or equipment suspected to be contaminated; delay decontamination and cleanup until instructions are received from Radiation Authority.

### PROTECTIVE CLOTHING

- Positive pressure self-contained breathing apparatus (SCBA) and structural firefighters' protective clothing will provide adequate protection against internal radiation exposure, but not external radiation exposure.

### EVACUATION

**Large Spill**

- Consider initial downwind evacuation for at least 100 meters (330 feet).

**Fire**

- When a large quantity of this material is involved in a major fire, consider an initial evacuation distance of 300 meters (1000 feet) in all directions.

## EMERGENCY RESPONSE

### FIRE

- Presence of radioactive material will not influence the fire control processes and should not influence selection of techniques.
- Move containers from fire area if you can do it without risk.
- Do not move damaged packages; move undamaged packages out of fire zone.

**Small Fire**

- Dry chemical, $CO_2$, water spray or regular foam.

**Large Fire**

- Water spray, fog (flooding amounts).
- Dike fire-control water for later disposal.

### SPILL OR LEAK

- Do not touch damaged packages or spilled material.
- Damp surfaces on undamaged or slightly damaged packages are seldom an indication of packaging failure. Most packaging for liquid content have inner containers and/or inner absorbent materials.
- Cover liquid spill with sand, earth or other non-combustible absorbent material.

### FIRST AID

- Ensure that medical personnel are aware of the material(s) involved, take precautions to protect themselves.
- Call 911 or emergency medical service.
- Medical problems take priority over radiological concerns.
- Use first aid treatment according to the nature of the injury.
- Do not delay care and transport of a seriously injured person.
- Give artificial respiration if victim is not breathing.
- Administer oxygen if breathing is difficult.
- In case of contact with substance, immediately flush skin or eyes with running water for at least 20 minutes.
- Injured persons contaminated by contact with released material are not a serious hazard to health care personnel, equipment or facilities.

# GUIDE 164 RADIOACTIVE MATERIALS (SPECIAL FORM/ LOW TO HIGH LEVEL EXTERNAL RADIATION)

## POTENTIAL HAZARDS

### HEALTH

- Radiation presents minimal risk to transport workers, emergency response personnel and the public during transportation accidents. Packaging durability increases as potential hazard of radioactive content increases.
- Undamaged packages are safe; contents of damaged packages may cause external radiation exposure, and much higher external exposure if contents (source capsules) are released.
- Contamination and internal radiation hazards are not expected, but not impossible.
- Type A packages (cartons, boxes, drums, articles, etc.) identified as "Type A" by marking on packages or by shipping papers contain non-life-endangering amounts. Radioactive sources may be released if "Type A" packages are damaged in moderately severe accidents.
- Type B packages, and the rarely occurring Type C packages, (large and small, usually metal) contain the most hazardous amounts. They can be identified by package markings or by shipping papers. Life-threatening conditions may exist only if contents are released or package shielding fails. Because of design, evaluation and testing of packages, these conditions would be expected only for accidents of utmost severity.
- Radioactive White-I labels indicate radiation levels outside single, isolated, undamaged packages are very low (less than 0.005 mSv/h (0.5 mrem/h)).
- Radioactive Yellow-II and Yellow-III labeled packages have higher radiation levels. The transport index (TI) on the label identifies the maximum radiation level in mrem/h one meter from a single, isolated, undamaged package.
- Radiation from the package contents, usually in durable metal capsules, can be detected by most radiation instruments.
- Water from cargo fire control is not expected to cause pollution.

### FIRE OR EXPLOSION

- Packagings can burn completely without risk of content loss from sealed source capsule.
- Radioactivity does not change flammability or other properties of materials.
- Radioactive source capsules and Type B packages are designed and evaluated to withstand total engulfment in flames at temperatures of 800°C (1475°F) for a period of 30 minutes.

## PUBLIC SAFETY

- **CALL EMERGENCY RESPONSE Telephone Number on Shipping Paper first. If Shipping Paper not available or no answer, refer to appropriate telephone number listed on the inside back cover.**
- **Priorities for rescue, life-saving, first aid, fire control and other hazards are higher than the priority for measuring radiation levels.**
- Radiation Authority must be notified of accident conditions. Radiation Authority is usually responsible for decisions about radiological consequences and closure of emergencies.
- As an immediate precautionary measure, isolate spill or leak area for at least 25 meters (75 feet) in all directions.
- Stay upwind, uphill and/or upstream.
- Keep unauthorized personnel away.
- Delay final cleanup until instructions or advice is received from Radiation Authority.

### PROTECTIVE CLOTHING

- Positive pressure self-contained breathing apparatus (SCBA) and structural firefighters' protective clothing will provide adequate protection against internal radiation exposure, but not external radiation exposure.

### EVACUATION

**Large Spill**

- Consider initial downwind evacuation for at least 100 meters (330 feet).

**Fire**

- When a large quantity of this material is involved in a major fire, consider an initial evacuation distance of 300 meters (1000 feet) in all directions.

## EMERGENCY RESPONSE

### FIRE

- Presence of radioactive material will not influence the fire control processes and should not influence selection of techniques.
- Move containers from fire area if you can do it without risk.
- Do not move damaged packages; move undamaged packages out of fire zone.

**Small Fire**

- Dry chemical, $CO_2$, water spray or regular foam.

**Large Fire**

- Water spray, fog (flooding amounts).

### SPILL OR LEAK

- Do not touch damaged packages or spilled material.
- Damp surfaces on undamaged or slightly damaged packages are seldom an indication of packaging failure. Contents are seldom liquid. Content is usually a metal capsule, easily seen if released from package.
- If source capsule is identified as being out of package, **DO NOT TOUCH**. Stay away and await advice from Radiation Authority.

### FIRST AID

- Ensure that medical personnel are aware of the material(s) involved, take precautions to protect themselves.
- Call 911 or emergency medical service.
- Medical problems take priority over radiological concerns.
- Use first aid treatment according to the nature of the injury.
- Do not delay care and transport of a seriously injured person.
- Persons exposed to special form sources are not likely to be contaminated with radioactive material.
- Give artificial respiration if victim is not breathing.
- Administer oxygen if breathing is difficult.
- Injured persons contaminated by contact with released material are not a serious hazard to health care personnel, equipment or facilities.

# GUIDE 165 RADIOACTIVE MATERIALS (FISSILE/LOW TO HIGH LEVEL RADIATION)

## POTENTIAL HAZARDS

### HEALTH

- Radiation presents minimal risk to transport workers, emergency response personnel and the public during transportation accidents. Packaging durability increases as potential radiation and criticality hazards of the content increase.
- Undamaged packages are safe. Contents of damaged packages may cause higher external radiation exposure, or both external and internal radiation exposure if contents are released.
- Type AF or IF packages, identified by package markings, do not contain life-threatening amounts of material. External radiation levels are low and packages are designed, evaluated and tested to control releases and to prevent a fission chain reaction under severe transport conditions.
- Type B(U)F, B(M)F and CF packages (identified by markings on packages or shipping papers) contain potentially life-endangering amounts. Because of design, evaluation and testing of packages, fission chain reactions are prevented and releases are not expected to be life-endangering for all accidents except those of utmost severity.
- The rarely occurring "Special Arrangement" shipments may be of Type AF, BF or CF packages. Package type will be marked on packages, and shipment details will be on shipping papers.
- The transport index (TI) shown on labels or a shipping paper might not indicate the radiation level at one meter from a single, isolated, undamaged package; instead, it might relate to controls needed during transport because of the fissile properties of the materials. Alternatively, the fissile nature of the contents may be indicated by a criticality safety index (CSI) on a special FISSILE label or on the shipping paper.
- Some radioactive materials cannot be detected by commonly available instruments.
- Water from cargo fire control is not expected to cause pollution.

### FIRE OR EXPLOSION

- These materials are seldom flammable. Packages are designed to withstand fires without damage to contents.
- Radioactivity does not change flammability or other properties of materials.
- Type AF, IF, B(U)F, B(M)F and CF packages are designed and evaluated to withstand total engulfment in flames at temperatures of 800°C (1475°F) for a period of 30 minutes.

## PUBLIC SAFETY

- **CALL EMERGENCY RESPONSE Telephone Number on Shipping Paper first. If Shipping Paper not available or no answer, refer to appropriate telephone number listed on the inside back cover.**
- **Priorities for rescue, life-saving, first aid, fire control and other hazards are higher than the priority for measuring radiation levels.**
- Radiation Authority must be notified of accident conditions. Radiation Authority is usually responsible for decisions about radiological consequences and closure of emergencies.
- As an immediate precautionary measure, isolate spill or leak area for at least 25 meters (75 feet) in all directions. • Stay upwind, uphill and/or upstream. • Keep unauthorized personnel away.
- Detain or isolate uninjured persons or equipment suspected to be contaminated; delay decontamination and cleanup until instructions are received from Radiation Authority.

### PROTECTIVE CLOTHING

- Positive pressure self-contained breathing apparatus (SCBA) and structural firefighters' protective clothing will provide adequate protection against internal radiation exposure, but not external radiation exposure.

### EVACUATION

**Large Spill**

- Consider initial downwind evacuation for at least 100 meters (330 feet).

**Fire**

- When a large quantity of this material is involved in a major fire, consider an initial evacuation distance of 300 meters (1000 feet) in all directions.

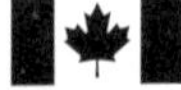

In Canada, an Emergency Response Assistance Plan (ERAP) may be required for this product. Please consult the shipping document and/or the ERAP Program Section (page 391).

## EMERGENCY RESPONSE

### FIRE

- Presence of radioactive material will not influence the fire control processes and should not influence selection of techniques.
- Move containers from fire area if you can do it without risk.
- Do not move damaged packages; move undamaged packages out of fire zone.

**Small Fire**

- Dry chemical, $CO_2$, water spray or regular foam.

**Large Fire**

- Water spray, fog (flooding amounts).

### SPILL OR LEAK

- Do not touch damaged packages or spilled material.
- Damp surfaces on undamaged or slightly damaged packages are seldom an indication of packaging failure. Most packaging for liquid content have inner containers and/or inner absorbent materials.

**Liquid Spill**

- Package contents are seldom liquid. If any radioactive contamination resulting from a liquid release is present, it probably will be low-level.

### FIRST AID

- Ensure that medical personnel are aware of the material(s) involved, take precautions to protect themselves.
- Call 911 or emergency medical service.
- Medical problems take priority over radiological concerns.
- Use first aid treatment according to the nature of the injury.
- Do not delay care and transport of a seriously injured person.
- Give artificial respiration if victim is not breathing.
- Administer oxygen if breathing is difficult.
- In case of contact with substance, immediately flush skin or eyes with running water for at least 20 minutes.
- Injured persons contaminated by contact with released material are not a serious hazard to health care personnel, equipment or facilities.

# GUIDE 166 RADIOACTIVE MATERIALS - CORROSIVE (URANIUM HEXAFLUORIDE/WATER-SENSITIVE)

## POTENTIAL HAZARDS

### HEALTH

- Radiation presents minimal risk to transport workers, emergency response personnel and the public during transportation accidents. Packaging durability increases as potential radiation and criticality hazards of the content increase.
- **Chemical hazard greatly exceeds radiation hazard.**
- Substance reacts with water and water vapor in air to form **toxic and corrosive hydrogen fluoride gas** and an extremely irritating and corrosive, white-colored, water-soluble residue.
- If inhaled, may be fatal. • Direct contact causes burns to skin, eyes, and respiratory tract.
- Low-level radioactive material; very low radiation hazard to people.
- Runoff from control of cargo fire may cause low-level pollution.

### FIRE OR EXPLOSION

- Substance does not burn. • The material may react violently with fuels.
- Product will decompose to produce toxic and/or corrosive fumes.
- Containers in protective overpacks (horizontal cylindrical shape with short legs for tie-downs), are identified with "AF", "B(U)F" or "H(U)" on shipping papers or by markings on the overpacks. They are designed and evaluated to withstand severe conditions including total engulfment in flames at temperatures of 800°C (1475°F) for a period of 30 minutes.
- Bare filled cylinders, identified with UN2978 as part of the marking (may also be marked H(U) or H(M)), may rupture in heat of engulfing fire; bare empty (except for residue) cylinders will not rupture in fires.
- Radioactivity does not change flammability or other properties of materials.

## PUBLIC SAFETY

- **CALL EMERGENCY RESPONSE Telephone Number on Shipping Paper first. If Shipping Paper not available or no answer, refer to appropriate telephone number listed on the inside back cover.**
- **Priorities for rescue, life-saving, first aid, fire control and other hazards are higher than the priority for measuring radiation levels.**
- Radiation Authority must be notified of accident conditions. Radiation Authority is usually responsible for decisions about radiological consequences and closure of emergencies.
- As an immediate precautionary measure, isolate spill or leak area for at least 25 meters (75 feet) in all directions.
- Stay upwind, uphill and/or upstream. • Keep unauthorized personnel away.
- Detain or isolate uninjured persons or equipment suspected to be contaminated; delay decontamination and cleanup until instructions are received from Radiation Authority.

### PROTECTIVE CLOTHING

- Wear positive pressure self-contained breathing apparatus (SCBA).
- Wear chemical protective clothing that is specifically recommended by the manufacturer. It may provide little or no thermal protection.
- Structural firefighters' protective clothing provides limited protection in fire situations ONLY; it is not effective in spill situations where direct contact with the substance is possible.

### EVACUATION

**Spill**

- See Table 1 - Initial Isolation and Protective Action Distances.

**Fire**

- When a large quantity of this material is involved in a major fire, consider an initial evacuation distance of 300 meters (1000 feet) in all directions.

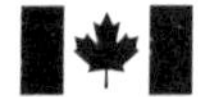

In Canada, an Emergency Response Assistance Plan (ERAP) may be required for this product. Please consult the shipping document and/or the ERAP Program Section (page 391).

## EMERGENCY RESPONSE

### FIRE

- DO NOT USE WATER OR FOAM ON MATERIAL ITSELF.
- Move containers from fire area if you can do it without risk.

**Small Fire**

- Dry chemical or $CO_2$.

**Large Fire**

- Water spray, fog or regular foam.
- Cool containers with flooding quantities of water until well after fire is out.
- If this is impossible, withdraw from area and let fire burn.
- ALWAYS stay away from tanks engulfed in fire.

### SPILL OR LEAK

- Do not touch damaged packages or spilled material.
- DO NOT GET WATER INSIDE CONTAINERS.
- Without fire or smoke, leak will be evident by visible and irritating vapors and residue forming at the point of release.
- Use fine water spray to reduce vapors; do not put water directly on point of material release from container.
- Residue buildup may self-seal small leaks.
- Dike far ahead of spill to collect runoff water.

### FIRST AID

- Ensure that medical personnel are aware of the material(s) involved, take precautions to protect themselves.
- Call 911 or emergency medical service.
- Medical problems take priority over radiological concerns.
- Use first aid treatment according to the nature of the injury.
- **In case of contact with Hydrofluoric acid (UN1790)**, flush with large amounts of water. For skin contact, if calcium gluconate gel is available, rinse 5 minutes, then apply gel. Otherwise, continue rinsing until medical treatment is available. For eyes, flush with water or a saline solution for 15 minutes.
- Do not delay care and transport of a seriously injured person.
- Give artificial respiration if victim is not breathing.
- Administer oxygen if breathing is difficult.
- In case of contact with substance, immediately flush skin or eyes with running water for at least 20 minutes.
- Effects of exposure (inhalation, ingestion or skin contact) to substance may be delayed.
- Keep victim calm and warm.

Page intentionally left blank

Page intentionally left blank

# GUIDE 168 CARBON MONOXIDE (REFRIGERATED LIQUID)

## POTENTIAL HAZARDS

### HEALTH

- **TOXIC; Extremely Hazardous.**
- Inhalation extremely dangerous; may be fatal.
- Contact with gas or liquefied gas may cause burns, severe injury and/or frostbite.
- Odorless, will not be detected by sense of smell.

### FIRE OR EXPLOSION

- **EXTREMELY FLAMMABLE.**
- May be ignited by heat, sparks or flames.
- Flame may be invisible.
- Containers may explode when heated.
- Vapor explosion and poison hazard indoors, outdoors or in sewers.
- Vapors from liquefied gas are initially heavier than air and spread along ground.
- Vapors may travel to source of ignition and flash back.
- Runoff may create fire or explosion hazard.

## PUBLIC SAFETY

- **CALL EMERGENCY RESPONSE Telephone Number on Shipping Paper first. If Shipping Paper not available or no answer, refer to appropriate telephone number listed on the inside back cover.**
- As an immediate precautionary measure, isolate spill or leak area for at least 100 meters (330 feet) in all directions.
- Keep unauthorized personnel away.
- Stay upwind, uphill and/or upstream.
- Many gases are heavier than air and will spread along ground and collect in low or confined areas (sewers, basements, tanks).
- Ventilate closed spaces before entering.

### PROTECTIVE CLOTHING

- Wear positive pressure self-contained breathing apparatus (SCBA).
- Wear chemical protective clothing that is specifically recommended by the manufacturer. It may provide little or no thermal protection.
- Structural firefighters' protective clothing provides limited protection in fire situations ONLY; it is not effective in spill situations where direct contact with the substance is possible.
- Always wear thermal protective clothing when handling refrigerated/cryogenic liquids.

### EVACUATION

**Spill**

- See Table 1 - Initial Isolation and Protective Action Distances.

**Fire**

- If tank, rail car or tank truck is involved in a fire, ISOLATE for 800 meters (1/2 mile) in all directions; also, consider initial evacuation for 800 meters (1/2 mile) in all directions.

## EMERGENCY RESPONSE

### FIRE

- **DO NOT EXTINGUISH A LEAKING GAS FIRE UNLESS LEAK CAN BE STOPPED.**

**Small Fire**

- Dry chemical, $CO_2$ or water spray.

**Large Fire**

- Water spray, fog or regular foam.
- Move containers from fire area if you can do it without risk.

**Fire involving Tanks**

- Fight fire from maximum distance or use unmanned hose holders or monitor nozzles.
- Cool containers with flooding quantities of water until well after fire is out.
- Do not direct water at source of leak or safety devices; icing may occur.
- Withdraw immediately in case of rising sound from venting safety devices or discoloration of tank.
- ALWAYS stay away from tanks engulfed in fire.

### SPILL OR LEAK

- ELIMINATE all ignition sources (no smoking, flares, sparks or flames in immediate area).
- All equipment used when handling the product must be grounded.
- Fully encapsulating, vapor-protective clothing should be worn for spills and leaks with no fire.
- Do not touch or walk through spilled material.
- Stop leak if you can do it without risk.
- Use water spray to reduce vapors or divert vapor cloud drift. Avoid allowing water runoff to contact spilled material.
- Do not direct water at spill or source of leak.
- If possible, turn leaking containers so that gas escapes rather than liquid.
- Prevent entry into waterways, sewers, basements or confined areas.
- Isolate area until gas has dispersed.

### FIRST AID

- Ensure that medical personnel are aware of the material(s) involved and take precautions to protect themselves.
- Move victim to fresh air.
- Call 911 or emergency medical service.
- Give artificial respiration if victim is not breathing.
- Administer oxygen if breathing is difficult.
- Remove and isolate contaminated clothing and shoes.
- In case of contact with substance, immediately flush skin or eyes with running water for at least 20 minutes.
- In case of contact with liquefied gas, thaw frosted parts with lukewarm water.
- Keep victim calm and warm.
- Keep victim under observation.
- Effects of contact or inhalation may be delayed.

# GUIDE 169 ALUMINUM (MOLTEN)

## POTENTIAL HAZARDS

### FIRE OR EXPLOSION

- Substance is transported in molten form at a temperature above 705°C (1300°F).
- Violent reaction with water; contact may cause an explosion or may produce a flammable gas.
- Will ignite combustible materials (wood, paper, oil, debris, etc.).
- Contact with nitrates or other oxidizers may cause an explosion.
- Contact with containers or other materials, including cold, wet or dirty tools, may cause an explosion.
- Contact with concrete will cause spalling and small pops.

### HEALTH

- Contact causes severe burns to skin and eyes.
- Fire may produce irritating and/or toxic gases.

## PUBLIC SAFETY

- **CALL EMERGENCY RESPONSE Telephone Number on Shipping Paper first. If Shipping Paper not available or no answer, refer to appropriate telephone number listed on the inside back cover.**
- As an immediate precautionary measure, isolate spill or leak area for at least 50 meters (150 feet) in all directions.
- Stay upwind, uphill and/or upstream.
- Keep unauthorized personnel away.
- Ventilate closed spaces before entering.

### PROTECTIVE CLOTHING

- Wear positive pressure self-contained breathing apparatus (SCBA).
- Wear flame-retardant structural firefighters' protective clothing, including faceshield, helmet and gloves, as this will provide limited thermal protection.

## EMERGENCY RESPONSE

### FIRE

- **Do Not Use Water, except in life-threatening situations and then only in a fine spray.**
- **Do not use halogenated extinguishing agents or foam.**
- Move combustibles out of path of advancing pool if you can do so without risk.
- Extinguish fires started by molten material by using appropriate method for the burning material; keep water, halogenated extinguishing agents and foam away from the molten material.

### SPILL OR LEAK

- Do not touch or walk through spilled material.
- Do not attempt to stop leak, due to danger of explosion.
- Keep combustibles (wood, paper, oil, etc.) away from spilled material.
- Substance is very fluid, spreads quickly, and may splash. Do not try to stop it with shovels or other objects.
- Dike far ahead of spill; use dry sand to contain the flow of material.
- Where possible allow molten material to solidify naturally.
- Avoid contact even after material solidifies. Molten, heated and cold aluminum look alike; do not touch unless you know it is cold.
- Clean up under the supervision of an expert after material has solidified.

### FIRST AID

- Ensure that medical personnel are aware of the material(s) involved and take precautions to protect themselves.
- Move victim to fresh air.
- Call 911 or emergency medical service.
- Give artificial respiration if victim is not breathing.
- Administer oxygen if breathing is difficult.
- For severe burns, immediate medical attention is required.
- Removal of solidified molten material from skin requires medical assistance.
- Remove and isolate contaminated clothing and shoes.
- In case of contact with substance, immediately flush skin or eyes with running water for at least 20 minutes.
- Keep victim calm and warm.

# GUIDE 170 METALS (POWDERS, DUSTS, SHAVINGS, BORINGS, TURNINGS, OR CUTTINGS, ETC.)

## POTENTIAL HAZARDS

### FIRE OR EXPLOSION

- May react violently or explosively on contact with water.
- Some are transported in flammable liquids.
- May be ignited by friction, heat, sparks or flames.
- Some of these materials will burn with intense heat.
- Dusts or fumes may form explosive mixtures in air.
- Containers may explode when heated.
- May re-ignite after fire is extinguished.

### HEALTH

- Oxides from metallic fires are a severe health hazard.
- Inhalation or contact with substance or decomposition products may cause severe injury or death.
- Fire may produce irritating, corrosive and/or toxic gases.
- Runoff from fire control or dilution water may cause pollution.

## PUBLIC SAFETY

- **CALL EMERGENCY RESPONSE Telephone Number on Shipping Paper first. If Shipping Paper not available or no answer, refer to appropriate telephone number listed on the inside back cover.**
- As an immediate precautionary measure, isolate spill or leak area in all directions for at least 50 meters (150 feet) for liquids and at least 25 meters (75 feet) for solids.
- Stay upwind, uphill and/or upstream.
- Keep unauthorized personnel away.

### PROTECTIVE CLOTHING

- Wear positive pressure self-contained breathing apparatus (SCBA).
- Structural firefighters' protective clothing will only provide limited protection.

### EVACUATION

**Large Spill**

- Consider initial downwind evacuation for at least 50 meters (160 feet).

**Fire**

- If tank, rail car or tank truck is involved in a fire, ISOLATE for 800 meters (1/2 mile) in all directions; also, consider initial evacuation for 800 meters (1/2 mile) in all directions.

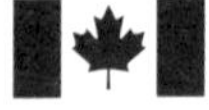

In Canada, an Emergency Response Assistance Plan (ERAP) may be required for this product. Please consult the shipping document and/or the ERAP Program Section (page 391).

## EMERGENCY RESPONSE

### FIRE

- **DO NOT USE WATER, FOAM OR $CO_2$.**
- Dousing metallic fires with water will generate hydrogen gas, an extremely dangerous explosion hazard, particularly if fire is in a confined environment (i.e., building, cargo hold, etc.).
- Use DRY sand, graphite powder, dry sodium chloride-based extinguishers, G-1® or Met-L-X® powder.
- Confining and smothering metal fires is preferable rather than applying water.
- Move containers from fire area if you can do it without risk.

**Fire involving Tanks or Car/Trailer Loads**

- If impossible to extinguish, protect surroundings and allow fire to burn itself out.

### SPILL OR LEAK

- ELIMINATE all ignition sources (no smoking, flares, sparks or flames in immediate area).
- Do not touch or walk through spilled material.
- Stop leak if you can do it without risk.
- Prevent entry into waterways, sewers, basements or confined areas.

### FIRST AID

- Ensure that medical personnel are aware of the material(s) involved and take precautions to protect themselves.
- Move victim to fresh air.
- Call 911 or emergency medical service.
- Give artificial respiration if victim is not breathing.
- Administer oxygen if breathing is difficult.
- Remove and isolate contaminated clothing and shoes.
- In case of contact with substance, immediately flush skin or eyes with running water for at least 20 minutes.
- Keep victim calm and warm.

# GUIDE 171 SUBSTANCES (LOW TO MODERATE HAZARD)

## POTENTIAL HAZARDS

### FIRE OR EXPLOSION

- Some may burn but none ignite readily.
- Containers may explode when heated.
- Some may be transported hot.
- For UN3508, be aware of possible short circuiting as this product is transported in a charged state.

### HEALTH

- Inhalation of material may be harmful.
- Contact may cause burns to skin and eyes.
- Inhalation of Asbestos dust may have a damaging effect on the lungs.
- Fire may produce irritating, corrosive and/or toxic gases.
- Some liquids produce vapors that may cause dizziness or suffocation.
- Runoff from fire control may cause pollution.

## PUBLIC SAFETY

- **CALL EMERGENCY RESPONSE Telephone Number on Shipping Paper first. If Shipping Paper not available or no answer, refer to appropriate telephone number listed on the inside back cover.**
- As an immediate precautionary measure, isolate spill or leak area in all directions for at least 50 meters (150 feet) for liquids and at least 25 meters (75 feet) for solids.
- Keep unauthorized personnel away.
- Stay upwind, uphill and/or upstream.

### PROTECTIVE CLOTHING

- Wear positive pressure self-contained breathing apparatus (SCBA).
- Structural firefighters' protective clothing will only provide limited protection.

### EVACUATION

**Spill**

- See Table 1 - Initial Isolation and Protective Action Distances for highlighted materials. For non-highlighted materials, increase, in the downwind direction, as necessary, the isolation distance shown under "PUBLIC SAFETY".

**Fire**

- If tank, rail car or tank truck is involved in a fire, ISOLATE for 800 meters (1/2 mile) in all directions; also, consider initial evacuation for 800 meters (1/2 mile) in all directions.

## EMERGENCY RESPONSE

### FIRE

**Small Fire**

- Dry chemical, $CO_2$, water spray or regular foam.

**Large Fire**

- Water spray, fog or regular foam.
- Do not scatter spilled material with high-pressure water streams.
- Move containers from fire area if you can do it without risk.
- Dike fire-control water for later disposal.

**Fire involving Tanks**

- Cool containers with flooding quantities of water until well after fire is out.
- Withdraw immediately in case of rising sound from venting safety devices or discoloration of tank.
- ALWAYS stay away from tanks engulfed in fire.

### SPILL OR LEAK

- Do not touch or walk through spilled material.
- Stop leak if you can do it without risk.
- Prevent dust cloud.
- Avoid inhalation of asbestos dust.

**Small Dry Spill**

- With clean shovel, place material into clean, dry container and cover loosely; move containers from spill area.

**Small Spill**

- Pick up with sand or other non-combustible absorbent material and place into containers for later disposal.

**Large Spill**

- Dike far ahead of liquid spill for later disposal.
- Cover powder spill with plastic sheet or tarp to minimize spreading.
- Prevent entry into waterways, sewers, basements or confined areas.

### FIRST AID

- Ensure that medical personnel are aware of the material(s) involved and take precautions to protect themselves.
- Move victim to fresh air.
- Call 911 or emergency medical service.
- Give artificial respiration if victim is not breathing.
- Administer oxygen if breathing is difficult.
- Remove and isolate contaminated clothing and shoes.
- In case of contact with substance, immediately flush skin or eyes with running water for at least 20 minutes.

# GUIDE 172 GALLIUM AND MERCURY

## POTENTIAL HAZARDS

### HEALTH

- Inhalation of vapors or contact with substance will result in contamination and potential harmful effects.
- Fire will produce irritating, corrosive and/or toxic gases.

### FIRE OR EXPLOSION

- Non-combustible, substance itself does not burn but may react upon heating to produce corrosive and/or toxic fumes.
- Runoff may pollute waterways.

## PUBLIC SAFETY

- **CALL EMERGENCY RESPONSE Telephone Number on Shipping Paper first. If Shipping Paper not available or no answer, refer to appropriate telephone number listed on the inside back cover.**
- As an immediate precautionary measure, isolate spill or leak area for at least 50 meters (150 feet) in all directions.
- Stay upwind, uphill and/or upstream.
- Keep unauthorized personnel away.

### PROTECTIVE CLOTHING

- Wear positive pressure self-contained breathing apparatus (SCBA).
- Structural firefighters' protective clothing will only provide limited protection.

### EVACUATION

**Large Spill**

- Consider initial downwind evacuation for at least 100 meters (330 feet).

**Fire**

- When any large container is involved in a fire, consider initial evacuation for 500 meters (1/3 mile) in all directions.

## EMERGENCY RESPONSE

### FIRE

- Use extinguishing agent suitable for type of surrounding fire.
- **Do not direct water at the heated metal.**

### SPILL OR LEAK

- Do not touch or walk through spilled material.
- Do not touch damaged containers or spilled material unless wearing appropriate protective clothing.
- Stop leak if you can do it without risk.
- Prevent entry into waterways, sewers, basements or confined areas.
- Do not use steel or aluminum tools or equipment.
- Cover with earth, sand or other non-combustible material followed with plastic sheet to minimize spreading or contact with rain.
- For mercury, use a mercury spill kit.
- Mercury spill areas may be subsequently treated with calcium sulphide/calcium sulfide or with sodium thiosulphate/sodium thiosulfate wash to neutralize any residual mercury.

### FIRST AID

- Ensure that medical personnel are aware of the material(s) involved and take precautions to protect themselves.
- Move victim to fresh air.
- Call 911 or emergency medical service.
- Give artificial respiration if victim is not breathing.
- Administer oxygen if breathing is difficult.
- Remove and isolate contaminated clothing and shoes.
- In case of contact with substance, immediately flush skin or eyes with running water for at least 20 minutes.
- Keep victim calm and warm.

# GUIDE 173 ADSORBED GASES - TOXIC*

## POTENTIAL HAZARDS

### HEALTH

- **TOXIC; may be fatal if inhaled or absorbed through skin.**
- Vapors may be irritating.
- Contact with gas may cause burns and injury.
- Fire will produce irritating, corrosive and/or toxic gases.
- Runoff from fire control may cause pollution.

### FIRE OR EXPLOSION

- Some gases may burn or be ignited by heat, sparks or flames but NOT readily due to low transportation pressures.
- May form explosive mixtures with air.
- Oxidizers may ignite combustibles (wood, paper, oil, clothing, etc.) but NOT readily due to low transportation pressures.
- Vapors may travel to source of ignition and flash back.
- Some of these materials may react violently with water.
- Cylinders exposed to fire may vent and release toxic and flammable gas through pressure relief devices.
- Runoff may create fire hazard.

## PUBLIC SAFETY

- **CALL Emergency Response Telephone Number on Shipping Paper first. If Shipping Paper not available or no answer, refer to appropriate telephone number listed on the inside back cover.**
- As an immediate precautionary measure, isolate spill or leak area for at least 100 meters (330 feet) in all directions.
- Keep unauthorized personnel away.
- Stay upwind, uphill and/or upstream.
- Many gases are heavier than air and will spread along ground and collect in low or confined areas (sewers, basements, tanks).
- Ventilate closed spaces before entering.

### PROTECTIVE CLOTHING

- Wear positive pressure self-contained breathing apparatus (SCBA).
- Wear chemical protective clothing that is specifically recommended by the manufacturer. It may provide little or no thermal protection.
- Structural firefighters' protective clothing provides limited protection in fire situations ONLY; it is not effective in spill situations where direct contact with the substance is possible.

### EVACUATION

**Spill**

- See Table 1 - Initial Isolation and Protective Action Distances.

**Fire**

- If several small packages (rail or trailer) are involved in a fire, ISOLATE for 1600 meters (1 mile) in all directions; also, consider initial evacuation for 1600 meters (1 mile) in all directions.

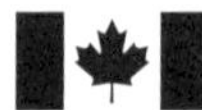

In Canada, an Emergency Response Assistance Plan (ERAP) may be required for this product. Please consult the shipping document and/or the ERAP Program Section (page 391).

* SOME SUBSTANCES MAY ALSO BE FLAMMABLE, CORROSIVE AND/OR OXIDIZING

## EMERGENCY RESPONSE

### FIRE

- **DO NOT EXTINGUISH A LEAKING GAS FIRE UNLESS LEAK CAN BE STOPPED.**

**Small Fire**

- Dry chemical, $CO_2$, water spray or alcohol-resistant foam.
- For UN3515, UN3518, UN3520, **use water only; no dry chemical, $CO_2$ or Halon®.**

**Large Fire**

- Water spray, fog or alcohol-resistant foam.
- Do not get water inside containers.
- Move containers from fire area if you can do it without risk.
- Damaged cylinders should be handled only by specialists.

**Fire involving Several Small Packages (rail or trailer)**

- Fight fire from maximum distance or use unmanned hose holders or monitor nozzles.
- Cool containers with flooding quantities of water until well after fire is out.
- Do not direct water at source of leak or safety devices.
- Withdraw immediately in case of rising sound from venting safety devices or discoloration of tank.
- ALWAYS stay away from tanks engulfed in fire.

### SPILL OR LEAK

- Some gases may be flammable. ELIMINATE all ignition sources (no smoking, flares, sparks or flames) from immediate area.
- For flammable gases, all equipment used when handling the product must be grounded.
- Fully encapsulating, vapor-protective clothing should be worn for spills and leaks with no fire.
- For oxidizing substances, keep combustibles (wood, paper, oil, etc.) away from spilled material.
- Do not touch or walk through spilled material.
- Stop leak if you can do it without risk.
- Do not direct water at spill or source of leak.
- Use water spray to reduce vapors or divert vapor cloud drift. Avoid allowing water runoff to contact spilled material.
- Prevent entry into waterways, sewers, basements or confined areas.
- Isolate area until gas has dispersed.

### FIRST AID

- Ensure that medical personnel are aware of the material(s) involved and take precautions to protect themselves.
- Move victim to fresh air. • Call 911 or emergency medical service.
- Give artificial respiration if victim is not breathing.
- **Do not use mouth-to-mouth method if victim ingested or inhaled the substance; give artificial respiration with the aid of a pocket mask equipped with a one-way valve or other proper respiratory medical device.**
- Administer oxygen if breathing is difficult.
- Remove and isolate contaminated clothing and shoes.
- In case of contact with substance, immediately flush skin or eyes with running water for at least 20 minutes.
- In case of burns, immediately cool affected skin for as long as possible with cold water. Do not remove clothing if adhering to skin.
- Keep victim calm and warm.
- Keep victim under observation.
- Effects of contact or inhalation may be delayed.

# GUIDE 174 ADSORBED GASES - FLAMMABLE OR OXIDIZING

## POTENTIAL HAZARDS

### FIRE OR EXPLOSION

- Some gases will be ignited by heat, sparks or flames but NOT readily due to low transportation pressure.
- Substance does not burn but will support combustion.
- Vapors may travel to source of ignition and flash back.
- Cylinders exposed to fire may vent and release flammable gas through pressure relief devices.
- Containers may explode when exposed to prolonged direct flame impingement.

### HEALTH

- Vapors may cause dizziness or asphyxiation without warning.
- Some may be irritating if inhaled at high concentrations.
- Contact with gas may cause burns and injury.
- Fire may produce irritating and/or toxic gases.

## PUBLIC SAFETY

- **CALL Emergency Response Telephone Number on Shipping Paper first. If Shipping Paper not available or no answer, refer to appropriate telephone number listed on the inside back cover.**
- As an immediate precautionary measure, isolate spill or leak area for at least 100 meters (330 feet) in all directions.
- Keep unauthorized personnel away.
- Stay upwind, uphill and/or upstream.
- Many gases are heavier than air and will spread along ground and collect in low or confined areas (sewers, basements, tanks).
- Ventilate closed spaces before entering.

### PROTECTIVE CLOTHING

- Wear positive pressure self-contained breathing apparatus (SCBA).
- Structural firefighters' protective clothing will only provide limited protection.

### EVACUATION

**Large Spill**

- Consider initial downwind evacuation for at least 800 meters (1/2 mile).

**Fire**

- If several small packages (rail or trailer) are involved in a fire, ISOLATE for 1600 meters (1 mile) in all directions; also, consider initial evacuation for 1600 meters (1 mile) in all directions.

## EMERGENCY RESPONSE

### FIRE

- **DO NOT EXTINGUISH A LEAKING GAS FIRE UNLESS LEAK CAN BE STOPPED.**
- Use extinguishing agent suitable for type of surrounding fire.

**Small Fire**

- Dry chemical or $CO_2$.

**Large Fire**

- Water spray or fog.
- Move containers from fire area if you can do it without risk.
- Damaged cylinders should be handled only by specialists.

**Fire involving Several Small Packages (rail or trailer)**

- Fight fire from maximum distance or use unmanned hose holders or monitor nozzles.
- Cool containers with flooding quantities of water until well after fire is out.
- Do not direct water at source of leak or safety devices.
- Withdraw immediately in case of rising sound from venting safety devices or discoloration of tank.
- ALWAYS stay away from tanks engulfed in fire.
- For massive fire, use unmanned hose holders or monitor nozzles; if this is impossible, withdraw from area and let fire burn.

### SPILL OR LEAK

- For flammable gases, ELIMINATE all ignition sources (no smoking, flares, sparks or flames) from immediate area.
- For oxidizing substances, keep combustibles (wood, paper, oil, etc.) away from spilled material.
- All equipment used when handling the product must be grounded.
- Do not touch or walk through spilled material.
- Stop leak if you can do it without risk.
- Use water spray to reduce vapors or divert vapor cloud drift. Avoid allowing water runoff to contact spilled material.
- Do not direct water at spill or source of leak.
- Prevent spreading of vapors through sewers, ventilation systems and confined areas.
- Ventilate the area.
- Isolate area until gas has dispersed.

### FIRST AID

- Ensure that medical personnel are aware of the material(s) involved and take precautions to protect themselves.
- Move victim to fresh air.
- Call 911 or emergency medical service.
- Give artificial respiration if victim is not breathing.
- Administer oxygen if breathing is difficult.
- Remove and isolate contaminated clothing and shoes.
- In case of burns, immediately cool affected skin for as long as possible with cold water. Do not remove clothing if adhering to skin.
- Keep victim calm and warm.

## NOTES

## INTRODUCTION TO GREEN TABLES - INITIAL ISOLATION AND PROTECTIVE ACTION DISTANCES

**Table 1** - Initial Isolation and Protective Action Distances suggests distances useful to protect people from vapors resulting from spills involving dangerous goods that are considered toxic by inhalation (TIH) (PIH in the US). This list includes certain chemical warfare agents and materials that produce toxic gases upon contact with water. Table 1 provides first responders with initial guidance until technically qualified emergency response personnel are available.

The **Initial Isolation Zone** defines an area SURROUNDING the incident in which persons may be exposed to dangerous (upwind) and life-threatening (downwind) concentrations of material. The **Protective Action Zone** defines an area DOWNWIND from the incident in which persons may become incapacitated and unable to take protective action and/or incur serious or irreversible health effects. Table 1 provides specific guidance for small and large spills occurring day or night.

Adjusting distances for a specific incident involves many interdependent variables and should be made only by personnel technically qualified to make such adjustments. For this reason, no precise guidance can be provided in this document to aid in adjusting the table distances; however, general guidance follows.

## Factors That May Change the Protective Action Distances

**The orange-bordered guide for a material** clearly indicates under the section EVACUATION – Fire, the evacuation distance required to protect against fragmentation hazard of a large container. If the material becomes involved in a **FIRE**, the toxic hazard may be less than the fire or explosion hazard. In these cases, the **Fire** hazard distance should be used.

Initial isolation and protective action distances in this guidebook are derived from historical data on transportation incidents and the use of statistical models. For worst-case scenarios involving the instantaneous release of the entire contents of a package (e.g., as a result of terrorism, sabotage or catastrophic accident) the distances may increase substantially. For such events, doubling of the initial isolation and protective action distances is appropriate in absence of other information.

If more than one tank car containing TIH materials involved in the incident is leaking, LARGE SPILL distances may need to be increased.

For a material with a protective action distance of 11.0+ km (7.0+ miles), the actual distance can be larger in certain atmospheric conditions. If the dangerous goods vapor plume is channeled in a valley or between many tall buildings, distances may be larger than shown in Table 1 due to less mixing of the plume with the atmosphere. Daytime spills in regions with known strong inversions or snow cover, or occurring near sunset, may require an increase of the protective action distance because airborne contaminants mix and disperse more slowly and may travel much farther downwind. In such cases, the nighttime protective action distance may be more appropriate. In addition, protective action distances may be larger for liquid spills when either the material or outdoor temperature exceeds 30°C (86°F).

Materials which react with water to produce large amounts of toxic gases are included in Table 1 - Initial Isolation and Protective Action Distances. Note that some water-reactive materials (WRM) which are also TIH (PIH in the US) (e.g., Bromine trifluoride (UN1746), Thionyl chloride (UN1836), etc.) produce additional TIH materials when spilled in water. For these materials, two entries are provided in Table 1 - Initial Isolation and Protective Action Distances (i.e., for spills on land and for spills in water). **If it is not clear whether the spill is on land or in water, or in cases where the spill occurs both on land and in water, choose the larger Protective Action Distance**.

Following Table 1, **Table 2** – Water-Reactive Materials Which Produce Toxic Gases lists materials that produce large amounts of Toxic Inhalation Hazard gases (TIH) when spilled in water as well as the toxic gases that are produced when spilled in water.

When a water-reactive TIH-producing material is spilled into a river or stream, the source of the toxic gas may move with the current and stretch from the spill point downstream for a substantial distance.

Finally, **Table 3** lists Initial Isolation and Protective Action Distances for Toxic Inhalation Hazard materials that may be more commonly encountered.

The selected materials are:

- Ammonia, anhydrous (UN1005)
- Chlorine (UN1017)
- Ethylene oxide (UN1040)
- Hydrogen chloride, anhydrous (UN1050) and Hydrogen chloride, refrigerated liquid (UN2186)
- Hydrogen fluoride, anhydrous (UN1052)
- Sulfur dioxide/Sulphur dioxide (UN1079)

The materials are presented in alphabetical order and provide Initial Isolation and Protective Action Distances for large spills (more than 208 liters or 55 US gallons) involving different container types (therefore different volume capacities) for day time and night time situations and for different wind speeds.

## PROTECTIVE ACTION DECISION FACTORS TO CONSIDER

The choice of protective actions for a given situation depends on a number of factors. For some cases, evacuation may be the best option; in others, sheltering in-place may be the best course. Sometimes, these two actions may be used in combination. In any emergency, officials need to quickly give the public instructions. The public will need continuing information and instructions while being evacuated or sheltered in-place.

Proper evaluation of the factors listed below will determine the effectiveness of evacuation or in-place protection (shelter in-place). The importance of these factors can vary with emergency conditions. In specific emergencies, other factors may need to be identified and considered as well. This list indicates what kind of information may be needed to make the initial decision.

### The Dangerous Goods

- Degree of health hazard
- Chemical and physical properties
- Amount involved
- Containment/control of release
- Rate of vapor movement

### The Population Threatened

- Location
- Number of people
- Time available to evacuate or shelter in-place
- Ability to control evacuation or shelter in-place
- Building types and availability
- Special institutions or populations, e.g., nursing homes, hospitals, prisons

### Weather Conditions

- Effect on vapor and cloud movement
- Potential for change
- Effect on evacuation or shelter in-place

## PROTECTIVE ACTIONS

**Protective Actions** are those steps taken to preserve the health and safety of emergency responders and the public during an incident involving releases of dangerous goods. Table 1 - Initial Isolation and Protective Action Distances (green-bordered pages) predicts the size of downwind areas which could be affected by a cloud of toxic gas. People in this area should be evacuated and/or sheltered in-place inside buildings.

**Isolate Hazard Area and Deny Entry** means to keep everybody away from the area if they are not directly involved in emergency response operations. Unprotected emergency responders should not be allowed to enter the isolation zone. This "isolation" task is done first to establish control over the area of operations. This is the first step for any protective actions that may follow. See Table 1 - Initial Isolation and Protective Action Distances (green-bordered pages) for more detailed information on specific materials.

**Evacuate** means to move all people from a threatened area to a safer place. To perform an evacuation, there must be enough time for people to be warned, to get ready, and to leave an area. If there is enough time, evacuation is the best protective action. Begin evacuating people nearby and those outdoors in direct view of the scene. When additional help arrives, expand the area to be evacuated downwind and crosswind to at least the extent recommended in this guidebook. Even after people move to the distances recommended, they may not be completely safe from harm. They should not be permitted to congregate at such distances. Send evacuees to a definite place, by a specific route, far enough away so they will not have to be moved again if the wind shifts.

**Shelter In-Place** means people should seek shelter inside a building and remain inside until the danger passes. **Sheltering in-place is used when evacuating the public would cause greater risk than staying where they are, or when an evacuation cannot be performed.** Direct the people inside to **close all doors and windows** and to **shut off all ventilating, heating and cooling systems.** In-place protection (shelter in-place) may not be the best option if (a) the vapors are flammable; (b) if it will take a long time for the gas to clear the area; or (c) if buildings cannot be closed tightly. Vehicles can offer some protection for a short period if the windows are closed and the ventilating systems are shut off. Vehicles are not as effective as buildings for in-place protection.

**It is vital to maintain communications with competent persons inside the building** so that they are advised about changing conditions. **Persons protected-in-place should be warned to stay far from windows** because of the danger from glass and projected metal fragments in a fire and/or explosion.

Every dangerous goods incident is different. Each will have special problems and concerns. Action to protect the public must be selected carefully. These pages can help with **initial** decisions on how to protect the public. Officials must continue to gather information and monitor the situation until the threat is removed.

## BACKGROUND ON TABLE 1 - INITIAL ISOLATION AND PROTECTIVE ACTION DISTANCES

Initial Isolation and Protective Action Distances in this guidebook were determined for small and large spills occurring during day or night. The overall analysis was statistical in nature and utilized state-of-the-art emission rate and dispersion models; statistical release data from the U.S. DOT HMIS (Hazardous Materials Information System) database; meteorological observations from over 120 locations in United States, Canada and Mexico; and the most current toxicological exposure guidelines.

For each chemical, thousands of hypothetical releases were modeled to account for the statistical variation in both release amount and atmospheric conditions. Based on this statistical sample, the $90^{th}$ percentile Protective Action Distance for each chemical and category was selected to appear in the Table. A brief description of the analysis is provided below. A detailed report outlining the methodology and data used in the generation of the Initial Isolation and Protective Action Distances may be obtained from the U.S. Department of Transportation, Pipeline and Hazardous Materials Safety Administration.

**Release amounts and emission rates** into the atmosphere were statistically modeled based on (1) data from the U.S. DOT HMIS database; (2) container types and sizes authorized for transport as specified in 49 CFR §172.101 and Part 173; (3) physical properties of the individual materials, and (4) atmospheric data from a historical database. The emission model calculated the release of vapor due to evaporation of pools on the ground, direct release of vapors from the container, or a combination of both, as would occur for liquefied gases which can flash to form both a vapor/aerosol mixture and an evaporating pool. In addition, the emission model also calculated the emission of toxic vapor by-products generated from spilling water-reactive materials in water. Spills that involve releases of approximately 208 liters for liquids (55 US gallons) and 300 kg for solids (660 lbs) or less are considered Small Spills, while spills that involve greater quantities are considered Large Spills. An exception to this is certain chemical warfare agents where Small Spills include releases up to 2 kg (4.4 lbs), and Large Spills include releases up to 25 kg (55 lbs). These agents are BZ, CX, GA, GB, GD, GF, HD, HL, HN1, HN2, HN3, L and VX.

**Downwind dispersion** of the vapor was estimated for each case modeled. Atmospheric parameters affecting the dispersion, and the emission rate, were selected in a statistical fashion from a database containing hourly meteorological data from 120 cities in the United States, Canada and Mexico. The dispersion calculation accounted for the time-dependent emission rate from the source as well as the density of the vapor plume (i.e., heavy gas effects). Since atmospheric mixing is less effective at dispersing vapor plumes during nighttime, day and night were separated in the analysis. In Table 1, "Day" refers to time periods after sunrise and before sunset, while "Night" includes all hours between sunset and sunrise.

**Toxicological short-term exposure guidelines** for the materials were applied to determine the downwind distance to which persons may become incapacitated and unable to take protective action or may incur serious health effects after a once-in-a-lifetime, or rare, exposure. When available, toxicological exposure guidelines were chosen from AEGL-2 or ERPG-2 emergency response guidelines, with AEGL-2 values being the first choice. For materials that do not have AEGL-2 or ERPG-2 values, emergency response guidelines estimated from lethal concentration limits derived from animal studies were used, as recommended by an independent panel of toxicological experts from industry and academia.

## HOW TO USE TABLE 1 - INITIAL ISOLATION AND PROTECTIVE ACTION DISTANCES

(1) The responder should already have:

- Identified the material by its ID Number and Name; (if an ID Number cannot be found, use the Name of Material index in the blue-bordered pages to locate that number.)
- Found the three-digit guide for that material in order to consult the emergency actions recommended jointly with this table;
- **Noted the wind direction.**

(2) Look in Table 1 (the green-bordered pages) for the ID Number and Name of the Material involved in the incident. Some ID Numbers have more than one shipping name listed - look for the specific name of the material. (If the shipping name is not known and Table 1 lists more than one name for the same ID Number, use the entry with the largest protective action distances.)

(3) Determine if the incident involves a SMALL or LARGE spill and if DAY or NIGHT. A SMALL SPILL consists of a release of less than 208 liters (55 US gallons). This generally corresponds to a spill from a single small package (e.g. a drum), a small cylinder, or a small leak from a large package. A LARGE SPILL consists of a release of more than 208 liters (55 US gallons). This usually involves a spill from a large package, or multiple spills from many small packages. DAY is any time after sunrise and before sunset. NIGHT is any time between sunset and sunrise.

(4) Look up the INITIAL ISOLATION DISTANCE. This distance defines the radius of a zone (Initial Isolation Zone) surrounding the spill in ALL DIRECTIONS. Within this zone, all public should be evacuated (protective clothing and respiratory protection is required in this zone). Persons should be directed to move out of the zone in a direction perpendicular to wind direction (crosswind), and away from the spill, to a minimum distance as prescribed by the Initial Isolation Distance.

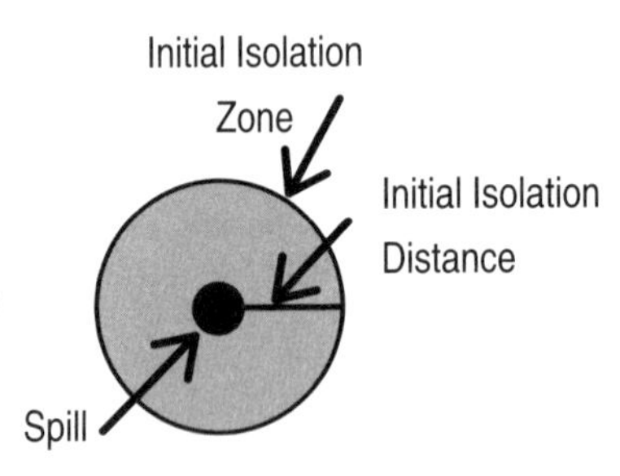


(5) Look up the initial PROTECTIVE ACTION DISTANCE. For a given material, spill size, and whether day or night, Table 1 gives the downwind distance—in kilometers and miles—from the spill/leak source for which protective actions should be considered. For practical purposes, the Protective Action Zone (i.e., the area in which people are at risk of harmful exposure) is a square, whose length and width are the same as the downwind

distance shown in Table 1. Protective actions are those steps taken to preserve the health and safety of emergency responders and the public. People in this area should be evacuated and/or sheltered-in-place.

(6) Initiate Protective Actions to the extent possible, beginning with those closest to the spill site and working away from the site in the downwind direction. When a water-reactive TIH (PIH in the US) producing material is spilled into a river or stream, the source of the toxic gas may move with the current or stretch from the spill point downstream for a substantial distance.

The shape of the area in which protective actions should be taken (the Protective Action Zone) is shown in this figure. The spill is located at the center of the small circle. The larger circle represents the INITIAL ISOLATION zone around the spill.

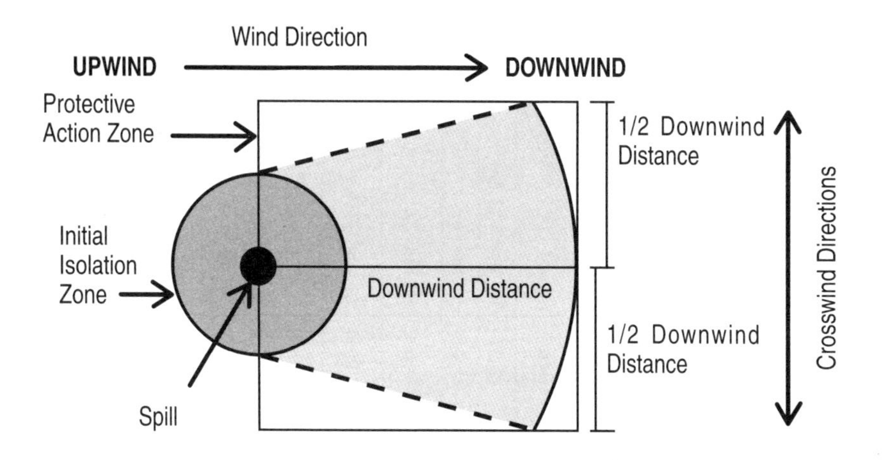


**NOTE 1: See "Introduction To Green Tables - Initial Isolation And Protective Action Distances" under "Factors That May Change the Protective Action Distances" (page 289)**

**NOTE 2: When a product in Table 1 has the mention "(when spilled in water)", refer to Table 2 – Water-Reactive Materials which Produce Toxic Gases for the list of gases produced when these materials are spilled in water.**

Call the emergency response telephone number listed on the shipping paper or the appropriate response agency as soon as possible for additional information on the material, safety precautions and mitigation procedures.

# TABLE 1 - INITIAL ISOLATION AND PROTECTIVE ACTION DISTANCES

| | | | SMALL SPILLS (From a small package or small leak from a large package) | | | | | | LARGE SPILLS (From a large package or from many small packages) | | | | | |
|---|---|---|---|---|---|---|---|---|---|---|---|---|---|---|
| | | | First **ISOLATE** in all Directions | | Then **PROTECT** persons Downwind during | | | | First **ISOLATE** in all Directions | | Then **PROTECT** persons Downwind during | | | |
| | | | | | **DAY** | | **NIGHT** | | | | **DAY** | | **NIGHT** | |
| **ID No.** | **Guide** | **NAME OF MATERIAL** | Meters | (Feet) | Kilometers | (Miles) | Kilometers | (Miles) | Meters | (Feet) | Kilometers | (Miles) | Kilometers | (Miles) |
| 1005<br>1005 | **125**<br>**125** | Ammonia, anhydrous<br>Anhydrous ammonia | 30 m | (100 ft) | 0.1 km | (0.1 mi) | 0.2 km | (0.1 mi) | **Refer to table 3** | | | | | |
| 1008<br>1008 | **125**<br>**125** | Boron trifluoride<br>Boron trifluoride, compressed | 30 m | (100 ft) | 0.1 km | (0.1 mi) | 0.7 km | (0.4 mi) | 400 m | (1250 ft) | 2.2 km | (1.4 mi) | 4.8 km | (3.0 mi) |
| 1016<br>1016 | **119**<br>**119** | Carbon monoxide<br>Carbon monoxide, compressed | 30 m | (100 ft) | 0.1 km | (0.1 mi) | 0.2 km | (0.1 mi) | 200 m | (600 ft) | 1.2 km | (0.7 mi) | 4.4 km | (2.8 mi) |
| 1017 | **124** | Chlorine | 60 m | (200 ft) | 0.3 km | (0.2 mi) | 1.1 km | (0.7 mi) | **Refer to table 3** | | | | | |
| 1026 | **119** | Cyanogen | 30 m | (100 ft) | 0.1 km | (0.1 mi) | 0.4 km | (0.3 mi) | 60 m | (200 ft) | 0.3 km | (0.2 mi) | 1.1 km | (0.7 mi) |
| 1040<br>1040 | **119P**<br>**119P** | Ethylene oxide<br>Ethylene oxide with Nitrogen | 30 m | (100 ft) | 0.1 km | (0.1 mi) | 0.2 km | (0.1 mi) | **Refer to table 3** | | | | | |
| 1045<br>1045 | **124**<br>**124** | Fluorine<br>Fluorine, compressed | 30 m | (100 ft) | 0.1 km | (0.1 mi) | 0.2 km | (0.1 mi) | 100 m | (300 ft) | 0.5 km | (0.3 mi) | 2.2 km | (1.4 mi) |
| 1048 | **125** | Hydrogen bromide, anhydrous | 30 m | (100 ft) | 0.1 km | (0.1 mi) | 0.2 km | (0.2 mi) | 150 m | (500 ft) | 0.9 km | (0.6 mi) | 2.6 km | (1.6 mi) |
| 1050 | **125** | Hydrogen chloride, anhydrous | 30 m | (100 ft) | 0.1 km | (0.1 mi) | 0.3 km | (0.2 mi) | **Refer to table 3** | | | | | |
| 1051 | **117** | AC **(when used as a weapon)** | 60 m | (200 ft) | 0.3 km | (0.2 mi) | 1.0 km | (0.6 mi) | 1000 m | (3000 ft) | 3.7 km | (2.3 mi) | 8.4 km | (5.3 mi) |
| 1051<br>1051<br>1051 | **117**<br>**117**<br>**117** | Hydrocyanic acid, aqueous solutions, with more than 20% Hydrogen cyanide<br>Hydrogen cyanide, anhydrous, stabilized<br>Hydrogen cyanide, stabilized | 60 m | (200 ft) | 0.2 km | (0.2 mi) | 0.9 km | (0.6 mi) | 300 m | (1000 ft) | 3.7 km | (0.7 mi) | 2.4 km | (1.5 mi) |

| | | | | | | | | | | | | | | |
|---|---|---|---|---|---|---|---|---|---|---|---|---|---|---|
| 1052 | **125** | Hydrogen fluoride, anhydrous | 30 m | (100 ft) | 0.1 km | (0.1 mi) | 0.4 km | (0.3 mi) | **Refer to table 3** | | | | | |
| 1053<br>1053 | **117**<br>**117** | Hydrogen sulfide<br>Hydrogen sulphide | 30 m | (100 ft) | 0.1 km | (0.1 mi) | 0.4 km | (0.3 mi) | 400 m | (1250 ft) | 2.1 km | (1.3 mi) | 5.4 km | (3.4 mi) |
| 1061 | **118** | Methylamine, anhydrous | 30 m | (100 ft) | 0.1 km | (0.1 mi) | 0.2 km | (0.1 mi) | 200 m | (600 ft) | 0.6 km | (0.4 mi) | 1.9 km | (1.2 mi) |
| 1062 | **123** | Methyl bromide | 30 m | (100 ft) | 0.1 km | (0.1 mi) | 0.1 km | (0.1 mi) | 150 m | (500 ft) | 0.3 km | (0.2 mi) | 0.7 km | (0.4 mi) |
| 1064 | **117** | Methyl mercaptan | 30 m | (100 ft) | 0.1 km | (0.1 mi) | 0.3 km | (0.2 mi) | 200 m | (600 ft) | 1.1 km | (0.7 mi) | 3.1 km | (1.9 mi) |
| 1067<br>1067 | **124**<br>**124** | Dinitrogen tetroxide<br>Nitrogen dioxide | 30 m | (100 ft) | 0.1 km | (0.1 mi) | 0.4 km | (0.3 mi) | 400 m | (1250 ft) | 1.2 km | (0.8 mi) | 3.0 km | (1.9 mi) |
| 1069 | **125** | Nitrosyl chloride | 30 m | (100 ft) | 0.2 km | (0.2 mi) | 1.0 km | (0.6 mi) | 500 m | (1500 ft) | 3.4 km | (2.1 mi) | 8.3 km | (5.2 mi) |
| 1076 | **125** | CG **(when used as a weapon)** | 150 m | (500 ft) | 0.8 km | (0.5 mi) | 3.2 km | (2.0 mi) | 1000 m | (3000 ft) | 7.5 km | (4.7 mi) | 11.0+ km | (7.0+ mi) |
| 1076 | **125** | DP **(when used as a weapon)** | 30 m | (100 ft) | 0.2 km | (0.1 mi) | 0.7 km | (0.4 mi) | 200 m | (600 ft) | 1.0 km | (0.7 mi) | 2.4 km | (1.5 mi) |
| 1076 | **125** | Phosgene | 100 m | 300 ft | 0.6 km | (0.4 mi) | 2.5 km | (1.5 mi) | 500 m | (1500 ft) | 3.0 km | (1.9 mi) | 9.0 km | (5.6 mi) |
| 1079<br>1079 | **125**<br>**125** | Sulfur dioxide<br>Sulphur dioxide | 100 m | (300 ft) | 0.7 km | (0.4 mi) | 2.2 km | (1.4 mi) | **Refer to table 3** | | | | | |
| 1082<br>1082 | **119P**<br>**119P** | Refrigerant gas R-1113<br>Trifluorochloroethylene, stabilized | 30 m | (100 ft) | 0.1 km | (0.1 mi) | 0.1 km | (0.1 mi) | 60 m | (200 ft) | 0.3 km | (0.2 mi) | 0.7 km | (0.5 mi) |
| 1092 | **131P** | Acrolein, stabilized | 100 m | (300 ft) | 1.3 km | (0.8 mi) | 3.4 km | (2.1 mi) | 500 m | (1500 ft) | 6.1 km | (3.8 mi) | 11.0 km | (6.8 mi) |
| 1093 | **131P** | Acrylonitrile, stabilized | 30 m | (100 ft) | 0.2 km | (0.2 mi) | 0.5 km | (0.4 mi) | 100 m | (300 ft) | 1.1 km | (0.7 mi) | 2.1 km | (1.3 mi) |
| 1098 | **131** | Allyl alcohol | 30 m | (100 ft) | 0.2 km | (0.1 mi) | 0.3 km | (0.2 mi) | 60 m | (200 ft) | 0.7 km | (0.5 mi) | 1.2 km | (0.7 mi) |
| 1135 | **131** | Ethylene chlorohydrin | 30 m | (100 ft) | 0.1 km | (0.1 mi) | 0.2 km | (0.1 mi) | 60 m | (200 ft) | 0.4 km | (0.3 mi) | 0.6 km | (0.4 mi) |
| 1143<br>1143 | **131P**<br>**131P** | Crotonaldehyde<br>Crotonaldehyde, stabilized | 30 m | (100 ft) | 0.1 km | (0.1 mi) | 0.2 km | (0.1 mi) | 60 m | (200 ft) | 0.5 km | (0.3 mi) | 0.8 km | (0.5 mi) |
| 1162 | **155** | Dimethyldichlorosilane **(when spilled in water)** | 30 m | (100 ft) | 0.1 km | (0.1 mi) | 0.2 km | (0.2 mi) | 60 m | (200 ft) | 0.5 km | (0.4 mi) | 1.7 km | (1.1 mi) |

**"+" means distance can be larger in certain atmospheric conditions**

# TABLE 1 - INITIAL ISOLATION AND PROTECTIVE ACTION DISTANCES

| | | | SMALL SPILLS (From a small package or small leak from a large package) | | | | | | LARGE SPILLS (From a large package or from many small packages) | | | | | |
|---|---|---|---|---|---|---|---|---|---|---|---|---|---|---|
| | | | First **ISOLATE** in all Directions | | Then **PROTECT** persons Downwind during | | | | First **ISOLATE** in all Directions | | Then **PROTECT** persons Downwind during | | | |
| | | | | | **DAY** | | **NIGHT** | | | | **DAY** | | **NIGHT** | |
| **ID No.** | **Guide** | **NAME OF MATERIAL** | Meters | (Feet) | Kilometers | (Miles) | Kilometers | (Miles) | Meters | (Feet) | Kilometers | (Miles) | Kilometers | (Miles) |
| 1163<br>1163 | **131**<br>**131** | 1,1-Dimethylhydrazine<br>Dimethylhydrazine, unsymmetrical | 30 m | (100 ft) | 0.2 km | (0.1 mi) | 0.5 km | (0.3 mi) | 100 m | (300 ft) | 1.0 km | (0.6 mi) | 1.8 km | (1.1 mi) |
| 1182 | **155** | Ethyl chloroformate | 30 m | (100 ft) | 0.1 km | (0.1 mi) | 0.1 km | (0.1 mi) | 60 m | (200 ft) | 0.3 km | (0.2 mi) | 0.5 km | (0.3 mi) |
| 1183 | **139** | Ethyldichlorosilane **(when spilled in water)** | 30 m | (100 ft) | 0.1 km | (0.1 mi) | 0.2 km | (0.2 mi) | 60 m | (200 ft) | 0.6 km | (0.4 mi) | 2.0 km | (1.2 mi) |
| 1185 | **131P** | Ethyleneimine, stabilized | 30 m | (100 ft) | 0.2 km | (0.1 mi) | 0.4 km | (0.3 mi) | 150 m | (500 ft) | 0.9 km | (0.6 mi) | 1.7 km | (1.1 mi) |
| 1196 | **155** | Ethyltrichlorosilane **(when spilled in water)** | 30 m | (100 ft) | 0.2 km | (0.1 mi) | 0.7 km | (0.4 mi) | 150 m | (500 ft) | 1.9 km | (1.2 mi) | 5.6 km | (3.5 mi) |
| 1238 | **155** | Methyl chloroformate | 30 m | (100 ft) | 0.2 km | (0.2 mi) | 0.6 km | (0.4 mi) | 150 m | (500 ft) | 1.1 km | (0.7 mi) | 2.1 km | (1.3 mi) |
| 1239 | **131** | Methyl chloromethyl ether | 60 m | (200 ft) | 0.5 km | (0.3 mi) | 1.4 km | (0.9 mi) | 300 m | (1000 ft) | 3.0 km | (1.9 mi) | 5.6 km | (3.5 mi) |
| 1242 | **139** | Methyldichlorosilane **(when spilled in water)** | 30 m | (100 ft) | 0.1 km | (0.1 mi) | 0.3 km | (0.2 mi) | 60 m | (200 ft) | 0.7 km | (0.5 mi) | 2.2 km | (1.4 mi) |
| 1244 | **131** | Methylhydrazine | 30 m | (100 ft) | 0.3 km | (0.2 mi) | 0.6 km | (0.4 mi) | 100 m | (300 ft) | 1.3 km | (0.8 mi) | 2.1 km | (1.3 mi) |
| 1250 | **155** | Methyltrichlorosilane **(when spilled in water)** | 30 m | (100 ft) | 0.1 km | (0.1 mi) | 0.3 km | (0.2 mi) | 60 m | (200 ft) | 0.8 km | (0.5 mi) | 2.4 km | (1.5 mi) |
| 1251 | **131P** | Methyl vinyl ketone, stabilized | 100 m | (300 ft) | 0.3 km | (0.2 mi) | 0.7 km | (0.4 mi) | 800 m | (2500 ft) | 1.5 km | (0.9 mi) | 2.6 km | (1.6 mi) |
| 1259 | **131** | Nickel carbonyl | 100 m | (300 ft) | 1.4 km | (0.9 mi) | 4.9 km | (3.0 mi) | 1000 m | (3000 ft) | 11.0+ km | (7.0+ mi) | 11.0+ km | (7.0+ mi) |
| 1295 | **139** | Trichlorosilane **(when spilled in water)** | 30 m | (100 ft) | 0.1 km | (0.1 mi) | 0.2 km | (0.2 mi) | 60 m | (200 ft) | 0.6 km | (0.4 mi) | 2.0 km | (1.3 mi) |

| | | | | | | | | | | | | | | |
|---|---|---|---|---|---|---|---|---|---|---|---|---|---|---|
| 1298 | **155** | Trimethylchlorosilane **(when spilled in water)** | 30 m | (100 ft) | 0.1 km | (0.1 mi) | 0.2 km | (0.1 mi) | 60 m | (200 ft) | 0.5 km | (0.3 mi) | 1.4 km | (0.9 mi) |
| 1305<br>1305 | **155P**<br>**155P** | Vinyltrichlorosilane **(when spilled in water)**<br>Vinyltrichlorosilane, stabilized **(when spilled in water)** | 30 m | (100 ft) | 0.1 km | (0.1 mi) | 0.2 km | (0.2 mi) | 60 m | (200 ft) | 0.6 km | (0.4 mi) | 1.8 km | (1.2 mi) |
| 1340<br>1340 | **139**<br>**139** | Phosphorus pentasulfide, free from yellow and white Phosphorus **(when spilled in water)**<br>Phosphorus pentasulphide, free from yellow and white Phosphorus **(when spilled in water)** | 30 m | (100 ft) | 0.1 km | (0.1 mi) | 0.2 km | (0.1 mi) | 60 m | (200 ft) | 0.3 km | (0.2 mi) | 1.3 km | (0.8 mi) |
| 1360 | **139** | Calcium phosphide **(when spilled in water)** | 30 m | (100 ft) | 0.2 km | (0.1 mi) | 0.6 km | (0.4 mi) | 300 m | (1000 ft) | 1.0 km | (0.7 mi) | 3.7 km | (2.3 mi) |
| 1380 | **135** | Pentaborane | 60 m | (200 ft) | 0.5 km | (0.4 mi) | 1.9 km | (1.2 mi) | 150 m | (500 ft) | 2.0 km | (1.3 mi) | 4.7 km | (3.0 mi) |
| 1384<br>1384<br>1384 | **135**<br>**135**<br>**135** | Sodium dithionite **(when spilled in water)**<br>Sodium hydrosulfite **(when spilled in water)**<br>Sodium hydrosulphite **(when spilled in water)** | 30 m | (100 ft) | 0.2 km | (0.1 mi) | 0.5 km | (0.3 mi) | 60 m | (200 ft) | 0.6 km | (0.4 mi) | 2.2 km | (1.4 mi) |
| 1397 | **139** | Aluminum phosphide **(when spilled in water)** | 60 m | (200 ft) | 0.2 km | (0.2 mi) | 0.9 km | (0.6 mi) | 500 m | (1500 ft) | 2.0 km | (1.2 mi) | 7.1 km | (4.4 mi) |
| 1419 | **139** | Magnesium aluminum phosphide **(when spilled in water)** | 60 m | (200 ft) | 0.2 km | (0.1 mi) | 0.8 km | (0.5 mi) | 500 m | (1500 ft) | 1.8 km | (1.2 mi) | 6.2 km | (3.9 mi) |

**"+" means distance can be larger in certain atmospheric conditions**

# TABLE 1 - INITIAL ISOLATION AND PROTECTIVE ACTION DISTANCES

| | | | SMALL SPILLS (From a small package or small leak from a large package) | | | LARGE SPILLS (From a large package or from many small packages) | | |
|---|---|---|---|---|---|---|---|---|
| | | | First **ISOLATE** in all Directions | Then **PROTECT** persons Downwind during | | First **ISOLATE** in all Directions | Then **PROTECT** persons Downwind during | |
| **ID No.** | **Guide** | **NAME OF MATERIAL** | Meters (Feet) | **DAY** Kilometers (Miles) | **NIGHT** Kilometers (Miles) | Meters (Feet) | **DAY** Kilometers (Miles) | **NIGHT** Kilometers (Miles) |
| 1432 | **139** | Sodium phosphide **(when spilled in water)** | 30 m (100 ft) | 0.2 km (0.1 mi) | 0.6 km (0.4 mi) | 300 m (1000 ft) | 1.3 km (0.8 mi) | 4.0 km (2.5 mi) |
| 1510 | **143** | Tetranitromethane | 30 m (100 ft) | 0.2 km (0.1 mi) | 0.3 km (0.2 mi) | 30 m (100 ft) | 0.4 km (0.3 mi) | 0.7 km (0.5 mi) |
| 1541 | **155** | Acetone cyanohydrin, stabilized **(when spilled in water)** | 30 m (100 ft) | 0.1 km (0.1 mi) | 0.1 km (0.1 mi) | 100 m (300 ft) | 0.3 km (0.2 mi) | 1.0 km (0.7 mi) |
| 1556 | **152** | MD **(when used as a weapon)** | 300 m (1000 ft) | 1.6 km (1.0 mi) | 4.3 km (2.7 mi) | 1000 m (3000 ft) | 11.0+ km (7.0+ mi) | 11.0+ km (7.0+ mi) |
| 1556 | **152** | Methyldichloroarsine | 100 m (300 ft) | 1.3 km (0.8 mi) | 2.0 km (1.3 mi) | 300 m (1000 ft) | 3.2 km (2.0 mi) | 4.2 km (2.6 mi) |
| 1556 | **152** | PD **(when used as a weapon)** | 60 m (200 ft) | 0.4 km (0.3 mi) | 0.4 km (0.3 mi) | 300 m (1000 ft) | 1.6 km (1.0 mi) | 1.6 km (1.0 mi) |
| 1560<br>1560 | **157**<br>**157** | Arsenic chloride<br>Arsenic trichloride | 30 m (100 ft) | 0.2 km (0.1 mi) | 0.3 km (0.2 mi) | 100 m (300 ft) | 1.0 km (0.6 mi) | 1.4 km (0.9 mi) |
| 1569 | **131** | Bromoacetone | 30 m (100 ft) | 0.4 km (0.3 mi) | 1.2 km (0.8 mi) | 150 m (500 ft) | 1.8 km (1.1 mi) | 3.4 km (2.1 mi) |
| 1580 | **154** | Chloropicrin | 60 m (200 ft) | 0.5 km (0.3 mi) | 1.2 km (0.8 mi) | 200 m (600 ft) | 2.2 km (1.4 mi) | 3.6 km (2.2 mi) |
| 1581<br>1581 | **123**<br>**123** | Chloropicrin and Methyl bromide mixture<br>Methyl bromide and Chloropicrin mixture | 30 m (100 ft) | 0.1 km (0.1 mi) | 0.6 km (0.4 mi) | 300 m (1000 ft) | 2.1 km (1.3 mi) | 5.9 km (3.7 mi) |
| 1582<br>1582 | **119**<br>**119** | Chloropicrin and Methyl chloride mixture<br>Methyl chloride and Chloropicrin mixture | 30 m (100 ft) | 0.1 km (0.1 mi) | 0.4 km (0.3 mi) | 60 m (200 ft) | 0.4 km (0.2 mi) | 1.7 km (1.1 mi) |
| 1583 | **154** | Chloropicrin mixture, n.o.s. | 60 m (200 ft) | 0.5 km (0.3 mi) | 1.2 km (0.8 mi) | 200 m (600 ft) | 2.2 km (1.4 mi) | 3.6 km (2.2 mi) |

| ID No. | Guide No. | Name of Material | Small spills: Isolate (m) | (ft) | Protect Day (km) | (mi) | Protect Night (km) | (mi) | Large spills: Isolate (m) | (ft) | Protect Day (km) | (mi) | Protect Night (km) | (mi) |
|---|---|---|---|---|---|---|---|---|---|---|---|---|---|---|
| 1589 | **125** | CK **(when used as a weapon)** | 800 m | (2500 ft) | 5.3 km | (3.2 mi) | 11.0+ km | (7.0+ mi) | 1000 m | (3000 ft) | 11.0+ km | (7.0+ mi) | 11.0+ km | (7.0+ mi) |
| 1589 | **125** | Cyanogen chloride, stabilized | 300 m | (1000 ft) | 1.8 km | (1.1 mi) | 6.2 km | (3.9 mi) | 1000 m | (3000 ft) | 9.4 km | (5.8 mi) | 11.0+ km | (7.0+ mi) |
| 1595<br>1595 | **156**<br>**156** | Dimethyl sulfate<br>Dimethyl sulphate | 30 m | (100 ft) | 0.2 km | (0.1 mi) | 0.2 km | (0.1 mi) | 60 m | (200 ft) | 0.5 km | (0.3 mi) | 0.6 km | (0.4 mi) |
| 1605 | **154** | Ethylene dibromide | 30 m | (100 ft) | 0.1 km | (0.1 mi) | 0.1 km | (0.1 mi) | 30 m | (100 ft) | 0.1 km | (0.1 mi) | 0.2 km | (0.1 mi) |
| 1612<br>1612 | **123**<br>**123** | Compressed gas and hexaethyl tetraphosphate mixture<br>Hexaethyl tetraphosphate and compressed gas mixture | 100 m | (300 ft) | 0.8 km | (0.5 mi) | 2.7 km | (1.7 mi) | 400 m | (1250 ft) | 3.5 km | (2.2 mi) | 8.1 km | (5.1 mi) |
| 1613<br>1613 | **154**<br>**154** | Hydrocyanic acid, aqueous solution, with not more than 20% Hydrogen cyanide<br>Hydrogen cyanide, aqueous solution, with not more than 20% Hydrogen cyanide | 30 m | (100 ft) | 0.1 km | (0.1 mi) | 0.1 km | (0.1 mi) | 100 m | (300 ft) | 0.5 km | (0.3 mi) | 1.1 km | (0.7 mi) |
| 1614 | **152** | Hydrogen cyanide, stabilized (absorbed) | 60 m | (200 ft) | 0.2 km | (0.1 mi) | 0.6 km | (0.4 mi) | 150 m | (500 ft) | 0.5 km | (0.4 mi) | 1.6 km | (1.0 mi) |
| 1647<br>1647 | **151**<br>**151** | Ethylene dibromide and Methyl bromide mixture, liquid<br>Methyl bromide and Ethylene dibromide mixture, liquid | 30 m | (100 ft) | 0.1 km | (0.1 mi) | 0.1 km | (0.1 mi) | 150 m | (500 ft) | 0.3 km | (0.2 mi) | 0.7 km | (0.4 mi) |
| 1660<br>1660 | **124**<br>**124** | Nitric oxide<br>Nitric oxide, compressed | 30 m | (100 ft) | 0.1 km | (0.1 mi) | 0.5 km | (0.4 mi) | 100 m | (300 ft) | 0.5 km | (0.4 mi) | 2.2 km | (1.4 mi) |
| 1670 | **157** | Perchloromethyl mercaptan | 30 m | (100 ft) | 0.2 km | (0.2 mi) | 0.3 km | (0.2 mi) | 100 m | (300 ft) | 0.6 km | (0.4 mi) | 1.1 km | (0.7 mi) |
| 1672 | **151** | Phenylcarbylamine chloride | 30 m | (100 ft) | 0.2 km | (0.1 mi) | 0.2 km | (0.1 mi) | 60 m | (200 ft) | 0.5 km | (0.3 mi) | 0.7 km | (0.4 mi) |
| 1680<br>1680 | **157**<br>**157** | Potassium cyanide **(when spilled in water)**<br>Potassium cyanide, solid **(when spilled in water)** | 30 m | (100 ft) | 0.1 km | (0.1 mi) | 0.2 km | (0.1 mi) | 100 m | (300 ft) | 0.3 km | (0.2 mi) | 1.2 km | (0.8 mi) |

**"+" means distance can be larger in certain atmospheric conditions**

## TABLE 1 - INITIAL ISOLATION AND PROTECTIVE ACTION DISTANCES

| | | | SMALL SPILLS (From a small package or small leak from a large package) | | | LARGE SPILLS (From a large package or from many small packages) | | |
|---|---|---|---|---|---|---|---|---|
| | | | First ISOLATE in all Directions | Then PROTECT persons Downwind during | | First ISOLATE in all Directions | Then PROTECT persons Downwind during | |
| ID No. | Guide | NAME OF MATERIAL | Meters (Feet) | DAY Kilometers (Miles) | NIGHT Kilometers (Miles) | Meters (Feet) | DAY Kilometers (Miles) | NIGHT Kilometers (Miles) |
| 1689<br>1689 | **157**<br>**157** | Sodium cyanide **(when spilled in water)**<br>Sodium cyanide, solid **(when spilled in water)** | 30 m (100 ft) | 0.1 km (0.1 mi) | 0.2 km (0.1 mi) | 100 m (300 ft) | 0.4 km (0.2 mi) | 1.4 km (0.9 mi) |
| 1694 | **159** | CA **(when used as a weapon)** | 30 m (100 ft) | 0.1 km (0.1 mi) | 0.4 km (0.3 mi) | 100 m (300 ft) | 0.5 km (0.4 mi) | 2.6 km (1.6 mi) |
| 1695 | **131** | Chloroacetone, stabilized | 30 m (100 ft) | 0.1 km (0.1 mi) | 0.2 km (0.1 mi) | 30 m (100 ft) | 0.4 km (0.3 mi) | 0.6 km (0.4 mi) |
| 1697 | **153** | CN **(when used as a weapon)** | 30 m (100 ft) | 0.1 km (0.1 mi) | 0.2 km (0.1 mi) | 60 m (200 ft) | 0.3 km (0.2 mi) | 1.2 km (0.8 mi) |
| 1698<br>1698 | **154**<br>**154** | Adamsite **(when used as a weapon)**<br>DM **(when used as a weapon)** | 30 m (100 ft) | 0.1 km (0.1 mi) | 0.3 km (0.2 mi) | 60 m (200 ft) | 0.3 km (0.2 mi) | 1.4 km (0.9 mi) |
| 1699 | **151** | DA **(when used as a weapon)** | 30 m (100 ft) | 0.2 km (0.1 mi) | 0.8 km (0.5 mi) | 300 m (1000 ft) | 1.9 km (1.2 mi) | 7.5 km (4.7 mi) |
| 1716 | **156** | Acetyl bromide **(when spilled in water)** | 30 m (100 ft) | 0.1 km (0.1 mi) | 0.2 km (0.1 mi) | 30 m (100 ft) | 0.4 km (0.2 mi) | 0.9 km (0.6 mi) |
| 1717 | **155** | Acetyl chloride **(when spilled in water)** | 30 m (100 ft) | 0.1 km (0.1 mi) | 0.3 km (0.2 mi) | 100 m (300 ft) | 0.9 km (0.6 mi) | 2.5 km (1.6 mi) |
| 1722<br>1722 | **155**<br>**155** | Allyl chlorocarbonate<br>Allyl chloroformate | 100 m (300 ft) | 0.3 km (0.2 mi) | 0.8 km (0.5 mi) | 400 m (1250 ft) | 1.4 km (0.9 mi) | 2.4 km (1.5 mi) |
| 1724 | **155** | Allyltrichlorosilane, stabilized **(when spilled in water)** | 30 m (100 ft) | 0.1 km (0.1 mi) | 0.2 km (0.2 mi) | 60 m (200 ft) | 0.5 km (0.4 mi) | 1.7 km (1.1 mi) |
| 1725 | **137** | Aluminum bromide, anhydrous **(when spilled in water)** | 30 m (100 ft) | 0.1 km (0.1 mi) | 0.1 km (0.1 mi) | 30 m (100 ft) | 0.1 km (0.1 mi) | 0.4 km (0.3 mi) |

| | | | | | | | | |
|---|---|---|---|---|---|---|---|---|
| 1726 | **137** | Aluminum chloride, anhydrous **(when spilled in water)** | 30 m (100 ft) | 0.1 km (0.1 mi) | 0.3 km (0.2 mi) | 60 m (200 ft) | 0.5 km (0.3 mi) | 2.0 km (1.2 mi) |
| 1728 | **155** | Amyltrichlorosilane **(when spilled in water)** | 30 m (100 ft) | 0.1 km (0.1 mi) | 0.2 km (0.2 mi) | 60 m (200 ft) | 0.5 km (0.3 mi) | 1.7 km (1.1 mi) |
| 1732 | **157** | Antimony pentafluoride **(when spilled in water)** | 30 m (100 ft) | 0.1 km (0.1 mi) | 0.5 km (0.3 mi) | 100 m (300 ft) | 1.0 km (0.7 mi) | 3.8 km (2.4 mi) |
| 1741 | **125** | Boron trichloride **(when spilled on land)** | 30 m (100 ft) | 0.1 km (0.1 mi) | 0.3 km (0.2 mi) | 100 m (300 ft) | 0.6 km (0.4 mi) | 1.3 km (0.8 mi) |
| 1741 | **125** | Boron trichloride **(when spilled in water)** | 30 m (100 ft) | 0.1 km (0.1 mi) | 0.4 km (0.3 mi) | 100 m (300 ft) | 1.1 km (0.7 mi) | 3.5 km (2.2 mi) |
| 1744<br>1744<br>1744 | **154**<br>**154**<br>**154** | Bromine<br>Bromine, solution<br>Bromine, solution (Inhalation Hazard Zone A) | 60 m (200 ft) | 0.8 km (0.5 mi) | 2.3 km (1.5 mi) | 300 m (1000 ft) | 3.7 km (2.3 mi) | 7.5 km (4.7 mi) |
| 1744 | **154** | Bromine, solution (Inhalation Hazard Zone B) | 30 m (100 ft) | 0.1 km (0.1 mi) | 0.2 km (0.1 mi) | 30 m (100 ft) | 0.3 km (0.2 mi) | 0.5 km (0.3 mi) |
| 1745 | **144** | Bromine pentafluoride **(when spilled on land)** | 60 m (200 ft) | 0.8 km (0.5 mi) | 2.4 km (1.5 mi) | 400 m (1250 ft) | 4.9 km (3.1 mi) | 10.2 km (6.4 mi) |
| 1745 | **144** | Bromine pentafluoride **(when spilled in water)** | 30 m (100 ft) | 0.1 km (0.1 mi) | 0.5 km (0.4 mi) | 100 m (300 ft) | 1.1 km (0.7 mi) | 3.9 km (2.5 mi) |
| 1746 | **144** | Bromine trifluoride **(when spilled on land)** | 30 m (100 ft) | 0.1 km (0.1 mi) | 0.2 km (0.1 mi) | 30 m (100 ft) | 0.3 km (0.2 mi) | 0.5 km (0.3 mi) |
| 1746 | **144** | Bromine trifluoride **(when spilled in water)** | 30 m (100 ft) | 0.1 km (0.1 mi) | 0.5 km (0.3 mi) | 100 m (300 ft) | 1.0 km (0.6 mi) | 3.7 km (2.3 mi) |
| 1747 | **155** | Butyltrichlorosilane **(when spilled in water)** | 30 m (100 ft) | 0.1 km (0.1 mi) | 0.2 km (0.2 mi) | 60 m (200 ft) | 0.5 km (0.3 mi) | 1.6 km (1.0 mi) |
| 1749 | **124** | Chlorine trifluoride | 60 m (200 ft) | 0.3 km (0.2 mi) | 1.1 km (0.7 mi) | 300 m (1000 ft) | 1.4 km (0.9 mi) | 4.1 km (2.6 mi) |

**"+" means distance can be larger in certain atmospheric conditions**

## TABLE 1 - INITIAL ISOLATION AND PROTECTIVE ACTION DISTANCES

| ID No. | Guide | NAME OF MATERIAL | SMALL SPILLS (From a small package or small leak from a large package) | | | | | | LARGE SPILLS (From a large package or from many small packages) | | | | | |
|---|---|---|---|---|---|---|---|---|---|---|---|---|---|---|
| | | | First ISOLATE in all Directions | | Then PROTECT persons Downwind during | | | | First ISOLATE in all Directions | | Then PROTECT persons Downwind during | | | |
| | | | | | DAY | | NIGHT | | | | DAY | | NIGHT | |
| | | | Meters | (Feet) | Kilometers | (Miles) | Kilometers | (Miles) | Meters | (Feet) | Kilometers | (Miles) | Kilometers | (Miles) |
| 1752 | **156** | Chloroacetyl chloride **(when spilled on land)** | 30 m | (100 ft) | 0.3 km | (0.2 mi) | 0.6 km | (0.4 mi) | 100 m | (300 ft) | 1.1 km | (0.7 mi) | 1.9 km | (1.2 mi) |
| 1752 | **156** | Chloroacetyl chloride **(when spilled in water)** | 30 m | (100 ft) | 0.1 km | (0.1 mi) | 0.1 km | (0.1 mi) | 30 m | (100 ft) | 0.3 km | (0.2 mi) | 0.8 km | (0.5 mi) |
| 1753 | **156** | Chlorophenyltrichlorosilane **(when spilled in water)** | 30 m | (100 ft) | 0.1 km | (0.1 mi) | 0.1 km | (0.1 mi) | 30 m | (100 ft) | 0.3 km | (0.2 mi) | 0.9 km | (0.6 mi) |
| 1754 | **137** | Chlorosulfonic acid (with or without sulfur trioxide mixture) **(when spilled on land)** | 30 m | (100 ft) | 0.1 km | (0.1 mi) | 0.1 km | (0.1 mi) | 30 m | (100 ft) | 0.2 km | (0.2 mi) | 0.3 km | (0.2 mi) |
| 1754 | **137** | Chlorosulfonic acid (with or without sulfur trioxide mixture) **(when spilled in water)** | 30 m | (100 ft) | 0.1 km | (0.1 mi) | 0.3 km | (0.2 mi) | 60 m | (200 ft) | 0.7 km | (0.4 mi) | 2.2 km | (1.4 mi) |
| 1754 | **137** | Chlorosulphonic acid (with or without sulphur trioxide mixture) **(when spilled on land)** | 30 m | (100 ft) | 0.1 km | (0.1 mi) | 0.1 km | (0.1 mi) | 30 m | (100 ft) | 0.2 km | (0.2 mi) | 0.3 km | (0.2 mi) |
| 1754 | **137** | Chlorosulphonic acid (with or without sulphur trioxide mixture) **(when spilled in water)** | 30 m | (100 ft) | 0.1 km | (0.1 mi) | 0.3 km | (0.2 mi) | 60 m | (200 ft) | 0.7 km | (0.4 mi) | 2.2 km | (1.4 mi) |
| 1758 | **137** | Chromium oxychloride **(when spilled in water)** | 30 m | (100 ft) | 0.1 km | (0.1 mi) | 0.1 km | (0.1 mi) | 30 m | (100 ft) | 0.2 km | (0.1 mi) | 0.7 km | (0.5 mi) |

| ID No. | Guide | Name of Material | | | | | | | | | | | | |
|---|---|---|---|---|---|---|---|---|---|---|---|---|---|---|
| 1762 | **156** | Cyclohexenyltrichlorosilane **(when spilled in water)** | 30 m | (100 ft) | 0.1 km | (0.1 mi) | 0.2 km | (0.1 mi) | 30 m | (100 ft) | 0.4 km | (0.3 mi) | 1.2 km | (0.8 mi) |
| 1763 | **156** | Cyclohexyltrichlorosilane **(when spilled in water)** | 30 m | (100 ft) | 0.1 km | (0.1 mi) | 0.2 km | (0.1 mi) | 30 m | (100 ft) | 0.4 km | (0.3 mi) | 1.3 km | (0.8 mi) |
| 1765 | **156** | Dichloroacetyl chloride **(when spilled in water)** | 30 m | (100 ft) | 0.1 km | (0.1 mi) | 0.1 km | (0.1 mi) | 30 m | (100 ft) | 0.3 km | (0.2 mi) | 0.9 km | (0.6 mi) |
| 1766 | **156** | Dichlorophenyltrichlorosilane **(when spilled in water)** | 30 m | (100 ft) | 0.1 km | (0.1 mi) | 0.2 km | (0.2 mi) | 60 m | (200 ft) | 0.6 km | (0.4 mi) | 1.9 km | (1.2 mi) |
| 1767 | **155** | Diethyldichlorosilane **(when spilled in water)** | 30 m | (100 ft) | 0.1 km | (0.1 mi) | 0.1 km | (0.1 mi) | 30 m | (100 ft) | 0.4 km | (0.2 mi) | 1.0 km | (0.6 mi) |
| 1769 | **156** | Diphenyldichlorosilane **(when spilled in water)** | 30 m | (100 ft) | 0.1 km | (0.1 mi) | 0.2 km | (0.1 mi) | 30 m | (100 ft) | 0.4 km | (0.2 mi) | 1.2 km | (0.8 mi) |
| 1771 | **156** | Dodecyltrichlorosilane **(when spilled in water)** | 30 m | (100 ft) | 0.1 km | (0.1 mi) | 0.2 km | (0.1 mi) | 60 m | (200 ft) | 0.5 km | (0.3 mi) | 1.3 km | (0.8 mi) |
| 1777<br>1777 | **137**<br>**137** | Fluorosulfonic acid **(when spilled in water)**<br>Fluorosulphonic acid **(when spilled in water)** | 30 m | (100 ft) | 0.1 km | (0.1 mi) | 0.1 km | (0.1 mi) | 30 m | (100 ft) | 0.2 km | (0.2 mi) | 0.7 km | (0.5 mi) |
| 1781 | **156** | Hexadecyltrichlorosilane **(when spilled in water)** | 30 m | (100 ft) | 0.1 km | (0.1 mi) | 0.1 km | (0.1 mi) | 30 m | (100 ft) | 0.2 km | (0.1 mi) | 0.6 km | (0.4 mi) |
| 1784 | **156** | Hexyltrichlorosilane **(when spilled in water)** | 30 m | (100 ft) | 0.1 km | (0.1 mi) | 0.2 km | (0.1 mi) | 30 m | (100 ft) | 0.4 km | (0.3 mi) | 1.4 km | (0.9 mi) |
| 1799 | **156** | Nonyltrichlorosilane **(when spilled in water)** | 30 m | (100 ft) | 0.1 km | (0.1 mi) | 0.2 km | (0.1 mi) | 60 m | (200 ft) | 0.5 km | (0.3 mi) | 1.4 km | (0.9 mi) |
| 1800 | **156** | Octadecyltrichlorosilane **(when spilled in water)** | 30 m | (100 ft) | 0.1 km | (0.1 mi) | 0.2 km | (0.1 mi) | 30 m | (100 ft) | 0.4 km | (0.3 mi) | 1.4 km | (0.9 mi) |

**"+" means distance can be larger in certain atmospheric conditions**

# TABLE 1 - INITIAL ISOLATION AND PROTECTIVE ACTION DISTANCES

| | | | SMALL SPILLS (From a small package or small leak from a large package) | | | | | | LARGE SPILLS (From a large package or from many small packages) | | | | | |
|---|---|---|---|---|---|---|---|---|---|---|---|---|---|---|
| | | | First ISOLATE in all Directions | | Then PROTECT persons Downwind during | | | | First ISOLATE in all Directions | | Then PROTECT persons Downwind during | | | |
| | | | | | DAY | | NIGHT | | | | DAY | | NIGHT | |
| ID No. | Guide | NAME OF MATERIAL | Meters | (Feet) | Kilometers | (Miles) | Kilometers | (Miles) | Meters | (Feet) | Kilometers | (Miles) | Kilometers | (Miles) |
| 1801 | **156** | Octyltrichlorosilane **(when spilled in water)** | 30 m | (100 ft) | 0.1 km | (0.1 mi) | 0.2 km | (0.1 mi) | 60 m | (200 ft) | 0.5 km | (0.3 mi) | 1.5 km | (0.9 mi) |
| 1804 | **156** | Phenyltrichlorosilane **(when spilled in water)** | 30 m | (100 ft) | 0.1 km | (0.1 mi) | 0.2 km | (0.1 mi) | 30 m | (100 ft) | 0.4 km | (0.3 mi) | 1.4 km | (0.9 mi) |
| 1806 | **137** | Phosphorus pentachloride **(when spilled in water)** | 30 m | (100 ft) | 0.1 km | (0.1 mi) | 0.2 km | (0.2 mi) | 30 m | (100 ft) | 0.4 km | (0.3 mi) | 1.4 km | (0.9 mi) |
| 1808 | **137** | Phosphorus tribromide **(when spilled in water)** | 30 m | (100 ft) | 0.1 km | (0.1 mi) | 0.3 km | (0.2 mi) | 30 m | (100 ft) | 0.4 km | (0.3 mi) | 1.3 km | (0.9 mi) |
| 1809 | **137** | Phosphorus trichloride **(when spilled on land)** | 30 m | (100 ft) | 0.2 km | (0.1 mi) | 0.5 km | (0.4 mi) | 100 m | (300 ft) | 1.1 km | (0.7 mi) | 2.2 km | (1.4 mi) |
| 1809 | **137** | Phosphorus trichloride **(when spilled in water)** | 30 m | (100 ft) | 0.1 km | (0.1 mi) | 0.3 km | (0.2 mi) | 60 m | (200 ft) | 0.7 km | (0.5 mi) | 2.3 km | (1.4 mi) |
| 1810 | **137** | Phosphorus oxychloride **(when spilled on land)** | 30 m | (100 ft) | 0.3 km | (0.2 mi) | 0.6 km | (0.4 mi) | 100 m | (300 ft) | 1.0 km | (0.6 mi) | 1.8 km | (1.1 mi) |
| 1810 | **137** | Phosphorus oxychloride **(when spilled in water)** | 30 m | (100 ft) | 0.1 km | (0.1 mi) | 0.2 km | (0.2 mi) | 60 m | (200 ft) | 0.6 km | (0.4 mi) | 2.0 km | (1.3 mi) |
| 1815 | **132** | Propionyl chloride **(when spilled in water)** | 30 m | (100 ft) | 0.1 km | (0.1 mi) | 0.1 km | (0.1 mi) | 30 m | (100 ft) | 0.3 km | (0.2 mi) | 0.7 km | (0.4 mi) |
| 1816 | **155** | Propyltrichlorosilane **(when spilled in water)** | 30 m | (100 ft) | 0.1 km | (0.1 mi) | 0.2 km | (0.2 mi) | 60 m | (200 ft) | 0.6 km | (0.4 mi) | 1.8 km | (1.1 mi) |
| 1818 | **157** | Silicon tetrachloride **(when spilled in water)** | 30 m | (100 ft) | 0.1 km | (0.1 mi) | 0.3 km | (0.2 mi) | 60 m | (200 ft) | 0.8 km | (0.5 mi) | 2.5 km | (1.6 mi) |

| | | | | | | | | | | | | | | |
|---|---|---|---|---|---|---|---|---|---|---|---|---|---|---|
| 1828 | **137** | Sulfur chlorides **(when spilled on land)** | 30 m | (100 ft) | 0.1 km | (0.1 mi) | 0.1 km | (0.1 mi) | 60 m | (200 ft) | 0.3 km | (0.2 mi) | 0.4 km | (0.3 mi) |
| 1828 | **137** | Sulfur chlorides **(when spilled in water)** | 30 m | (100 ft) | 0.1 km | (0.1 mi) | 0.2 km | (0.1 mi) | 30 m | (100 ft) | 0.3 km | (0.2 mi) | 1.1 km | (0.7 mi) |
| 1828 | **137** | Sulphur chlorides **(when spilled on land)** | 30 m | (100 ft) | 0.1 km | (0.1 mi) | 0.1 km | (0.1 mi) | 60 m | (200 ft) | 0.3 km | (0.2 mi) | 0.4 km | (0.3 mi) |
| 1828 | **137** | Sulphur chlorides **(when spilled in water)** | 30 m | (100 ft) | 0.1 km | (0.1 mi) | 0.2 km | (0.1 mi) | 30 m | (100 ft) | 0.3 km | (0.2 mi) | 1.1 km | (0.7 mi) |
| 1829<br>1829 | **137**<br>**137** | Sulfur trioxide, stabilized<br>Sulphur trioxide, stabilized | 60 m | (200 ft) | 0.4 km | (0.2 mi) | 1.0 km | (0.6 mi) | 300 m | (1000 ft) | 2.9 km | (1.8 mi) | 5.7 km | (3.6 mi) |
| 1831<br>1831<br><br><br>1831<br>1831 | **137**<br>**137**<br><br><br>**137**<br>**137** | Sulfuric acid, fuming<br>Sulfuric acid, fuming, with not less than 30% free Sulfur trioxide<br>Sulphuric acid, fuming<br>Sulphuric acid, fuming, with not less than 30% free Sulphur trioxide | 60 m | (200 ft) | 0.4 km | (0.2 mi) | 1.0 km | (0.6 mi) | 300 m | (1000 ft) | 2.9 km | (1.8 mi) | 5.7 km | (3.6 mi) |
| 1834 | **137** | Sulfuryl chloride **(when spilled on land)** | 30 m | (100 ft) | 0.2 km | (0.1 mi) | 0.4 km | (0.3 mi) | 60 m | (200 ft) | 0.8 km | (0.5 mi) | 1.5 km | (1.0 mi) |
| 1834 | **137** | Sulfuryl chloride **(when spilled in water)** | 30 m | (100 ft) | 0.1 km | (0.1 mi) | 0.2 km | (0.1 mi) | 60 m | (200 ft) | 0.5 km | (0.3 mi) | 1.6 km | (1.0 mi) |
| 1834 | **137** | Sulphuryl chloride **(when spilled on land)** | 30 m | (100 ft) | 0.2 km | (0.1 mi) | 0.4 km | (0.3 mi) | 60 m | (200 ft) | 0.8 km | (0.5 mi) | 1.5 km | (1.0 mi) |
| 1834 | **137** | Sulphuryl chloride **(when spilled in water)** | 30 m | (100 ft) | 0.1 km | (0.1 mi) | 0.2 km | (0.1 mi) | 60 m | (200 ft) | 0.5 km | (0.3 mi) | 1.6 km | (1.0 mi) |
| 1836 | **137** | Thionyl chloride **(when spilled on land)** | 30 m | (100 ft) | 0.2 km | (0.2 mi) | 0.6 km | (0.4 mi) | 60 m | (200 ft) | 0.7 km | (0.5 mi) | 1.5 km | (0.9 mi) |

**"+" means distance can be larger in certain atmospheric conditions**

## TABLE 1 - INITIAL ISOLATION AND PROTECTIVE ACTION DISTANCES

| | | | SMALL SPILLS (From a small package or small leak from a large package) | | | LARGE SPILLS (From a large package or from many small packages) | | |
|---|---|---|---|---|---|---|---|---|
| | | | First **ISOLATE** in all Directions | Then **PROTECT** persons Downwind during | | First **ISOLATE** in all Directions | Then **PROTECT** persons Downwind during | |
| ID No. | Guide | NAME OF MATERIAL | Meters (Feet) | **DAY** Kilometers (Miles) | **NIGHT** Kilometers (Miles) | Meters (Feet) | **DAY** Kilometers (Miles) | **NIGHT** Kilometers (Miles) |
| 1836 | **137** | Thionyl chloride **(when spilled in water)** | 100 m (300 ft) | 0.9 km (0.6 mi) | 2.4 km (1.5 mi) | 600 m (2000 ft) | 7.9 km (4.9 mi) | 11.0+ km (7.0+ mi) |
| 1838 | **137** | Titanium tetrachloride **(when spilled on land)** | 30 m (100 ft) | 0.1 km (0.1 mi) | 0.1 km (0.1 mi) | 30 m (100 ft) | 0.1 km (0.1 mi) | 0.2 km (0.1 mi) |
| 1838 | **137** | Titanium tetrachloride **(when spilled in water)** | 30 m (100 ft) | 0.1 km (0.1 mi) | 0.2 km (0.1 mi) | 60 m (200 ft) | 0.5 km (0.3 mi) | 1.6 km (1.0 mi) |
| 1859<br>1859 | **125**<br>**125** | Silicon tetrafluoride<br>Silicon tetrafluoride, compressed | 30 m (100 ft) | 0.2 km (0.1 mi) | 0.7 km (0.5 mi) | 100 m (300 ft) | 0.5 km (0.3 mi) | 1.8 km (1.1 mi) |
| 1892 | **151** | ED **(when used as a weapon)** | 150 m (500 ft) | 2.0 km (1.2 mi) | 2.9 km (1.8 mi) | 1000 m (3000 ft) | 10.4 km (6.5 mi) | 11.0+ km (7.0+ mi) |
| 1892 | **151** | Ethyldichloroarsine | 150 m (500 ft) | 1.4 km (0.9 mi) | 2.1 km (1.3 mi) | 400 m (1250 ft) | 4.6 km (2.9 mi) | 6.3 km (3.9 mi) |
| 1898 | **156** | Acetyl iodide **(when spilled in water)** | 30 m (100 ft) | 0.1 km (0.1 mi) | 0.2 km (0.2 mi) | 30 m (100 ft) | 0.4 km (0.3 mi) | 1.0 km (0.7 mi) |
| 1911<br>1911<br>1911 | **119**<br>**119**<br>**119** | Diborane<br>Diborane, compressed<br>Diborane mixtures | 60 m (200 ft) | 0.3 km (0.2 mi) | 1.0 km (0.6 mi) | 200 m (600 ft) | 1.3 km (0.8 mi) | 4.0 km (2.5 mi) |
| 1923<br>1923<br>1923 | **135**<br>**135**<br>**135** | Calcium dithionite **(when spilled in water)**<br>Calcium hydrosulfite **(when spilled in water)**<br>Calcium hydrosulphite **(when spilled in water)** | 30 m (100 ft) | 0.2 km (0.1 mi) | 0.5 km (0.4 mi) | 60 m (200 ft) | 0.6 km (0.4 mi) | 2.2 km (1.4 mi) |

| ID No. | Guide No. | Name of Material | Small spills: Isolate | | Small spills: Day | | Small spills: Night | | Large spills: Isolate | | Large spills: Day | | Large spills: Night | |
|---|---|---|---|---|---|---|---|---|---|---|---|---|---|---|
| 1929<br>1929<br>1929 | **135**<br>**135**<br>**135** | Potassium dithionite **(when spilled in water)**<br>Potassium hydrosulfite **(when spilled in water)**<br>Potassium hydrosulphite **(when spilled in water)** | 30 m | (100 ft) | 0.1 km | (0.1 mi) | 0.5 km | (0.3 mi) | 60 m | (200 ft) | 0.6 km | (0.4 mi) | 2.0 km | (1.2 mi) |
| 1931<br>1931<br>1931 | **171**<br>**171**<br>**171** | Zinc dithionite **(when spilled in water)**<br>Zinc hydrosulfite **(when spilled in water)**<br>Zinc hydrosulphite **(when spilled in water)** | 30 m | (100 ft) | 0.1 km | (0.1 mi) | 0.5 km | (0.3 mi) | (60 m) | (200 ft) | 0.6 km | (0.4 mi) | 2.0 km | (1.3 mi) |
| 1953<br>1953 | **119**<br>**119** | Compressed gas, poisonous, flammable, n.o.s.<br>Compressed gas, poisonous, flammable, n.o.s. (Inhalation Hazard Zone A) | 150 m | (500 ft) | 1.0 km | (0.6 mi) | 3.8 km | (2.4 mi) | 1000 m | (3000 ft) | 5.6 km | (3.5 mi) | 10.2 km | (6.3 mi) |
| 1953 | **119** | Compressed gas, poisonous, flammable, n.o.s. (Inhalation Hazard Zone B) | 30 m | (100 ft) | 0.1 km | (0.1 mi) | 0.4 km | (0.2 mi) | 200 m | (600 ft) | 1.2 km | (0.8 mi) | 2.6 km | (1.6 mi) |
| 1953 | **119** | Compressed gas, poisonous, flammable, n.o.s. (Inhalation Hazard Zone C) | 30 m | (100 ft) | 0.1 km | (0.1 mi) | 0.3 km | (0.2 mi) | 150 m | (500 ft) | 0.9 km | (0.6 mi) | 2.4 km | (1.5 mi) |
| 1953 | **119** | Compressed gas, poisonous, flammable, n.o.s. (Inhalation Hazard Zone D) | 30 m | (100 ft) | 0.1 km | (0.1 mi) | 0.2 km | (0.1 mi) | 100 m | (300 ft) | 0.7 km | (0.5 mi) | 1.9 km | (1.2 mi) |
| 1953<br>1953 | **119**<br>**119** | Compressed gas, toxic, flammable, n.o.s.<br>Compressed gas, toxic, flammable, n.o.s. (Inhalation Hazard Zone A) | 150 m | (500 ft) | 1.0 km | (0.6 mi) | 3.8 km | (2.4 mi) | 1000 m | (3000 ft) | 5.6 km | (3.5 mi) | 10.2 km | (6.3 mi) |

**"+" means distance can be larger in certain atmospheric conditions**

## TABLE 1 - INITIAL ISOLATION AND PROTECTIVE ACTION DISTANCES

| ID No. | Guide | NAME OF MATERIAL | SMALL SPILLS (From a small package or small leak from a large package) First ISOLATE in all Directions Meters (Feet) | SMALL SPILLS Then PROTECT persons Downwind during DAY Kilometers (Miles) | SMALL SPILLS Then PROTECT persons Downwind during NIGHT Kilometers (Miles) | LARGE SPILLS (From a large package or from many small packages) First ISOLATE in all Directions Meters (Feet) | LARGE SPILLS Then PROTECT persons Downwind during DAY Kilometers (Miles) | LARGE SPILLS Then PROTECT persons Downwind during NIGHT Kilometers (Miles) |
|---|---|---|---|---|---|---|---|---|
| 1953 | **119** | Compressed gas, toxic, flammable, n.o.s. (Inhalation Hazard Zone B) | 30 m (100 ft) | 0.1 km (0.1 mi) | 0.4 km (0.2 mi) | 200 m (600 ft) | 1.2 km (0.8 mi) | 2.6 km (1.6 mi) |
| 1953 | **119** | Compressed gas, toxic, flammable, n.o.s. (Inhalation Hazard Zone C) | 30 m (100 ft) | 0.1 km (0.1 mi) | 0.3 km (0.2 mi) | 150 m (500 ft) | 0.9 km (0.6 mi) | 2.4 km (1.5 mi) |
| 1953 | **119** | Compressed gas, toxic, flammable, n.o.s. (Inhalation Hazard Zone D) | 30 m (100 ft) | 0.1 km (0.1 mi) | 0.2 km (0.1 mi) | 100 m (300 ft) | 0.7 km (0.5 mi) | 1.9 km (1.2 mi) |
| 1955<br>1955 | **123**<br>**123** | Compressed gas, poisonous, n.o.s.<br>Compressed gas, poisonous, n.o.s. (Inhalation Hazard Zone A) | 100 m (300 ft) | 0.5 km (0.3 mi) | 2.5 km (1.6 mi) | 1000 m (3000 ft) | 5.6 km (3.5 mi) | 10.2 km (6.3 mi) |
| 1955 | **123** | Compressed gas, poisonous, n.o.s. (Inhalation Hazard Zone B) | 30 m (100 ft) | 0.2 km (0.1 mi) | 0.8 km (0.5 mi) | 300 m (1000 ft) | 1.4 km (0.9 mi) | 4.1 km (2.6 mi) |
| 1955 | **123** | Compressed gas, poisonous, n.o.s. (Inhalation Hazard Zone C) | 30 m (100 ft) | 0.1 km (0.1 mi) | 0.3 km (0.2 mi) | 150 m (500 ft) | 0.9 km (0.6 mi) | 2.4 km (1.5 mi) |
| 1955 | **123** | Compressed gas, poisonous, n.o.s. (Inhalation Hazard Zone D) | 30 m (100 ft) | 0.1 km (0.1 mi) | 0.2 km (0.1 mi) | 100 m (300 ft) | 0.7 km (0.5 mi) | 1.9 km (1.2 mi) |

| | | | | | | | | | | | | | | |
|---|---|---|---|---|---|---|---|---|---|---|---|---|---|---|
| 1955 | **123** | Compressed gas, toxic, n.o.s. | | | | | | | | | | | | |
| 1955 | **123** | Compressed gas, toxic, n.o.s. (Inhalation Hazard Zone A) | 100 m | (300 ft) | 0.5 km | (0.3 mi) | 2.5 km | (1.6 mi) | 1000 m | (3000 ft) | 5.6 km | (3.5 mi) | 10.2 km | (6.3 mi) |
| 1955 | **123** | Compressed gas, toxic, n.o.s. (Inhalation Hazard Zone B) | 30 m | (100 ft) | 0.2 km | (0.1 mi) | 0.8 km | (0.5 mi) | 300 m | (1000 ft) | 1.4 km | (0.9 mi) | 4.1 km | (2.6 mi) |
| 1955 | **123** | Compressed gas, toxic, n.o.s. (Inhalation Hazard Zone C) | 30 m | (100 ft) | 0.1 km | (0.1 mi) | 0.3 km | (0.2 mi) | 150 m | (500 ft) | 0.9 km | (0.6 mi) | 2.4 km | (1.5 mi) |
| 1955 | **123** | Compressed gas, toxic, n.o.s. (Inhalation Hazard Zone D) | 30 m | (100 ft) | 0.1 km | (0.1 mi) | 0.2 km | (0.1 mi) | 100 m | (300 ft) | 0.7 km | (0.5 mi) | 1.9 km | (1.2 mi) |
| 1955 | **123** | Organic phosphate compound mixed with compressed gas | | | | | | | | | | | | |
| 1955 | **123** | Organic phosphate mixed with compressed gas | 100 m | (300 ft) | 1.0 km | (0.7 mi) | 3.4 km | (2.1 mi) | 500 m | (1500 ft) | 4.4 km | (2.7 mi) | 9.6 km | (6.0 mi) |
| 1955 | **123** | Organic phosphorus compound mixed with compressed gas | | | | | | | | | | | | |
| 1967 | **123** | Insecticide gas, poisonous, n.o.s. | | | | | | | | | | | | |
| 1967 | **123** | Insecticide gas, toxic, n.o.s. | 100 m | (300 ft) | 1.0 km | (0.7 mi) | 3.4 km | (2.1 mi) | 500 m | (1500 ft) | 4.4 km | (2.7 mi) | 9.6 km | (6.0 mi) |
| 1967 | **123** | Parathion and compressed gas mixture | | | | | | | | | | | | |
| 1975 | **124** | Dinitrogen tetroxide and Nitric oxide mixture | | | | | | | | | | | | |
| 1975 | **124** | Nitric oxide and Dinitrogen tetroxide mixture | | | | | | | | | | | | |
| 1975 | **124** | Nitric oxide and Nitrogen dioxide mixture | | | | | | | | | | | | |
| 1975 | **124** | Nitric oxide and Nitrogen tetroxide mixture | 30 m | (100 ft) | 0.1 km | (0.1 mi) | 0.5 km | (0.4 mi) | 100 m | (300 ft) | 0.5 km | (0.4 mi) | 2.2 km | (1.4 mi) |
| 1975 | **124** | Nitrogen dioxide and Nitric oxide mixture | | | | | | | | | | | | |
| 1975 | **124** | Nitrogen tetroxide and Nitric oxide mixture | | | | | | | | | | | | |

**"+" means distance can be larger in certain atmospheric conditions**

# TABLE 1 - INITIAL ISOLATION AND PROTECTIVE ACTION DISTANCES

| | | | SMALL SPILLS (From a small package or small leak from a large package) | | | LARGE SPILLS (From a large package or from many small packages) | | |
|---|---|---|---|---|---|---|---|---|
| | | | First **ISOLATE** in all Directions | Then **PROTECT** persons Downwind during | | First **ISOLATE** in all Directions | Then **PROTECT** persons Downwind during | |
| **ID No.** | **Guide** | **NAME OF MATERIAL** | Meters (Feet) | **DAY** Kilometers (Miles) | **NIGHT** Kilometers (Miles) | Meters (Feet) | **DAY** Kilometers (Miles) | **NIGHT** Kilometers (Miles) |
| 1994 | **131** | Iron pentacarbonyl | 100 m (300 ft) | 0.9 km (0.6 mi) | 2.0 km (1.2 mi) | 400 m (1250 ft) | 4.5 km (2.8 mi) | 7.4 km (4.6 mi) |
| 2004 | **135** | Magnesium diamide **(when spilled in water)** | 30 m (100 ft) | 0.1 km (0.1 mi) | 0.5 km (0.3 mi) | 60 m (200 ft) | 0.6 km (0.4 mi) | 2.1 km (1.4 mi) |
| 2011 | **139** | Magnesium phosphide **(when spilled in water)** | 60 m (200 ft) | 0.2 km (0.1 mi) | 0.8 km (0.5 mi) | 400 m (1250 ft) | 1.7 km (1.1 mi) | 5.7 km (3.6 mi) |
| 2012 | **139** | Potassium phosphide **(when spilled in water)** | 30 m (100 ft) | 0.1 km (0.1 mi) | 0.6 km (0.4 mi) | 300 m (1000 ft) | 1.2 km (0.7 mi) | 3.8 km (2.4 mi) |
| 2013 | **139** | Strontium phosphide **(when spilled in water)** | 30 m (100 ft) | 0.1 km (0.1 mi) | 0.5 km (0.4 mi) | 300 m (1000 ft) | 1.1 km (0.7 mi) | 3.7 km (2.3 mi) |
| 2032 | **157** | Nitric acid, red fuming | 30 m (100 ft) | 0.1 km (0.1 mi) | 0.1 km (0.1 mi) | 150 m (500 ft) | 0.2 km (0.2 mi) | 0.4 km (0.3 mi) |
| 2186 | **125** | Hydrogen chloride, refrigerated liquid | 30 m (100 ft) | 0.1 km (0.1 mi) | 0.3 km (0.2 mi) | **Refer to table 3** | | |
| 2188 | **119** | Arsine | 150 m (500 ft) | 1.0 km (0.6 mi) | 3.8 km (2.4 mi) | 1000 m (3000 ft) | 5.6 km (3.5 mi) | 10.2 km (6.3 mi) |
| 2188 | **119** | SA **(when used as a weapon)** | 300 m (1000 ft) | 1.9 km (1.2 mi) | 5.7 km (3.6 mi) | 1000 m (3000 ft) | 8.9 km (5.6 mi) | 11.0+ km (7.0+ mi) |
| 2189 | **119** | Dichlorosilane | 30 m (100 ft) | 0.1 km (0.1 mi) | 0.4 km (0.2 mi) | 200 m (600 ft) | 1.2 km (0.8 mi) | 2.6 km (1.6 mi) |
| 2190<br>2190 | **124**<br>**124** | Oxygen difluoride<br>Oxygen difluoride, compressed | 300 m (1000 ft) | 1.6 km (1.0 mi) | 6.7 km (4.2 mi) | 1000 m (3000 ft) | 9.8 km (6.1 mi) | 11.0+ km (7.0+ mi) |
| 2191<br>2191 | **123**<br>**123** | Sulfuryl fluoride<br>Sulphuryl fluoride | 30 m (100 ft) | 0.1 km (0.1 mi) | 0.5 km (0.3 mi) | 300 m (1000 ft) | 1.9 km (1.2 mi) | 4.4 km (2.7 mi) |
| 2192 | **119** | Germane | 150 m (500 ft) | 0.7 km (0.5 mi) | 3.0 km (1.9 mi) | 500 m (1500 ft) | 2.9 km (1.8 mi) | 6.7 km (4.2 mi) |

| ID No. | Guide No. | Name of Material | | | | | | | | | | | | |
|---|---|---|---|---|---|---|---|---|---|---|---|---|---|---|
| 2194 | **125** | Selenium hexafluoride | 200 m | (600 ft) | 1.1 km | (0.7 mi) | 3.4 km | (2.1 mi) | 600 m | (2000 ft) | 3.4 km | (2.1 mi) | 7.8 km | (4.9 mi) |
| 2195 | **125** | Tellurium hexafluoride | 600 m | (2000 ft) | 3.6 km | (2.2 mi) | 8.6 km | (5.4 mi) | 1000 m | (3000 ft) | 11.0+ km | (7.0+ mi) | 11.0+ km | (7.0+ mi) |
| 2196 | **125** | Tungsten hexafluoride | 30 m | (100 ft) | 0.2 km | (0.1 mi) | 0.7 km | (0.5 mi) | 150 m | (500 ft) | 0.9 km | (0.6 mi) | 2.8 km | (1.8 mi) |
| 2197 | **125** | Hydrogen iodide, anhydrous | 30 m | (100 ft) | 0.1 km | (0.1 mi) | 0.3 km | (0.2 mi) | 150 m | (500 ft) | 0.9 km | (0.6 mi) | 2.4 km | (1.5 mi) |
| 2198<br>2198 | **125**<br>**125** | Phosphorus pentafluoride<br>Phosphorus pentafluoride, compressed | 30 m | (100 ft) | 0.2 km | (0.1 mi) | 0.8 km | (0.5 mi) | 150 m | (500 ft) | 0.8 km | (0.5 mi) | 2.9 km | (1.8 mi) |
| 2199 | **119** | Phosphine | 60 m | (200 ft) | 0.2 km | (0.2 mi) | 1.0 km | (0.6 mi) | 300 m | (1000 ft) | 1.3 km | (0.8 mi) | 3.8 km | (2.4 mi) |
| 2202 | **117** | Hydrogen selenide, anhydrous | 300 m | (1000 ft) | 1.7 km | (1.1 mi) | 5.9 km | (3.7 mi) | 1000 m | (3000 ft) | 11.0+ km | (7.0+ mi) | 11.0+ km | (7.0+ mi) |
| 2204<br>2204 | **119**<br>**119** | Carbonyl sulfide<br>Carbonyl sulphide | 30 m | (100 ft) | 0.1 km | (0.1 mi) | 0.3 km | (0.2 mi) | 300 m | (1000 ft) | 1.3 km | (0.8 mi) | 3.2 km | (2.0 mi) |
| 2232<br>2232 | **153**<br>**153** | Chloroacetaldehyde<br>2-Chloroethanal | 30 m | (100 ft) | 0.2 km | (0.1 mi) | 0.3 km | (0.2 mi) | 60 m | (200 ft) | 0.6 km | (0.4 mi) | 1.1 km | (0.7 mi) |
| 2285 | **156** | Isocyanatobenzotrifluorides | 30 m | (100 ft) | 0.1 km | (0.1 mi) | 0.2 km | (0.1 mi) | 30 m | (100 ft) | 0.4 km | (0.3 mi) | 0.6 km | (0.4 mi) |
| 2308<br>2308<br>2308<br>2308 | **157**<br>**157**<br>**157**<br>**157** | Nitrosylsulfuric acid, liquid **(when spilled in water)**<br>Nitrosylsulfuric acid, solid **(when spilled in water)**<br>Nitrosylsulphuric acid, liquid **(when spilled in water)**<br>Nitrosylsulphuric acid, solid **(when spilled in water)** | 30 m | (100 ft) | 0.1 km | (0.1 mi) | 0.4 km | (0.3 mi) | 300 m | (1000 ft) | 1.0 km | (0.6 mi) | 2.8 km | (1.8 mi) |
| 2334 | **131** | Allylamine | 30 m | (100 ft) | 0.2 km | (0.1 mi) | 0.5 km | (0.3 mi) | 150 m | (500 ft) | 1.4 km | (0.9 mi) | 2.5 km | (1.6 mi) |
| 2337 | **131** | Phenyl mercaptan | 30 m | (100 ft) | 0.1 km | (0.1 mi) | 0.1 km | (0.1 mi) | 30 m | (100 ft) | 0.3 km | (0.2 mi) | 0.4 km | (0.2 mi) |
| 2353 | **132** | Butyryl chloride **(when spilled in water)** | 30 m | (100 ft) | 0.1 km | (0.1 mi) | 0.1 km | (0.1 mi) | 30 m | (100 ft) | 0.3 km | (0.2 mi) | 0.9 km | (0.6 mi) |

**"+" means distance can be larger in certain atmospheric conditions**

## TABLE 1 - INITIAL ISOLATION AND PROTECTIVE ACTION DISTANCES

| ID No. | Guide | NAME OF MATERIAL | SMALL SPILLS (From a small package or small leak from a large package) First ISOLATE in all Directions Meters (Feet) | SMALL SPILLS Then PROTECT persons Downwind during DAY Kilometers (Miles) | SMALL SPILLS Then PROTECT persons Downwind during NIGHT Kilometers (Miles) | LARGE SPILLS (From a large package or from many small packages) First ISOLATE in all Directions Meters (Feet) | LARGE SPILLS Then PROTECT persons Downwind during DAY Kilometers (Miles) | LARGE SPILLS Then PROTECT persons Downwind during NIGHT Kilometers (Miles) |
|---|---|---|---|---|---|---|---|---|
| 2382 | **131** | Dimethylhydrazine, symmetrical | 30 m (100 ft) | 0.2 km (0.1 mi) | 0.3 km (0.2 mi) | 60 m (200 ft) | 0.7 km (0.5 mi) | 1.3 km (0.8 mi) |
| 2395 | **132** | Isobutyryl chloride **(when spilled in water)** | 30 m (100 ft) | 0.1 km (0.1 mi) | 0.1 km (0.1 mi) | 30 m (100 ft) | 0.2 km (0.2 mi) | 0.6 km (0.4 mi) |
| 2407 | **155** | Isopropyl chloroformate | 30 m (100 ft) | 0.1 km (0.1 mi) | 0.2 km (0.2 mi) | 60 m (200 ft) | 0.5 km (0.3 mi) | 0.9 km (0.5 mi) |
| 2417<br>2417 | **125**<br>**125** | Carbonyl fluoride<br>Carbonyl fluoride, compressed | 100 m (300 ft) | 0.6 km (0.4 mi) | 2.2 km (1.4 mi) | 600 m (2000 ft) | 3.6 km (2.2 mi) | 8.1 km (5.1 mi) |
| 2418<br>2418 | **125**<br>**125** | Sulfur tetrafluoride<br>Sulphur tetrafluoride | 100 m (300 ft) | 0.5 km (0.3 mi) | 2.4 km (1.5 mi) | 400 m (1250 ft) | 2.1 km (1.3 mi) | 6.0 km (3.8 mi) |
| 2420 | **125** | Hexafluoroacetone | 100 m (300 ft) | 0.6 km (0.4 mi) | 2.6 km (1.6 mi) | 1000 m (3000 ft) | 11.0+ km (7.0+ mi) | 11.0+ km (7.0+ mi) |
| 2421 | **124** | Nitrogen trioxide | 60 m (200 ft) | 0.3 km (0.2 mi) | 1.1 km (0.7 mi) | 150 m (500 ft) | 0.9 km (0.6 mi) | 3.0 km (1.9 mi) |
| 2434 | **156** | Dibenzyldichlorosilane **(when spilled in water)** | 30 m (100 ft) | 0.1 km (0.1 mi) | 0.1 km (0.1 mi) | 30 m (100 ft) | 0.2 km (0.1 mi) | 0.6 km (0.4 mi) |
| 2435 | **156** | Ethylphenyldichlorosilane **(when spilled in water)** | 30 m (100 ft) | 0.1 km (0.1 mi) | 0.1 km (0.1 mi) | 30 m (100 ft) | 0.3 km (0.2 mi) | 1.0 km (0.6 mi) |
| 2437 | **156** | Methylphenyldichlorosilane **(when spilled in water)** | 30 m (100 ft) | 0.1 km (0.1 mi) | 0.2 km (0.1 mi) | 30 m (100 ft) | 0.4 km (0.3 mi) | 1.3 km (0.8 mi) |
| 2438 | **132** | Trimethylacetyl chloride | 60 m (200 ft) | 0.5 km (0.3 mi) | 1.0 km (0.6 mi) | 150 m (500 ft) | 2.0 km (1.3 mi) | 3.2 km (2.0 mi) |
| 2442 | **156** | Trichloroacetyl chloride | 30 m (100 ft) | 0.2 km (0.1 mi) | 0.3 km (0.2 mi) | 60 m (200 ft) | 0.6 km (0.4 mi) | 1.0 km (0.7 mi) |
| 2474 | **157** | Thiophosgene | 60 m (200 ft) | 0.6 km (0.4 mi) | 1.7 km (1.1 mi) | 200 m (600 ft) | 2.2 km (1.4 mi) | 4.1 km (2.5 mi) |

| ID No. | Guide | Name of Material | | | | | | | | | | | | | | |
|---|---|---|---|---|---|---|---|---|---|---|---|---|---|---|---|---|
| 2477 | **131** | Methyl isothiocyanate | 30 m | (100 ft) | 0.1 km | (0.1 mi) | 0.1 km | (0.1 mi) | 30 m | (100 ft) | 0.2 km | (0.2 mi) | 0.3 km | (0.2 mi) |
| 2478 | **155** | Isocyanate solution, flammable, poisonous, n.o.s. | 60 m | (200 ft) | 0.8 km | (0.5 mi) | 1.8 km | (1.1 mi) | 400 m | (1250 ft) | 4.3 km | (2.7 mi) | 7.0 km | (4.3 mi) |
| 2478 | **155** | Isocyanate solution, flammable, toxic, n.o.s. | | | | | | | | | | | | |
| 2478 | **155** | Isocyanates, flammable, poisonous, n.o.s. | | | | | | | | | | | | |
| 2478 | **155** | Isocyanates, flammable, toxic, n.o.s. | | | | | | | | | | | | |
| 2480 | **155** | Methyl isocyanate | 150 m | (500 ft) | 1.5 km | (1.0 mi) | 4.4 km | (2.8 mi) | 1000 m | (3000 ft) | 11.0+ km | (7.0+ mi) | 11.0+ km | (7.0+ mi) |
| 2481 | **155** | Ethyl isocyanate | 150 m | (500 ft) | 2.0 km | (1.2 mi) | 5.1 km | (3.2 mi) | 1000 m | (3000 ft) | 11.0+ km | (7.0+ mi) | 11.0+ km | (7.0+ mi) |
| 2482 | **155** | n-Propyl isocyanate | 100 m | (300 ft) | 1.3 km | (0.8 mi) | 2.7 km | (1.7 mi) | 600 m | (2000 ft) | 7.1 km | (4.4 mi) | 10.8 km | (6.7 mi) |
| 2483 | **155** | Isopropyl isocyanate | 100 m | (300 ft) | 1.4 km | (0.9 mi) | 3.0 km | (1.9 mi) | 800 m | (2500 ft) | 8.4 km | (5.2 mi) | 11.0+ km | (7.0+ mi) |
| 2484 | **155** | tert-Butyl isocyanate | 60 m | (200 ft) | 0.8 km | (0.5 mi) | 1.8 km | (1.1 mi) | 400 m | (1250 ft) | 4.3 km | (2.7 mi) | 7.0 km | (4.3 mi) |
| 2485 | **155** | n-Butyl isocyanate | 60 m | (200 ft) | 0.6 km | (0.4 mi) | 1.2 km | (0.7 mi) | 200 m | (600 ft) | 2.6 km | (1.6 mi) | 4.0 km | (2.5 mi) |
| 2486 | **155** | Isobutyl isocyanate | 60 m | (200 ft) | 0.6 km | (0.4 mi) | 1.1 km | (0.7 mi) | 200 m | (600 ft) | 2.5 km | (1.6 mi) | 4.0 km | (2.5 mi) |
| 2487 | **155** | Phenyl isocyanate | 60 m | (200 ft) | 0.8 km | (0.5 mi) | 1.3 km | (0.8 mi) | 300 m | (1000 ft) | 3.1 km | (1.9 mi) | 4.6 km | (2.9 mi) |
| 2488 | **155** | Cyclohexyl isocyanate | 30 m | (100 ft) | 0.3 km | (0.2 mi) | 0.4 km | (0.2 mi) | 100 m | (300 ft) | 0.9 km | (0.6 mi) | 1.3 km | (0.8 mi) |
| 2495 | **144** | Iodine pentafluoride **(when spilled in water)** | 30 m | (100 ft) | 0.1 km | (0.1 mi) | 0.5 km | (0.4 mi) | 100 m | (300 ft) | 1.1 km | (0.7 mi) | 4.1 km | (2.6 mi) |
| 2521 | **131P** | Diketene, stabilized | 30 m | (100 ft) | 0.1 km | (0.1 mi) | 0.1 km | (0.1 mi) | 30 m | (100 ft) | 0.3 km | (0.2 mi) | 0.4 km | (0.3 mi) |
| 2534 | **119** | Methylchlorosilane | 30 m | (100 ft) | 0.1 km | (0.1 mi) | 0.3 km | (0.2 mi) | 100 m | (300 ft) | 0.6 km | (0.4 mi) | 1.4 km | (0.9 mi) |
| 2548 | **124** | Chlorine pentafluoride | 100 m | (300 ft) | 0.5 km | (0.3 mi) | 2.5 km | (1.6 mi) | 800 m | (2500 ft) | 5.2 km | (3.3 mi) | 11.0+ km | (7.0+ mi) |

**"+" means distance can be larger in certain atmospheric conditions**

# TABLE 1 - INITIAL ISOLATION AND PROTECTIVE ACTION DISTANCES

| | | | SMALL SPILLS (From a small package or small leak from a large package) | | | | LARGE SPILLS (From a large package or from many small packages) | | | |
|---|---|---|---|---|---|---|---|---|---|---|
| | | | First ISOLATE in all Directions | Then PROTECT persons Downwind during | | | First ISOLATE in all Directions | Then PROTECT persons Downwind during | | |
| ID No. | Guide | NAME OF MATERIAL | Meters (Feet) | DAY Kilometers (Miles) | | NIGHT Kilometers (Miles) | Meters (Feet) | DAY Kilometers (Miles) | | NIGHT Kilometers (Miles) |
| 2600<br>2600 | **119**<br>**119** | Carbon monoxide and Hydrogen mixture, compressed<br>Hydrogen and Carbon monoxide mixture, compressed | 30 m (100 ft) | 0.1 km (0.1 mi) | | 0.2 km (0.1 mi) | 200 m (600 ft) | 1.2 km (0.7 mi) | | 4.4 km (2.8 mi) |
| 2605 | **155** | Methoxymethyl isocyanate | 30 m (100 ft) | 0.3 km (0.2 mi) | | 0.5 km (0.3 mi) | 100 m (300 ft) | 1.0 km (0.7 mi) | | 1.5 km (1.0 mi) |
| 2606 | **155** | Methyl orthosilicate | 30 m (100 ft) | 0.2 km (0.1 mi) | | 0.3 km (0.2 mi) | 60 m (200 ft) | 0.6 km (0.4 mi) | | 0.9 km (0.6 mi) |
| 2644 | **151** | Methyl iodide | 30 m (100 ft) | 0.1 km (0.1 mi) | | 0.2 km (0.1 mi) | 60 m (200 ft) | 0.3 km (0.2 mi) | | 0.6 km (0.4 mi) |
| 2646 | **151** | Hexachlorocyclopentadiene | 30 m (100 ft) | 0.1 km (0.1 mi) | | 0.1 km (0.1 mi) | 30 m (100 ft) | 0.3 km (0.2 mi) | | 0.4 km (0.2 mi) |
| 2668 | **131** | Chloroacetonitrile | 30 m (100 ft) | 0.1 km (0.1 mi) | | 0.1 km (0.1 mi) | 30 m (100 ft) | 0.3 km (0.2 mi) | | 0.4 km (0.2 mi) |
| 2676 | **119** | Stibine | 60 m (200 ft) | 0.3 km (0.2 mi) | | 1.6 km (1.0 mi) | 200 m (600 ft) | 1.2 km (0.8 mi) | | 4.2 km (2.6 mi) |
| 2691 | **137** | Phosphorus pentabromide **(when spilled in water)** | 30 m (100 ft) | 0.1 km (0.1 mi) | | 0.1 km (0.1 mi) | 30 m (100 ft) | 0.2 km (0.1 mi) | | 0.7 km (0.4 mi) |
| 2692 | **157** | Boron tribromide **(when spilled on land)** | 30 m (100 ft) | 0.1 km (0.1 mi) | | 0.2 km (0.1 mi) | 30 m (100 ft) | 0.2 km (0.1 mi) | | 0.4 km (0.3 mi) |
| 2692 | **157** | Boron tribromide **(when spilled in water)** | 30 m (100 ft) | 0.1 km (0.1 mi) | | 0.3 km (0.2 mi) | 60 m (200 ft) | 0.5 km (0.3 mi) | | 1.7 km (1.1 mi) |
| 2740 | **155** | n-Propyl chloroformate | 30 m (100 ft) | 0.1 km (0.1 mi) | | 0.3 km (0.2 mi) | 60 m (200 ft) | 0.5 km (0.4 mi) | | 1.0 km (0.6 mi) |
| 2742 | **155** | sec-Butyl chloroformate | 30 m (100 ft) | 0.1 km (0.1 mi) | | 0.2 km (0.1 mi) | 30 m (100 ft) | 0.4 km (0.2 mi) | | 0.5 km (0.3 mi) |

| | | | | | | | | | | | | | | |
|---|---|---|---|---|---|---|---|---|---|---|---|---|---|---|
| 2742<br>2742 | **155**<br>**155** | Chloroformates, poisonous, corrosive, flammable, n.o.s.<br>Chloroformates, toxic, corrosive, flammable, n.o.s. | 30 m | (100 ft) | 0.1 km | (0.1 mi) | 0.2 km | (0.1 mi) | 30 m | (100 ft) | 0.4 km | (0.2 mi) | 0.5 km | (0.4 mi) |
| 2742 | **155** | Isobutyl chloroformate | 30 m | (100 ft) | 0.1 km | (0.1 mi) | 0.1 km | (0.1 mi) | 30 m | (100 ft) | 0.3 km | (0.2 mi) | 0.4 km | (0.3 mi) |
| 2743 | **155** | n-Butyl chloroformate | 30 m | (100 ft) | 0.1 km | (0.1 mi) | 0.1 km | (0.1 mi) | 30 m | (100 ft) | 0.3 km | (0.2 mi) | 0.4 km | (0.3 mi) |
| 2806 | **138** | Lithium nitride **(when spilled in water)** | 30 m | (100 ft) | 0.1 km | (0.1 mi) | 0.4 km | (0.3 mi) | 60 m | (200 ft) | 0.6 km | (0.4 mi) | 1.9 km | (1.2 mi) |
| 2810<br>2810 | **153**<br>**153** | Buzz **(when used as a weapon)**<br>BZ **(when used as a weapon)** | 60 m | (200 ft) | 0.4 km | (0.2 mi) | 1.7 km | (1.1 mi) | 400 m | (1250 ft) | 2.2 km | (1.4 mi) | 8.1 km | (5.0 mi) |
| 2810 | **153** | CS **(when used as a weapon)** | 30 m | (100 ft) | 0.1 km | (0.1 mi) | 0.6 km | (0.4 mi) | 100 m | (300 ft) | 0.4 km | (0.3 mi) | 1.9 km | (1.2 mi) |
| 2810 | **153** | DC **(when used as a weapon)** | 30 m | (100 ft) | 0.1 km | (0.1 mi) | 0.6 km | (0.4 mi) | 60 m | (200 ft) | 0.4 km | (0.3 mi) | 1.8 km | (1.1 mi) |
| 2810 | **153** | GA **(when used as a weapon)** | 30 m | (100 ft) | 0.2 km | (0.1 mi) | 0.2 km | (0.1 mi) | 100 m | (300 ft) | 0.5 km | (0.4 mi) | 0.6 km | (0.4 mi) |
| 2810 | **153** | GB **(when used as a weapon)** | 60 m | (200 ft) | 0.4 km | (0.3 mi) | 1.1 km | (0.7 mi) | 400 m | (1250 ft) | 2.1 km | (1.3 mi) | 4.9 km | (3.0 mi) |
| 2810 | **153** | GD **(when used as a weapon)** | 60 m | (200 ft) | 0.4 km | (0.3 mi) | 0.7 km | (0.5 mi) | 300 m | (1000 ft) | 1.8 km | (1.1 mi) | 2.7 km | (1.7 mi) |
| 2810 | **153** | GF **(when used as a weapon)** | 30 m | (100 ft) | 0.2 km | (0.2 mi) | 0.3 km | (0.2 mi) | 150 m | (500 ft) | 0.8 km | (0.5 mi) | 1.0 km | (0.6 mi) |
| 2810<br>2810 | **153**<br>**153** | H **(when used as a weapon)**<br>HD **(when used as a weapon)** | 30 m | (100 ft) | 0.1 km | (0.1 mi) | 0.1 km | (0.1 mi) | 60 m | (200 ft) | 0.3 km | (0.2 mi) | 0.4 km | (0.3 mi) |
| 2810 | **153** | HL **(when used as a weapon)** | 30 m | (100 ft) | 0.1 km | (0.1 mi) | 0.3 km | (0.2 mi) | 100 m | (300 ft) | 0.5 km | (0.3 mi) | 1.0 km | (0.6 mi) |
| 2810 | **153** | HN-1 **(when used as a weapon)** | 60 m | (200 ft) | 0.3 km | (0.2 mi) | 0.5 km | (0.3 mi) | 200 m | (600 ft) | 1.1 km | (0.7 mi) | 1.8 km | (1.1 mi) |
| 2810 | **153** | HN-2 **(when used as a weapon)** | 60 m | (200 ft) | 0.3 km | (0.2 mi) | 0.6 km | (0.4 mi) | 300 m | (1000 ft) | 1.3 km | (0.8 mi) | 2.1 km | (1.3 mi) |
| 2810 | **153** | HN-3 **(when used as a weapon)** | 30 m | (100 ft) | 0.1 km | (0.1 mi) | 0.1 km | (0.1 mi) | 60 m | (200 ft) | 0.3 km | (0.2 mi) | 0.3 km | (0.2 mi) |

**"+" means distance can be larger in certain atmospheric conditions**

## TABLE 1 - INITIAL ISOLATION AND PROTECTIVE ACTION DISTANCES

| | | | SMALL SPILLS (From a small package or small leak from a large package) | | | LARGE SPILLS (From a large package or from many small packages) | | |
|---|---|---|---|---|---|---|---|---|
| | | | First ISOLATE in all Directions | Then PROTECT persons Downwind during | | First ISOLATE in all Directions | Then PROTECT persons Downwind during | |
| ID No. | Guide | NAME OF MATERIAL | Meters (Feet) | DAY Kilometers (Miles) | NIGHT Kilometers (Miles) | Meters (Feet) | DAY Kilometers (Miles) | NIGHT Kilometers (Miles) |
| 2810<br>2810 | **153**<br>**153** | L (Lewisite) **(when used as a weapon)**<br>Lewisite **(when used as a weapon)** | 30 m (100 ft) | 0.1 km (0.1 mi) | 0.3 km (0.2 mi) | 100 m (300 ft) | 0.5 km (0.3 mi) | 1.0 km (0.6 mi) |
| 2810 | **153** | Mustard **(when used as a weapon)** | 30 m (100 ft) | 0.1 km (0.1 mi) | 0.1 km (0.1 mi) | 60 m (200 ft) | 0.3 km (0.2 mi) | 0.4 km (0.3 mi) |
| 2810 | **153** | Mustard Lewisite **(when used as a weapon)** | 30 m (100 ft) | 0.1 km (0.1 mi) | 0.3 km (0.2 mi) | 100 m (300 ft) | 0.5 km (0.3 mi) | 1.0 km (0.6 mi) |
| 2810 | **153** | Sarin **(when used as a weapon)** | 60 m (200 ft) | 0.4 km (0.3 mi) | 1.1 km (0.7 mi) | 400 m (1250 ft) | 2.1 km (1.3 mi) | 4.9 km (3.0 mi) |
| 2810 | **153** | Soman **(when used as a weapon)** | 60 m (200 ft) | 0.4 km (0.3 mi) | 0.7 km (0.5 mi) | 300 m (1000 ft) | 1.8 km (1.1 mi) | 2.7 km (1.7 mi) |
| 2810 | **153** | Tabun **(when used as a weapon)** | 30 m (100 ft) | 0.2 km (0.1 mi) | 0.2 km (0.1 mi) | 100 m (300 ft) | 0.5 km (0.4 mi) | 0.6 km (0.4 mi) |
| 2810 | **153** | Thickened GD **(when used as a weapon)** | 60 m (200 ft) | 0.4 km (0.3 mi) | 0.7 km (0.5 mi) | 300 m (1000 ft) | 1.8 km (1.1 mi) | 2.7 km (1.7 mi) |
| 2810 | **153** | VX **(when used as a weapon)** | 30 m (100 ft) | 0.1 km (0.1 mi) | 0.1 km (0.1 mi) | 60 m (200 ft) | 0.4 km (0.2 mi) | 0.3 km (0.2 mi) |
| 2811 | **154** | CX **(when used as a weapon)** | 60 m (200 ft) | 0.2 km (0.2 mi) | 1.1 km (0.7 mi) | 200 m (600 ft) | 1.2 km (0.7 mi) | 5.1 km (3.2 mi) |
| 2826 | **155** | Ethyl chlorothioformate | 30 m (100 ft) | 0.1 km (0.1 mi) | 0.2 km (0.1 mi) | 30 m (100 ft) | 0.4 km (0.2 mi) | 0.5 km (0.4 mi) |
| 2845 | **135** | Ethyl phosphonous dichloride, anhydrous | 30 m (100 ft) | 0.3 km (0.2 mi) | 0.7 km (0.5 mi) | 100 m (300 ft) | 1.3 km (0.8 mi) | 2.3 km (1.4 mi) |

| ID No. | Guide | Name of Material | | | | | | | | | | | | |
|---|---|---|---|---|---|---|---|---|---|---|---|---|---|---|
| 2845 | **135** | Methyl phosphonous dichloride | 30 m | (100 ft) | 0.4 km | (0.2 mi) | 1.0 km | (0.7 mi) | 150 m | (500 ft) | 1.9 km | (1.2 mi) | 3.5 km | (2.2 mi) |
| 2901 | **124** | Bromine chloride | 100 m | (300 ft) | 0.5 km | (0.3 mi) | 1.8 km | (1.1 mi) | 800 m | (2500 ft) | 4.5 km | (2.8 mi) | 10.0 km | (6.2 mi) |
| 2927 | **154** | Ethyl phosphonothioic dichloride, anhydrous | 30 m | (100 ft) | 0.1 km | (0.1 mi) | 0.1 km | (0.1 mi) | 30 m | (100 ft) | 0.2 km | (0.1 mi) | 0.2 km | (0.1 mi) |
| 2927 | **154** | Ethyl phosphorodichloridate | 30 m | (100 ft) | 0.1 km | (0.1 mi) | 0.1 km | (0.1 mi) | 30 m | (100 ft) | 0.3 km | (0.2 mi) | 0.3 km | (0.2 mi) |
| 2977<br>2977 | **166**<br>**166** | Radioactive material, Uranium hexafluoride, fissile **(when spilled in water)**<br>Uranium hexafluoride, radioactive material, fissile **(when spilled in water)** | 30 m | (100 ft) | 0.1 km | (0.1 mi) | 0.4 km | (0.3 mi) | 60 m | (200 ft) | 0.5 km | (0.3 mi) | 2.1 km | (1.4 mi) |
| 2978<br>2978 | **166**<br>**166** | Radioactive material, Uranium hexafluoride, non fissile or fissile-excepted **(when spilled in water)**<br>Uranium hexafluoride, radioactive material, non fissile or fissile-excepted **(when spilled in water)** | 30 m | (100 ft) | 0.1 km | (0.1 mi) | 0.4 km | (0.3 mi) | 60 m | (200 ft) | 0.5 km | (0.3 mi) | 2.1 km | (1.4 mi) |
| 2985 | **155** | Chlorosilanes, flammable, corrosive, n.o.s. **(when spilled in water)** | 30 m | (100 ft) | 0.1 km | (0.1 mi) | 0.2 km | (0.1 mi) | 60 m | (200 ft) | 0.5 km | (0.3 mi) | 1.6 km | (1.0 mi) |
| 2986 | **155** | Chlorosilanes, corrosive, flammable, n.o.s. **(when spilled in water)** | 30 m | (100 ft) | 0.1 km | (0.1 mi) | 0.2 km | (0.1 mi) | 60 m | (200 ft) | 0.5 km | (0.3 mi) | 1.6 km | (1.0 mi) |
| 2987 | **156** | Chlorosilanes, corrosive, n.o.s. **(when spilled in water)** | 30 m | (100 ft) | 0.1 km | (0.1 mi) | 0.2 km | (0.1 mi) | 60 m | (200 ft) | 0.5 km | (0.3 mi) | 1.6 km | (1.0 mi) |
| 2988 | **139** | Chlorosilanes, water-reactive, flammable, corrosive, n.o.s. **(when spilled in water)** | 30 m | (100 ft) | 0.1 km | (0.1 mi) | 0.2 km | (0.1 mi) | 60 m | (200 ft) | 0.5 km | (0.3 mi) | 1.6 km | (1.0 mi) |

**"+" means distance can be larger in certain atmospheric conditions**

# TABLE 1 - INITIAL ISOLATION AND PROTECTIVE ACTION DISTANCES

| ID No. | Guide | NAME OF MATERIAL | SMALL SPILLS (From a small package or small leak from a large package) — First ISOLATE in all Directions, Meters (Feet) | SMALL SPILLS — Then PROTECT persons Downwind during DAY, Kilometers (Miles) | SMALL SPILLS — Then PROTECT persons Downwind during NIGHT, Kilometers (Miles) | LARGE SPILLS (From a large package or from many small packages) — First ISOLATE in all Directions, Meters (Feet) | LARGE SPILLS — Then PROTECT persons Downwind during DAY, Kilometers (Miles) | LARGE SPILLS — Then PROTECT persons Downwind during NIGHT, Kilometers (Miles) |
|---|---|---|---|---|---|---|---|---|
| 3023 | **131** | 2-Methyl-2-heptanethiol | 30 m (100 ft) | 0.1 km (0.1 mi) | 0.2 km (0.1 mi) | 60 m (200 ft) | 0.5 km (0.3 mi) | 0.7 km (0.4 mi) |
| 3048 | **157** | Aluminum phosphide pesticide **(when spilled in water)** | 60 m (200 ft) | 0.2 km (0.2 mi) | 0.9 km (0.6 mi) | 500 m (1500 ft) | 2.0 km (1.2 mi) | 7.0 km (4.4 mi) |
| 3049<br>3049 | **138**<br>**138** | Metal alkyl halides, water-reactive, n.o.s. **(when spilled in water)**<br>Metal aryl halides, water-reactive, n.o.s. **(when spilled in water)** | 30 m (100 ft) | 0.1 km (0.1 mi) | 0.2 km (0.1 mi) | 60 m (200 ft) | 0.4 km (0.3 mi) | 1.3 km (0.8 mi) |
| 3052<br>3052 | **135**<br>**135** | Aluminum alkyl halides, liquid **(when spilled in water)**<br>Aluminum alkyl halides, solid **(when spilled in water)** | 30 m (100 ft) | 0.1 km (0.1 mi) | 0.2 km (0.1 mi) | 60 m (200 ft) | 0.4 km (0.3 mi) | 1.3 km (0.8 mi) |
| 3057 | **125** | Trifluoroacetyl chloride | 30 m (100 ft) | 0.2 km (0.1 mi) | 0.9 km (0.6 mi) | 600 m (2000 ft) | 4.0 km (2.5 mi) | 9.5 km (5.9 mi) |
| 3079 | **131P** | Methacrylonitrile, stabilized | 30 m (100 ft) | 0.3 km (0.2 mi) | 0.7 km (0.4 mi) | 150 m (500 ft) | 1.4 km (0.9 mi) | 2.5 km (1.6 mi) |
| 3083 | **124** | Perchloryl fluoride | 30 m (100 ft) | 0.2 km (0.2 mi) | 1.1 km (0.7 mi) | 800 m (2500 ft) | 4.5 km (2.8 mi) | 9.6 km (6.0 mi) |
| 3160<br>3160 | **119**<br>**119** | Liquefied gas, poisonous, flammable, n.o.s.<br>Liquefied gas, poisonous, flammable, n.o.s. (Inhalation Hazard Zone A) | 150 m (500 ft) | 1.0 km (0.6 mi) | 3.8 km (2.4 mi) | 1000 m (3000 ft) | 5.6 km (3.5 mi) | 10.2 km (6.3 mi) |

| ID No. | Guide | Name of Material | Small Spills: Isolate in all Directions | | Small Spills: Protect Day | | Small Spills: Protect Night | | Large Spills: Isolate in all Directions | | Large Spills: Protect Day | | Large Spills: Protect Night | |
|---|---|---|---|---|---|---|---|---|---|---|---|---|---|---|
| 3160 | **119** | Liquefied gas, poisonous, flammable, n.o.s. (Inhalation Hazard Zone B) | 30 m | (100 ft) | 0.1 km | (0.1 mi) | 0.4 km | (0.2 mi) | 200 m | (600 ft) | 1.2 km | (0.8 mi) | 2.6 km | (1.6 mi) |
| 3160 | **119** | Liquefied gas, poisonous, flammable, n.o.s. (Inhalation Hazard Zone C) | 30 m | (100 ft) | 0.1 km | (0.1 mi) | 0.3 km | (0.2 mi) | 150 m | (500 ft) | 0.9 km | (0.6 mi) | 2.4 km | (1.5 mi) |
| 3160 | **119** | Liquefied gas, poisonous, flammable, n.o.s. (Inhalation Hazard Zone D) | 30 m | (100 ft) | 0.1 km | (0.1 mi) | 0.2 km | (0.1 mi) | 100 m | (300 ft) | 0.7 km | (0.5 mi) | 1.9 km | (1.2 mi) |
| 3160<br>3160 | **119**<br>**119** | Liquefied gas, toxic, flammable, n.o.s.<br>Liquefied gas, toxic, flammable, n.o.s. (Inhalation Hazard Zone A) | 150 m | (500 ft) | 1.0 km | (0.6 mi) | 3.8 km | (2.4 mi) | 1000 m | (3000 ft) | 5.6 km | (3.5 mi) | 10.2 km | (6.3 mi) |
| 3160 | **119** | Liquefied gas, toxic, flammable, n.o.s. (Inhalation Hazard Zone B) | 30 m | (100 ft) | 0.1 km | (0.1 mi) | 0.4 km | (0.2 mi) | 200 m | (600 ft) | 1.2 km | (0.8 mi) | 2.6 km | (1.6 mi) |
| 3160 | **119** | Liquefied gas, toxic, flammable, n.o.s. (Inhalation Hazard Zone C) | 30 m | (100 ft) | 0.1 km | (0.1 mi) | 0.3 km | (0.2 mi) | 150 m | (500 ft) | 0.9 km | (0.6 mi) | 2.4 km | (1.5 mi) |
| 3160 | **119** | Liquefied gas, toxic, flammable, n.o.s. (Inhalation Hazard Zone D) | 30 m | (100 ft) | 0.1 km | (0.1 mi) | 0.2 km | (0.1 mi) | 100 m | (300 ft) | 0.7 km | (0.5 mi) | 1.9 km | (1.2 mi) |
| 3162<br>3162 | **123**<br>**123** | Liquefied gas, poisonous, n.o.s.<br>Liquefied gas, poisonous, n.o.s. (Inhalation Hazard Zone A) | 100 m | (300 ft) | 0.5 km | (0.3 mi) | 2.5 km | (1.6 mi) | 1000 m | (3000 ft) | 5.6 km | (3.5 mi) | 10.2 km | (6.3 mi) |
| 3162 | **123** | Liquefied gas, poisonous, n.o.s. (Inhalation Hazard Zone B) | 30 m | (100 ft) | 0.2 km | (0.1 mi) | 0.8 km | (0.5 mi) | 300 m | (1000 ft) | 1.4 km | (0.9 mi) | 4.1 km | (2.6 mi) |
| 3162 | **123** | Liquefied gas, poisonous, n.o.s. (Inhalation Hazard Zone C) | 30 m | (100 ft) | 0.1 km | (0.1 mi) | 0.3 km | (0.2 mi) | 150 m | (500 ft) | 0.9 km | (0.6 mi) | 2.4 km | (1.5 mi) |

**"+" means distance can be larger in certain atmospheric conditions**

# TABLE 1 - INITIAL ISOLATION AND PROTECTIVE ACTION DISTANCES

| ID No. | Guide | NAME OF MATERIAL | SMALL SPILLS (From a small package or small leak from a large package) — First ISOLATE in all Directions: Meters (Feet) | SMALL SPILLS — Then PROTECT persons Downwind during DAY: Kilometers (Miles) | SMALL SPILLS — Then PROTECT persons Downwind during NIGHT: Kilometers (Miles) | LARGE SPILLS (From a large package or from many small packages) — First ISOLATE in all Directions: Meters (Feet) | LARGE SPILLS — Then PROTECT persons Downwind during DAY: Kilometers (Miles) | LARGE SPILLS — Then PROTECT persons Downwind during NIGHT: Kilometers (Miles) |
|---|---|---|---|---|---|---|---|---|
| 3162 | **123** | Liquefied gas, poisonous, n.o.s. (Inhalation Hazard Zone D) | 30 m (100 ft) | 0.1 km (0.1 mi) | 0.2 km (0.1 mi) | 100 m (300 ft) | 0.7 km (0.5 mi) | 1.9 km (1.2 mi) |
| 3162<br>3162 | **123**<br>**123** | Liquefied gas, toxic, n.o.s.<br>Liquefied gas, toxic, n.o.s. (Inhalation Hazard Zone A) | 100 m (300 ft) | 0.5 km (0.3 mi) | 2.5 km (1.6 mi) | 1000 m (3000 ft) | 5.6 km (3.5 mi) | 10.2 km (6.3 mi) |
| 3162 | **123** | Liquefied gas, toxic, n.o.s. (Inhalation Hazard Zone B) | 30 m (100 ft) | 0.2 km (0.1 mi) | 0.8 km (0.5 mi) | 300 m (1000 ft) | 1.4 km (0.9 mi) | 4.1 km (2.6 mi) |
| 3162 | **123** | Liquefied gas, toxic, n.o.s. (Inhalation Hazard Zone C) | 30 m (100 ft) | 0.1 km (0.1 mi) | 0.3 km (0.2 mi) | 150 m (500 ft) | 0.9 km (0.6 mi) | 2.4 km (1.5 mi) |
| 3162 | **123** | Liquefied gas, toxic, n.o.s. (Inhalation Hazard Zone D) | 30 m (100 ft) | 0.1 km (0.1 mi) | 0.2 km (0.1 mi) | 100 m (300 ft) | 0.7 km (0.5 mi) | 1.9 km (1.2 mi) |
| 3246<br>3246 | **156**<br>**156** | Methanesulfonyl chloride<br>Methanesulphonyl chloride | 30 m (100 ft) | 0.2 km (0.1 mi) | 0.3 km (0.2 mi) | 60 m (200 ft) | 0.6 km (0.4 mi) | 0.8 km (0.5 mi) |
| 3275<br>3275 | **131**<br>**131** | Nitriles, poisonous, flammable, n.o.s.<br>Nitriles, toxic, flammable, n.o.s. | 30 m (100 ft) | 0.3 km (0.2 mi) | 0.7 km (0.4 mi) | 150 m (500 ft) | 1.4 km (0.9 mi) | 2.5 km (1.6 mi) |
| 3276<br>3276<br>3276<br>3276<br>3276<br>3276 | **151**<br>**151**<br>**151**<br>**151**<br>**151**<br>**151** | Nitriles, liquid, poisonous, n.o.s.<br>Nitriles, liquid, toxic, n.o.s.<br>Nitriles, poisonous, liquid, n.o.s.<br>Nitriles, poisonous, n.o.s.<br>Nitriles, toxic, liquid, n.o.s.<br>Nitriles, toxic, n.o.s. | 30 m (100 ft) | 0.3 km (0.2 mi) | 0.7 km (0.4 mi) | 150 m (500 ft) | 1.4 km (0.9 mi) | 2.5 km (1.6 mi) |

| ID No. | Guide No. | Name of Material | | | | | | | | | | | | |
|---|---|---|---|---|---|---|---|---|---|---|---|---|---|---|
| 3278 | **151** | Organophosphorus compound, liquid, poisonous, n.o.s. | 30 m | (100 ft) | 0.4 km | (0.2 mi) | 1.0 km | (0.7 mi) | 150 m | (500 ft) | 1.9 km | (1.2 mi) | 3.5 km | (2.2 mi) |
| 3278 | **151** | Organophosphorus compound, liquid, toxic, n.o.s. | | | | | | | | | | | | |
| 3278 | **151** | Organophosphorus compound, poisonous, liquid, n.o.s. | | | | | | | | | | | | |
| 3278 | **151** | Organophosphorus compound, poisonous, n.o.s. | | | | | | | | | | | | |
| 3278 | **151** | Organophosphorus compound, toxic, liquid, n.o.s. | | | | | | | | | | | | |
| 3278 | **151** | Organophosphorus compound, toxic, n.o.s. | | | | | | | | | | | | |
| 3279 | **131** | Organophosphorus compound, poisonous, flammable, n.o.s. | 30 m | (100 ft) | 0.4 km | (0.2 mi) | 1.0 km | (0.7 mi) | 150 m | (500 ft) | 1.9 km | (1.2 mi) | 3.5 km | (2.2 mi) |
| 3279 | **131** | Organophosphorus compound, toxic, flammable, n.o.s. | | | | | | | | | | | | |
| 3280 | **151** | Organoarsenic compound, liquid, n.o.s. | 30 m | (100 ft) | 0.2 km | (0.1 mi) | 0.7 km | (0.5 mi) | 150 m | (500 ft) | 1.5 km | (1.0 mi) | 3.5 km | (2.2 mi) |
| 3280 | **151** | Organoarsenic compound, n.o.s. | | | | | | | | | | | | |
| 3281 | **151** | Metal carbonyls, liquid, n.o.s. | 100 m | (300 ft) | 1.4 km | (0.9 mi) | 4.9 km | (3.0 mi) | 1000 m | (3000 ft) | 11.0+ km | (7.0+ mi) | 11.0+ km | (7.0+ mi) |
| 3281 | **151** | Metal carbonyls, n.o.s. | | | | | | | | | | | | |
| 3294 | **131** | Hydrogen cyanide, solution in alcohol, with not more than 45% Hydrogen cyanide | 30 m | (100 ft) | 0.1 km | (0.1 mi) | 0.3 km | (0.2 mi) | 200 m | (600 ft) | 0.5 km | (0.3 mi) | 1.9 km | (1.2 mi) |
| 3300 | **119P** | Carbon dioxide and Ethylene oxide mixture, with more than 87% Ethylene oxide | 30 m | (100 ft) | 0.1 km | (0.1 mi) | 0.2 km | (0.1 mi) | 100 m | (300 ft) | 0.7 km | (0.5 mi) | 1.9 km | (1.2 mi) |
| 3300 | **119P** | Ethylene oxide and Carbon dioxide mixture, with more than 87% Ethylene oxide | | | | | | | | | | | | |

**"+" means distance can be larger in certain atmospheric conditions**

# TABLE 1 - INITIAL ISOLATION AND PROTECTIVE ACTION DISTANCES

| | | | SMALL SPILLS (From a small package or small leak from a large package) | | | LARGE SPILLS (From a large package or from many small packages) | | |
|---|---|---|---|---|---|---|---|---|
| | | | First ISOLATE in all Directions | Then PROTECT persons Downwind during | | First ISOLATE in all Directions | Then PROTECT persons Downwind during | |
| ID No. | Guide | NAME OF MATERIAL | Meters (Feet) | DAY Kilometers (Miles) | NIGHT Kilometers (Miles) | Meters (Feet) | DAY Kilometers (Miles) | NIGHT Kilometers (Miles) |
| 3303 | **124** | Compressed gas, poisonous, oxidizing, n.o.s. | | | | | | |
| 3303 | **124** | Compressed gas, poisonous, oxidizing, n.o.s. (Inhalation Hazard Zone A) | 100 m (300 ft) | 0.5 km (0.3 mi) | 2.5 km (1.6 mi) | 800 m (2500 ft) | 5.2 km (3.3 mi) | 11.0+ km (7.0+ mi) |
| 3303 | **124** | Compressed gas, poisonous, oxidizing, n.o.s. (Inhalation Hazard Zone B) | 60 m (200 ft) | 0.3 km (0.2 mi) | 1.1 km (0.7 mi) | 800 m (2500 ft) | 4.5 km (2.8 mi) | 9.6 km (6.0 mi) |
| 3303 | **124** | Compressed gas, poisonous, oxidizing, n.o.s. (Inhalation Hazard Zone C) | 30 m (100 ft) | 0.1 km (0.1 mi) | 0.3 km (0.2 mi) | 150 m (500 ft) | 0.9 km (0.6 mi) | 2.4 km (1.5 mi) |
| 3303 | **124** | Compressed gas, poisonous, oxidizing, n.o.s. (Inhalation Hazard Zone D) | 30 m (100 ft) | 0.1 km (0.1 mi) | 0.2 km (0.1 mi) | 100 m (300 ft) | 0.7 km (0.5 mi) | 1.9 km (1.2 mi) |
| 3303 | **124** | Compressed gas, toxic, oxidizing, n.o.s. | | | | | | |
| 3303 | **124** | Compressed gas, toxic, oxidizing, n.o.s. (Inhalation Hazard Zone A) | 100 m (300 ft) | 0.5 km (0.3 mi) | 2.5 km (1.6 mi) | 800 m (2500 ft) | 5.2 km (3.3 mi) | 11.0+ km (7.0+ mi) |
| 3303 | **124** | Compressed gas, toxic, oxidizing, n.o.s. (Inhalation Hazard Zone B) | 60 m (200 ft) | 0.3 km (0.2 mi) | 1.1 km (0.7 mi) | 800 m (2500 ft) | 4.5 km (2.8 mi) | 9.6 km (6.0 mi) |

| ID No. | Guide No. | Name of Material | | | | | | | | | | | | |
|---|---|---|---|---|---|---|---|---|---|---|---|---|---|---|
| 3303 | **124** | Compressed gas, toxic, oxidizing, n.o.s. (Inhalation Hazard Zone C) | 30 m | (100 ft) | 0.1 km | (0.1 mi) | 0.3 km | (0.2 mi) | 150 m | (500 ft) | 0.9 km | (0.6 mi) | 2.4 km | (1.5 mi) |
| 3303 | **124** | Compressed gas, toxic, oxidizing, n.o.s. (Inhalation Hazard Zone D) | 30 m | (100 ft) | 0.1 km | (0.1 mi) | 0.2 km | (0.1 mi) | 100 m | (300 ft) | 0.7 km | (0.5 mi) | 1.9 km | (1.2 mi) |
| 3304<br>3304 | **123**<br>**123** | Compressed gas, poisonous, corrosive, n.o.s.<br>Compressed gas, poisonous, corrosive, n.o.s. (Inhalation Hazard Zone A) | 100 m | (300 ft) | 0.6 km | (0.4 mi) | 2.5 km | (1.5 mi) | 500 m | (1500 ft) | 3.0 km | (1.9 mi) | 9.0 km | (5.6 mi) |
| 3304 | **123** | Compressed gas, poisonous, corrosive, n.o.s. (Inhalation Hazard Zone B) | 30 m | (100 ft) | 0.2 km | (0.2 mi) | 1.0 km | (0.6 mi) | 400 m | (1250 ft) | 2.2 km | (1.4 mi) | 4.8 km | (3.0 mi) |
| 3304 | **123** | Compressed gas, poisonous, corrosive, n.o.s. (Inhalation Hazard Zone C) | 30 m | (100 ft) | 0.1 km | (0.1 mi) | 0.4 km | (0.3 mi) | 150 m | (500 ft) | 0.9 km | (0.6 mi) | 2.6 km | (1.6 mi) |
| 3304 | **123** | Compressed gas, poisonous, corrosive, n.o.s. (Inhalation Hazard Zone D) | 30 m | (100 ft) | 0.1 km | (0.1 mi) | 0.2 km | (0.1 mi) | 150 m | (500 ft) | 0.7 km | (0.5 mi) | 1.9 km | (1.2 mi) |
| 3304<br>3304 | **123**<br>**123** | Compressed gas, toxic, corrosive, n.o.s.<br>Compressed gas, toxic, corrosive, n.o.s. (Inhalation Hazard Zone A) | 100 m | (300 ft) | 0.6 km | (0.4 mi) | 2.5 km | (1.5 mi) | 500 m | (1500 ft) | 3.0 km | (1.9 mi) | 9.0 km | (5.6 mi) |
| 3304 | **123** | Compressed gas, toxic, corrosive, n.o.s. (Inhalation Hazard Zone B) | 30 m | (100 ft) | 0.2 km | (0.2 mi) | 1.0 km | (0.6 mi) | 400 m | (1250 ft) | 2.2 km | (1.4 mi) | 4.8 km | (3.0 mi) |
| 3304 | **123** | Compressed gas, toxic, corrosive, n.o.s. (Inhalation Hazard Zone C) | 30 m | (100 ft) | 0.1 km | (0.1 mi) | 0.4 km | (0.3 mi) | 150 m | (500 ft) | 0.9 km | (0.6 mi) | 2.6 km | (1.6 mi) |

**"+" means distance can be larger in certain atmospheric conditions**

## TABLE 1 - INITIAL ISOLATION AND PROTECTIVE ACTION DISTANCES

| ID No. | Guide | NAME OF MATERIAL | SMALL SPILLS (From a small package or small leak from a large package) | | | LARGE SPILLS (From a large package or from many small packages) | | |
|---|---|---|---|---|---|---|---|---|
| | | | First ISOLATE in all Directions | Then PROTECT persons Downwind during | | First ISOLATE in all Directions | Then PROTECT persons Downwind during | |
| | | | Meters (Feet) | DAY Kilometers (Miles) | NIGHT Kilometers (Miles) | Meters (Feet) | DAY Kilometers (Miles) | NIGHT Kilometers (Miles) |
| 3304 | **123** | Compressed gas, toxic, corrosive, n.o.s. (Inhalation Hazard Zone D) | 30 m (100 ft) | 0.1 km (0.1 mi) | 0.2 km (0.1 mi) | 150 m (500 ft) | 0.7 km (0.5 mi) | 1.9 km (1.2 mi) |
| 3305<br>3305 | **119**<br>**119** | Compressed gas, poisonous, flammable, corrosive, n.o.s.<br>Compressed gas, poisonous, flammable, corrosive, n.o.s. (Inhalation Hazard Zone A) | 150 m (500 ft) | 1.0 km (0.6 mi) | 3.8 km (2.4 mi) | 1000 m (3000 ft) | 5.6 km (3.5 mi) | 10.2 km (6.3 mi) |
| 3305 | **119** | Compressed gas, poisonous, flammable, corrosive, n.o.s. (Inhalation Hazard Zone B) | 30 m (100 ft) | 0.1 km (0.1 mi) | 0.4 km (0.2 mi) | 200 m (600 ft) | 1.2 km (0.8 mi) | 2.6 km (1.6 mi) |
| 3305 | **119** | Compressed gas, poisonous, flammable, corrosive, n.o.s. (Inhalation Hazard Zone C) | 30 m (100 ft) | 0.1 km (0.1 mi) | 0.3 km (0.2 mi) | 150 m (500 ft) | 0.9 km (0.6 mi) | 2.4 km (1.5 mi) |
| 3305 | **119** | Compressed gas, poisonous, flammable, corrosive, n.o.s. (Inhalation Hazard Zone D) | 30 m (100 ft) | 0.1 km (0.1 mi) | 0.2 km (0.1 mi) | 100 m (300 ft) | 0.7 km (0.5 mi) | 1.9 km (1.2 mi) |
| 3305<br>3305 | **119**<br>**119** | Compressed gas, toxic, flammable, corrosive, n.o.s.<br>Compressed gas, toxic, flammable, corrosive, n.o.s. (Inhalation Hazard Zone A) | 150 m (500 ft) | 1.0 km (0.6 mi) | 3.8 km (2.4 mi) | 1000 m (3000 ft) | 5.6 km (3.5 mi) | 10.2 km (6.3 mi) |

| | | | | | | | | | | | | | | |
|---|---|---|---|---|---|---|---|---|---|---|---|---|---|---|
| 3305 | **119** | Compressed gas, toxic, flammable, corrosive, n.o.s. (Inhalation Hazard Zone B) | 30 m | (100 ft) | 0.1 km | (0.1 mi) | 0.4 km | (0.2 mi) | 200 m | (600 ft) | 1.2 km | (0.8 mi) | 2.6 km | (1.6 mi) |
| 3305 | **119** | Compressed gas, toxic, flammable, corrosive, n.o.s. (Inhalation Hazard Zone C) | 30 m | (100 ft) | 0.1 km | (0.1 mi) | 0.3 km | (0.2 mi) | 150 m | (500 ft) | 0.9 km | (0.6 mi) | 2.4 km | (1.5 mi) |
| 3305 | **119** | Compressed gas, toxic, flammable, corrosive, n.o.s. (Inhalation Hazard Zone D) | 30 m | (100 ft) | 0.1 km | (0.1 mi) | 0.2 km | (0.1 mi) | 100 m | (300 ft) | 0.7 km | (0.5 mi) | 1.9 km | (1.2 mi) |
| 3306 | **124** | Compressed gas, poisonous, oxidizing, corrosive, n.o.s. | | | | | | | | | | | | |
| 3306 | **124** | Compressed gas, poisonous, oxidizing, corrosive, n.o.s. (Inhalation Hazard Zone A) | 100 m | (300 ft) | 0.5 km | (0.3 mi) | 2.5 km | (1.6 mi) | 800 m | (2500 ft) | 5.2 km | (3.3 mi) | 11.0+ km | (7.0+ mi) |
| 3306 | **124** | Compressed gas, poisonous, oxidizing, corrosive, n.o.s. (Inhalation Hazard Zone B) | 60 m | (200 ft) | 0.3 km | (0.2 mi) | 1.1 km | (0.7 mi) | 800 m | (2500 ft) | 4.5 km | (2.8 mi) | 9.6 km | (6.0 mi) |
| 3306 | **124** | Compressed gas, poisonous, oxidizing, corrosive, n.o.s. (Inhalation Hazard Zone C) | 30 m | (100 ft) | 0.1 km | (0.1 mi) | 0.3 km | (0.2 mi) | 150 m | (500 ft) | 0.9 km | (0.6 mi) | 2.4 km | (1.5 mi) |
| 3306 | **124** | Compressed gas, poisonous, oxidizing, corrosive, n.o.s. (Inhalation Hazard Zone D) | 30 m | (100 ft) | 0.1 km | (0.1 mi) | 0.2 km | (0.1 mi) | 100 m | (300 ft) | 0.7 km | (0.5 mi) | 1.9 km | (1.2 mi) |
| 3306 | **124** | Compressed gas, toxic, oxidizing, corrosive, n.o.s. | | | | | | | | | | | | |
| 3306 | **124** | Compressed gas, toxic, oxidizing, corrosive, n.o.s. (Inhalation Hazard Zone A) | 100 m | (300 ft) | 0.5 km | (0.3 mi) | 2.5 km | (1.6 mi) | 800 m | (2500 ft) | 5.2 km | (3.3 mi) | 11.0+ km | (7.0+ mi) |
| 3306 | **124** | Compressed gas, toxic, oxidizing, corrosive, n.o.s. (Inhalation Hazard Zone B) | 60 m | (200 ft) | 0.3 km | (0.2 mi) | 1.1 km | (0.7 mi) | 800 m | (2500 ft) | 4.5 km | (2.8 mi) | 9.6 km | (6.0 mi) |

**"+" means distance can be larger in certain atmospheric conditions**

## TABLE 1 - INITIAL ISOLATION AND PROTECTIVE ACTION DISTANCES

| | | | SMALL SPILLS (From a small package or small leak from a large package) | | | LARGE SPILLS (From a large package or from many small packages) | | |
|---|---|---|---|---|---|---|---|---|
| | | | First ISOLATE in all Directions | Then PROTECT persons Downwind during | | First ISOLATE in all Directions | Then PROTECT persons Downwind during | |
| ID No. | Guide | NAME OF MATERIAL | Meters (Feet) | DAY Kilometers (Miles) | NIGHT Kilometers (Miles) | Meters (Feet) | DAY Kilometers (Miles) | NIGHT Kilometers (Miles) |
| 3306 | **124** | Compressed gas, toxic, oxidizing, corrosive, n.o.s. (Inhalation Hazard Zone C) | 30 m (100 ft) | 0.1 km (0.1 mi) | 0.3 km (0.2 mi) | 150 m (500 ft) | 0.9 km (0.6 mi) | 2.4 km (1.5 mi) |
| 3306 | **124** | Compressed gas, toxic, oxidizing, corrosive, n.o.s. (Inhalation Hazard Zone D) | 30 m (100 ft) | 0.1 km (0.1 mi) | 0.2 km (0.1 mi) | 100 m (300 ft) | 0.7 km (0.5 mi) | 1.9 km (1.2 mi) |
| 3307 | **124** | Liquefied gas, poisonous, oxidizing, n.o.s. | | | | | | |
| 3307 | **124** | Liquefied gas, poisonous, oxidizing, n.o.s. (Inhalation Hazard Zone A) | 100 m (300 ft) | 0.5 km (0.3 mi) | 2.5 km (1.6 mi) | 800 m (2500 ft) | 5.2 km (3.3 mi) | 11.0+ km (7.0+ mi) |
| 3307 | **124** | Liquefied gas, poisonous, oxidizing, n.o.s. (Inhalation Hazard Zone B) | 60 m (200 ft) | 0.3 km (0.2 mi) | 1.1 km (0.7 mi) | 800 m (2500 ft) | 4.5 km (2.8 mi) | 9.6 km (6.0 mi) |
| 3307 | **124** | Liquefied gas, poisonous, oxidizing, n.o.s. (Inhalation Hazard Zone C) | 30 m (100 ft) | 0.1 km (0.1 mi) | 0.3 km (0.2 mi) | 150 m (500 ft) | 0.9 km (0.6 mi) | 2.4 km (1.5 mi) |
| 3307 | **124** | Liquefied gas, poisonous, oxidizing, n.o.s. (Inhalation Hazard Zone D) | 30 m (100 ft) | 0.1 km (0.1 mi) | 0.2 km (0.1 mi) | 100 m (300 ft) | 0.7 km (0.5 mi) | 1.9 km (1.2 mi) |

| ID No. | Guide No. | Name of Material | | | | | | | | | | | | |
|---|---|---|---|---|---|---|---|---|---|---|---|---|---|---|
| 3307 | **124** | Liquefied gas, toxic, oxidizing, n.o.s. | | | | | | | | | | | | |
| 3307 | **124** | Liquefied gas, toxic, oxidizing, n.o.s. (Inhalation Hazard Zone A) | 100 m | (300 ft) | 0.5 km | (0.3 mi) | 2.5 km | (1.6 mi) | 800 m | (2500 ft) | 5.2 km | (3.3 mi) | 11.0+ km | (7.0+ mi) |
| 3307 | **124** | Liquefied gas, toxic, oxidizing, n.o.s. (Inhalation Hazard Zone B) | 60 m | (200 ft) | 0.3 km | (0.2 mi) | 1.1 km | (0.7 mi) | 800 m | (2500 ft) | 4.5 km | (2.8 mi) | 9.6 km | (6.0 mi) |
| 3307 | **124** | Liquefied gas, toxic, oxidizing, n.o.s. (Inhalation Hazard Zone C) | 30 m | (100 ft) | 0.1 km | (0.1 mi) | 0.3 km | (0.2 mi) | 150 m | (500 ft) | 0.9 km | (0.6 mi) | 2.4 km | (1.5 mi) |
| 3307 | **124** | Liquefied gas, toxic, oxidizing, n.o.s. (Inhalation Hazard Zone D) | 30 m | (100 ft) | 0.1 km | (0.1 mi) | 0.2 km | (0.1 mi) | 100 m | (300 ft) | 0.7 km | (0.5 mi) | 1.9 km | (1.2 mi) |
| 3308 | **123** | Liquefied gas, poisonous, corrosive, n.o.s. | | | | | | | | | | | | |
| 3308 | **123** | Liquefied gas, poisonous, corrosive, n.o.s. (Inhalation Hazard Zone A) | 100 m | (300 ft) | 0.6 km | (0.4 mi) | 2.5 km | (1.5 mi) | 500 m | (1500 ft) | 3.0 km | (1.9 mi) | 9.0 km | (5.6 mi) |
| 3308 | **123** | Liquefied gas, poisonous, corrosive, n.o.s. (Inhalation Hazard Zone B) | 30 m | (100 ft) | 0.2 km | (0.2 mi) | 1.0 km | (0.6 mi) | 400 m | (1250 ft) | 2.2 km | (1.4 mi) | 4.8 km | (3.0 mi) |
| 3308 | **123** | Liquefied gas, poisonous, corrosive, n.o.s. (Inhalation Hazard Zone C) | 30 m | (100 ft) | 0.1 km | (0.1 mi) | 0.4 km | (0.3 mi) | 150 m | (500 ft) | 0.9 km | (0.6 mi) | 2.6 km | (1.6 mi) |
| 3308 | **123** | Liquefied gas, poisonous, corrosive, n.o.s. (Inhalation Hazard Zone D) | 30 m | (100 ft) | 0.1 km | (0.1 mi) | 0.2 km | (0.1 mi) | 150 m | (500 ft) | 0.7 km | (0.5 mi) | 1.9 km | (1.2 mi) |

**"+" means distance can be larger in certain atmospheric conditions**

# TABLE 1 - INITIAL ISOLATION AND PROTECTIVE ACTION DISTANCES

| ID No. | Guide | NAME OF MATERIAL | SMALL SPILLS (From a small package or small leak from a large package) First ISOLATE in all Directions Meters (Feet) | SMALL SPILLS Then PROTECT persons Downwind during DAY Kilometers (Miles) | SMALL SPILLS Then PROTECT persons Downwind during NIGHT Kilometers (Miles) | LARGE SPILLS (From a large package or from many small packages) First ISOLATE in all Directions Meters (Feet) | LARGE SPILLS Then PROTECT persons Downwind during DAY Kilometers (Miles) | LARGE SPILLS Then PROTECT persons Downwind during NIGHT Kilometers (Miles) |
|---|---|---|---|---|---|---|---|---|
| 3308<br>3308 | **123**<br>**123** | Liquefied gas, toxic, corrosive, n.o.s.<br>Liquefied gas, toxic, corrosive, n.o.s. (Inhalation Hazard Zone A) | 100 m (300 ft) | 0.6 km (0.4 mi) | 2.5 km (1.5 mi) | 500 m (1500 ft) | 3.0 km (1.9 mi) | 9.0 km (5.6 mi) |
| 3308 | **123** | Liquefied gas, toxic, corrosive, n.o.s. (Inhalation Hazard Zone B) | 30 m (100 ft) | 0.2 km (0.2 mi) | 1.0 km (0.6 mi) | 400 m (1250 ft) | 2.2 km (1.4 mi) | 4.8 km (3.0 mi) |
| 3308 | **123** | Liquefied gas, toxic, corrosive, n.o.s. (Inhalation Hazard Zone C) | 30 m (100 ft) | 0.1 km (0.1 mi) | 0.4 km (0.3 mi) | 150 m (500 ft) | 0.9 km (0.6 mi) | 2.6 km (1.6 mi) |
| 3308 | **123** | Liquefied gas, toxic, corrosive, n.o.s. (Inhalation Hazard Zone D) | 30 m (100 ft) | 0.1 km (0.1 mi) | 0.2 km (0.1 mi) | 150 m (500 ft) | 0.7 km (0.5 mi) | 1.9 km (1.2 mi) |
| 3309<br>3309 | **119**<br>**119** | Liquefied gas, poisonous, flammable, corrosive, n.o.s.<br>Liquefied gas, poisonous, flammable, corrosive, n.o.s. (Inhalation Hazard Zone A) | 150 m (500 ft) | 1.0 km (0.6 mi) | 3.8 km (2.4 mi) | 1000 m (3000 ft) | 5.6 km (3.5 mi) | 10.2 km (6.3 mi) |
| 3309 | **119** | Liquefied gas, poisonous, flammable, corrosive, n.o.s. (Inhalation Hazard Zone B) | 30 m (100 ft) | 0.1 km (0.1 mi) | 0.4 km (0.2 mi) | 200 m (600 ft) | 1.2 km (0.8 mi) | 2.6 km (1.6 mi) |

| ID No. | Guide No. | Name of Material | Small Spills: Isolate | | Small Spills: Protect Day | | Small Spills: Protect Night | | Large Spills: Isolate | | Large Spills: Protect Day | | Large Spills: Protect Night | |
|---|---|---|---|---|---|---|---|---|---|---|---|---|---|---|
| 3309 | **119** | Liquefied gas, poisonous, flammable, corrosive, n.o.s. (Inhalation Hazard Zone C) | 30 m | (100 ft) | 0.1 km | (0.1 mi) | 0.3 km | (0.2 mi) | 150 m | (500 ft) | 0.9 km | (0.6 mi) | 2.4 km | (1.5 mi) |
| 3309 | **119** | Liquefied gas, poisonous, flammable, corrosive, n.o.s. (Inhalation Hazard Zone D) | 30 m | (100 ft) | 0.1 km | (0.1 mi) | 0.2 km | (0.1 mi) | 100 m | (300 ft) | 0.7 km | (0.5 mi) | 1.9 km | (1.2 mi) |
| 3309<br>3309 | **119**<br>**119** | Liquefied gas, toxic, flammable, corrosive, n.o.s.<br>Liquefied gas, toxic, flammable, corrosive, n.o.s. (Inhalation Hazard Zone A) | 150 m | (500 ft) | 1.0 km | (0.6 mi) | 3.8 km | (2.4 mi) | 1000 m | (3000 ft) | 5.6 km | (3.5 mi) | 10.2 km | (6.3 mi) |
| 3309 | **119** | Liquefied gas, toxic, flammable, corrosive, n.o.s. (Inhalation Hazard Zone B) | 30 m | (100 ft) | 0.1 km | (0.1 mi) | 0.4 km | (0.2 mi) | 200 m | (600 ft) | 1.2 km | (0.8 mi) | 2.6 km | (1.6 mi) |
| 3309 | **119** | Liquefied gas, toxic, flammable, corrosive, n.o.s. (Inhalation Hazard Zone C) | 30 m | (100 ft) | 0.1 km | (0.1 mi) | 0.3 km | (0.2 mi) | 150 m | (500 ft) | 0.9 km | (0.6 mi) | 2.4 km | (1.5 mi) |
| 3309 | **119** | Liquefied gas, toxic, flammable, corrosive, n.o.s. (Inhalation Hazard Zone D) | 30 m | (100 ft) | 0.1 km | (0.1 mi) | 0.2 km | (0.1 mi) | 100 m | (300 ft) | 0.7 km | (0.5 mi) | 1.9 km | (1.2 mi) |
| 3310<br>3310 | **124**<br>**124** | Liquefied gas, poisonous, oxidizing, corrosive, n.o.s.<br>Liquefied gas, poisonous, oxidizing, corrosive, n.o.s. (Inhalation Hazard Zone A) | 100 m | (300 ft) | 0.5 km | (0.3 mi) | 2.5 km | (1.6 mi) | 800 m | (2500 ft) | 5.2 km | (3.3 mi) | 11.0+ km | (7.0+ mi) |
| 3310 | **124** | Liquefied gas, poisonous, oxidizing, corrosive, n.o.s. (Inhalation Hazard Zone B) | 60 m | (200 ft) | 0.3 km | (0.2 mi) | 1.1 km | (0.7 mi) | 800 m | (2500 ft) | 4.5 km | (2.8 mi) | 9.6 km | (6.0 mi) |
| 3310 | **124** | Liquefied gas, poisonous, oxidizing, corrosive, n.o.s. (Inhalation Hazard Zone C) | 30 m | (100 ft) | 0.1 km | (0.1 mi) | 0.3 km | (0.2 mi) | 150 m | (500 ft) | 0.9 km | (0.6 mi) | 2.4 km | (1.5 mi) |

**"+" means distance can be larger in certain atmospheric conditions**

# TABLE 1 - INITIAL ISOLATION AND PROTECTIVE ACTION DISTANCES

| ID No. | Guide | NAME OF MATERIAL | SMALL SPILLS (From a small package or small leak from a large package) First ISOLATE in all Directions Meters (Feet) | Then PROTECT persons Downwind during DAY Kilometers (Miles) | NIGHT Kilometers (Miles) | LARGE SPILLS (From a large package or from many small packages) First ISOLATE in all Directions Meters (Feet) | Then PROTECT persons Downwind during DAY Kilometers (Miles) | NIGHT Kilometers (Miles) |
|---|---|---|---|---|---|---|---|---|
| 3310 | **124** | Liquefied gas, poisonous, oxidizing, corrosive, n.o.s. (Inhalation Hazard Zone D) | 30 m (100 ft) | 0.1 km (0.1 mi) | 0.2 km (0.1 mi) | 100 m (300 ft) | 0.7 km (0.5 mi) | 1.9 km (1.2 mi) |
| 3310 | **124** | Liquefied gas, toxic, oxidizing, corrosive, n.o.s. | | | | | | |
| 3310 | **124** | Liquefied gas, toxic, oxidizing, corrosive, n.o.s. (Inhalation Hazard Zone A) | 100 m (300 ft) | 0.5 km (0.3 mi) | 2.5 km (1.6 mi) | 800 m (2500 ft) | 5.2 km (3.3 mi) | 11.0+ km (7.0+ mi) |
| 3310 | **124** | Liquefied gas, toxic, oxidizing, corrosive, n.o.s. (Inhalation Hazard Zone B) | 60 m (200 ft) | 0.3 km (0.2 mi) | 1.1 km (0.7 mi) | 800 m (2500 ft) | 4.5 km (2.8 mi) | 9.6 km (6.0 mi) |
| 3310 | **124** | Liquefied gas, toxic, oxidizing, corrosive, n.o.s. (Inhalation Hazard Zone C) | 30 m (100 ft) | 0.1 km (0.1 mi) | 0.3 km (0.2 mi) | 150 m (500 ft) | 0.9 km (0.6 mi) | 2.4 km (1.5 mi) |
| 3310 | **124** | Liquefied gas, toxic, oxidizing, corrosive, n.o.s. (Inhalation Hazard Zone D) | 30 m (100 ft) | 0.1 km (0.1 mi) | 0.2 km (0.1 mi) | 100 m (300 ft) | 0.7 km (0.5 mi) | 1.9 km (1.2 mi) |
| 3318 | **125** | Ammonia solution, with more than 50% Ammonia | 30 m (100 ft) | 0.1 km (0.1 mi) | 0.2 km (0.1 mi) | 150 m (500 ft) | 0.7 km (0.5 mi) | 1.9 km (1.2 mi) |
| 3355 | **119** | Insecticide gas, poisonous, flammable, n.o.s. | | | | | | |
| 3355 | **119** | Insecticide gas, poisonous, flammable, n.o.s. (Inhalation Hazard Zone A) | 150 m (500 ft) | 1.0 km (0.6 mi) | 3.8 km (2.4 mi) | 1000 m (3000 ft) | 5.6 km (3.5 mi) | 10.2. km (6.3 mi) |

| ID No. | Guide | Name of Material | | | | | | | | | | | | |
|---|---|---|---|---|---|---|---|---|---|---|---|---|---|---|
| 3355 | **119** | Insecticide gas, poisonous, flammable, n.o.s. (Inhalation Hazard Zone B) | 30 m | (100 ft) | 0.1 km | (0.1 mi) | 0.4 km | (0.2 mi) | 200 m | 600 ft | 1.2 km | (0.8 mi) | 2.6 km | (1.6 mi) |
| 3355 | **119** | Insecticide gas, poisonous, flammable, n.o.s. (Inhalation Hazard Zone C) | 30 m | (100 ft) | 0.1 km | (0.1 mi) | 0.3 km | (0.2 mi) | 150 m | (500 ft) | 0.9 km | (0.6 mi) | 2.4 km | (1.5 mi) |
| 3355 | **119** | Insecticide gas, poisonous, flammable, n.o.s. (Inhalation Hazard Zone D) | 30 m | (100 ft) | 0.1 km | (0.1 mi) | 0.2 km | (0.1 mi) | 100 m | (300 ft) | 0.7 km | (0.5 mi) | 1.9 km | (1.2 mi) |
| 3355<br>3355 | **119**<br>**119** | Insecticide gas, toxic, flammable, n.o.s.<br>Insecticide gas, toxic, flammable, n.o.s. (Inhalation Hazard Zone A) | 150 m | (500 ft) | 1.0 km | (0.6 mi) | 3.8 km | (2.4 mi) | 1000 m | (3000 ft) | 5.6 km | (3.5 mi) | 10.2 km | (6.3 mi) |
| 3355 | **119** | Insecticide gas, toxic, flammable, n.o.s. (Inhalation Hazard Zone B) | 30 m | (100 ft) | 0.1 km | (0.1 mi) | 0.4 km | (0.2 mi) | 200 m | (600 ft) | 1.2 km | (0.8 mi) | 2.6 km | (1.6 mi) |
| 3355 | **119** | Insecticide gas, toxic, flammable, n.o.s. (Inhalation Hazard Zone C) | 30 m | (100 ft) | 0.1 km | (0.1 mi) | 0.3 km | (0.2 mi) | 150 m | (500 ft) | 0.9 km | (0.6 mi) | 2.4 km | (1.5 mi) |
| 3355 | **119** | Insecticide gas, toxic, flammable, n.o.s. (Inhalation Hazard Zone D) | 30 m | (100 ft) | 0.1 km | (0.1 mi) | 0.2 km | (0.1 mi) | 100 m | (300 ft) | 0.7 km | (0.5 mi) | 1.9 km | (1.2 mi) |
| 3361<br>3361 | **156**<br>**156** | Chlorosilanes, poisonous, corrosive, n.o.s. **(when spilled in water)**<br>Chlorosilanes, toxic, corrosive, n.o.s. **(when spilled in water)** | 30 m | (100 ft) | 0.1 km | (0.1 mi) | 0.2 km | (0.1 mi) | 60 m | (200 ft) | 0.5 km | (0.3 mi) | 1.6 km | (1.0 mi) |

**"+" means distance can be larger in certain atmospheric conditions**

# TABLE 1 - INITIAL ISOLATION AND PROTECTIVE ACTION DISTANCES

| ID No. | Guide | NAME OF MATERIAL | SMALL SPILLS (From a small package or small leak from a large package): First ISOLATE in all Directions, Meters (Feet) | SMALL SPILLS: Then PROTECT persons Downwind during DAY, Kilometers (Miles) | SMALL SPILLS: Then PROTECT persons Downwind during NIGHT, Kilometers (Miles) | LARGE SPILLS (From a large package or from many small packages): First ISOLATE in all Directions, Meters (Feet) | LARGE SPILLS: Then PROTECT persons Downwind during DAY, Kilometers (Miles) | LARGE SPILLS: Then PROTECT persons Downwind during NIGHT, Kilometers (Miles) |
|---|---|---|---|---|---|---|---|---|
| 3362<br>3362 | **155**<br>**155** | Chlorosilanes, poisonous, corrosive, flammable, n.o.s. **(when spilled in water)**<br>Chlorosilanes, toxic, corrosive, flammable, n.o.s. **(when spilled in water)** | 30 m (100 ft) | 0.1 km (0.1 mi) | 0.2 km (0.1 mi) | 60 m (200 ft) | 0.5 km (0.3 mi) | 1.6 km (1.0 mi) |
| 3381<br>3381 | **151**<br>**151** | Poisonous by inhalation liquid, n.o.s. (Inhalation Hazard Zone A)<br>Toxic by inhalation liquid, n.o.s. (Inhalation Hazard Zone A) | 30 m (100 ft) | 0.4 km (0.3 mi) | 1.2 km (0.8 mi) | 200 m (600 ft) | 2.5 km (1.6 mi) | 4.0 km (2.5 mi) |
| 3382<br>3382 | **151**<br>**151** | Poisonous by inhalation liquid, n.o.s. (Inhalation Hazard Zone B)<br>Toxic by inhalation liquid, n.o.s. (Inhalation Hazard Zone B) | 30 m (100 ft) | 0.1 km (0.1 mi) | 0.2 km (0.1 mi) | 60 m (200 ft) | 0.5 km (0.3 mi) | 0.7 km (0.4 mi) |
| 3383<br>3383 | **131**<br>**131** | Poisonous by inhalation liquid, flammable, n.o.s. (Inhalation Hazard Zone A)<br>Toxic by inhalation liquid, flammable, n.o.s. (Inhalation Hazard Zone A) | 60 m (200 ft) | 0.5 km (0.3 mi) | 1.4 km (0.9 mi) | 150 m (500 ft) | 2.0 km (1.3 mi) | 4.7 km (3.0 mi) |

| ID No. | Guide No. | Name of Material | | | | | | | | | | | | |
|---|---|---|---|---|---|---|---|---|---|---|---|---|---|---|
| 3384<br>3384 | **131**<br>**131** | Poisonous by inhalation liquid, flammable, n.o.s. (Inhalation Hazard Zone B)<br>Toxic by inhalation liquid, flammable, n.o.s. (Inhalation Hazard Zone B) | 30 m | (100 ft) | 0.2 km | (0.1 mi) | 0.2 km | (0.1 mi) | 60 m | (200 ft) | 0.5 km | (0.3 mi) | 0.8 km | (0.5 mi) |
| 3385<br>3385 | **139**<br>**139** | Poisonous by inhalation liquid, water-reactive, n.o.s. (Inhalation Hazard Zone A)<br>Toxic by inhalation liquid, water-reactive, n.o.s. (Inhalation Hazard Zone A) | 30 m | (100 ft) | 0.4 km | (0.3 mi) | 1.2 km | (0.8 mi) | 200 m | (600 ft) | 2.5 km | (1.6 mi) | 4.0 km | (2.5 mi) |
| 3386<br>3386 | **139**<br>**139** | Poisonous by inhalation liquid, water-reactive, n.o.s. (Inhalation Hazard Zone B)<br>Toxic by inhalation liquid, water-reactive, n.o.s. (Inhalation Hazard Zone B) | 30 m | (100 ft) | 0.1 km | (0.1 mi) | 0.2 km | (0.1 mi) | 60 m | (200 ft) | 0.5 km | (0.3 mi) | 0.7 km | (0.4 mi) |
| 3387<br>3387 | **142**<br>**142** | Poisonous by inhalation liquid, oxidizing, n.o.s. (Inhalation Hazard Zone A)<br>Toxic by inhalation liquid, oxidizing, n.o.s. (Inhalation Hazard Zone A) | 30 m | (100 ft) | 0.4 km | (0.3 mi) | 1.2 km | (0.8 mi) | 200 m | (600 ft) | 2.5 km | (1.6 mi) | 4.0 km | (2.5 mi) |
| 3388<br>3388 | **142**<br>**142** | Poisonous by inhalation liquid, oxidizing, n.o.s. (Inhalation Hazard Zone B)<br>Toxic by inhalation liquid, oxidizing, n.o.s. (Inhalation Hazard Zone B) | 30 m | (100 ft) | 0.1 km | (0.1 mi) | 0.2 km | (0.1 mi) | 30 m | (100 ft) | 0.3 km | (0.2 mi) | 0.5 km | (0.3 mi) |

**"+" means distance can be larger in certain atmospheric conditions**

## TABLE 1 - INITIAL ISOLATION AND PROTECTIVE ACTION DISTANCES

| | | | SMALL SPILLS (From a small package or small leak from a large package) | | | | | | LARGE SPILLS (From a large package or from many small packages) | | | | | |
|---|---|---|---|---|---|---|---|---|---|---|---|---|---|---|
| | | | First **ISOLATE** in all Directions | | Then **PROTECT** persons Downwind during | | | | First **ISOLATE** in all Directions | | Then **PROTECT** persons Downwind during | | | |
| | | | | | **DAY** | | **NIGHT** | | | | **DAY** | | **NIGHT** | |
| **ID No.** | **Guide** | **NAME OF MATERIAL** | Meters | (Feet) | Kilometers | (Miles) | Kilometers | (Miles) | Meters | (Feet) | Kilometers | (Miles) | Kilometers | (Miles) |
| 3389 | **154** | Poisonous by inhalation liquid, corrosive, n.o.s. (Inhalation Hazard Zone A) | 60 m | (200 ft) | 0.3 km | (0.2 mi) | 0.7 km | (0.4 mi) | 300 m | (1000 ft) | 1.5 km | (0.9 mi) | 2.6 km | (1.6 mi) |
| 3389 | **154** | Toxic by inhalation liquid, corrosive, n.o.s. (Inhalation Hazard Zone A) | | | | | | | | | | | | |
| 3390 | **154** | Poisonous by inhalation liquid, corrosive, n.o.s. (Inhalation Hazard Zone B) | 30 m | (100 ft) | 0.1 km | (0.1 mi) | 0.2 km | (0.1 mi) | 60 m | (200 ft) | 0.5 km | (0.3 mi) | 0.6 km | (0.4 mi) |
| 3390 | **154** | Toxic by inhalation liquid, corrosive, n.o.s. (Inhalation Hazard Zone B) | | | | | | | | | | | | |
| 3416 | **153** | CN **(when used as a weapon)** | 30 m | (100 ft) | 0.1 km | (0.1 mi) | 0.2 km | (0.1 mi) | 60 m | (200 ft) | 0.3 km | (0.2 mi) | 1.2 km | (0.8 mi) |
| 3456 | **157** | Nitrosylsulfuric acid, solid **(when spilled in water)** | 60 m | (200 ft) | 0.2 km | (0.1 mi) | 0.6 km | (0.4 mi) | 300 m | (1000 ft) | 0.8 km | (0.5 mi) | 2.8 km | (1.8 mi) |
| 3456 | **157** | Nitrosylsulphuric acid, solid **(when spilled in water)** | | | | | | | | | | | | |
| 3461 | **135** | Aluminum alkyl halides, solid **(when spilled in water)** | 30 m | (100 ft) | 0.1 km | (0.1 mi) | 0.2 km | (0.1 mi) | 60 m | (200 ft) | 0.4 km | (0.3 mi) | 1.3 km | (0.8 mi) |

| | | | | | | | | | | | | | | |
|---|---|---|---|---|---|---|---|---|---|---|---|---|---|---|
| 3488<br>3488 | **131**<br>**131** | Poisonous by inhalation liquid, flammable, corrosive, n.o.s. (Inhalation Hazard Zone A)<br>Toxic by inhalation liquid, flammable, corrosive, n.o.s. (Inhalation Hazard Zone A) | 100 m | (300 ft) | 0.9 km | (0.6 mi) | 2.0 km | (1.2 mi) | 400 m | (1250 ft) | 4.5 km | (2.8 mi) | 7.4 km | (4.6 mi) |
| 3489<br>3489 | **131**<br>**131** | Poisonous by inhalation liquid, flammable, corrosive, n.o.s. (Inhalation Hazard Zone B)<br>Toxic by inhalation liquid, flammable, corrosive, n.o.s. (Inhalation Hazard Zone B) | 30 m | (100 ft) | 0.2 km | (0.1 mi) | 0.2 km | (0.1 mi) | 60 m | (200 ft) | 0.5 km | (0.3 mi) | 0.8 km | (0.5 mi) |
| 3490<br>3490 | **155**<br>**155** | Poisonous by inhalation liquid, water-reactive, flammable, n.o.s. (Inhalation Hazard Zone A)<br>Toxic by inhalation liquid, water-reactive, flammable, n.o.s. (Inhalation Hazard Zone A) | 60 m | (200 ft) | 0.5 km | (0.3 mi) | 1.4 km | (0.9 mi) | 150 m | (500 ft) | 2.0 km | (1.3 mi) | 4.7 km | (3.0 mi) |
| 3491<br>3491 | **155**<br>**155** | Poisonous by inhalation liquid, water-reactive, flammable, n.o.s. (Inhalation Hazard Zone B)<br>Toxic by inhalation liquid, water-reactive, flammable, n.o.s. (Inhalation Hazard Zone B) | 30 m | (100 ft) | 0.2 km | (0.1 mi) | 0.2 km | (0.1 mi) | 60 m | (200 ft) | 0.5 km | (0.3 mi) | 0.8 km | (0.5 mi) |

**"+" means distance can be larger in certain atmospheric conditions**

# TABLE 1 - INITIAL ISOLATION AND PROTECTIVE ACTION DISTANCES

| ID No. | Guide | NAME OF MATERIAL | SMALL SPILLS (From a small package or small leak from a large package) First ISOLATE in all Directions Meters (Feet) | SMALL SPILLS Then PROTECT persons Downwind during DAY Kilometers (Miles) | SMALL SPILLS Then PROTECT persons Downwind during NIGHT Kilometers (Miles) | LARGE SPILLS (From a large package or from many small packages) First ISOLATE in all Directions Meters (Feet) | LARGE SPILLS Then PROTECT persons Downwind during DAY Kilometers (Miles) | LARGE SPILLS Then PROTECT persons Downwind during NIGHT Kilometers (Miles) |
|---|---|---|---|---|---|---|---|---|
| 3492<br>3492 | **131**<br>**131** | Poisonous by inhalation liquid, corrosive, flammable, n.o.s. (Inhalation Hazard Zone A)<br>Toxic by inhalation liquid, corrosive, flammable, n.o.s. (Inhalation Hazard Zone A) | 100 m (300 ft) | 0.9 km (0.6 mi) | 2.0 km (1.2 mi) | 400 m (1250 ft) | 4.5 km (2.8 mi) | 7.4 km (4.6 mi) |
| 3493<br>3493 | **131**<br>**131** | Poisonous by inhalation liquid, corrosive, flammable, n.o.s. (Inhalation Hazard Zone B)<br>Toxic by inhalation liquid, corrosive, flammable, n.o.s. (Inhalation Hazard Zone B) | 30 m (100 ft) | 0.2 km (0.1 mi) | 0.2 km (0.1 mi) | 60 m (200 ft) | 0.5 km (0.3 mi) | 0.8 km (0.5 mi) |
| 3494<br>3494 | **131**<br>**131** | Petroleum sour crude oil, flammable, poisonous<br>Petroleum sour crude oil, flammable, toxic | 30 m (100 ft) | 0.1 km (0.1 mi) | 0.2 km (0.1 mi) | 60 m (200 ft) | 0.5 km (0.3 mi) | 0.7 km (0.4 mi) |
| 3507 | **166** | Uranium hexafluoride, radioactive material, excepted package, less than 0.1 kg per package, non-fissile or fissile-excepted **(when spilled in water)** | 30 m (100 ft) | 0.1 km (0.1 mi) | 0.1 km (0.1 mi) | 30 m (100 ft) | 0.1 km (0.1 mi) | 0.1 km (0.1 mi) |
| 3512<br>3512 | **173**<br>**173** | Adsorbed gas, poisonous, n.o.s.<br>Adsorbed gas, poisonous, n.o.s. (Inhalation hazard zone A) | 30 m (100 ft) | 0.1 km (0.1 mi) | 0.2 km (0.1 mi) | 30 m (100 ft) | 0.1 km (0.1 mi) | 0.4 km (0.2 mi) |

| ID No. | Guide No. | Name of Material | | | | | | | | | | | | |
|---|---|---|---|---|---|---|---|---|---|---|---|---|---|---|
| 3512<br>3512<br>3512 | **173**<br>**173**<br>**173** | Adsorbed gas, poisonous, n.o.s. (Inhalation hazard zone B)<br>Adsorbed gas, poisonous, n.o.s. (Inhalation hazard zone C)<br>Adsorbed gas, poisonous, n.o.s. (Inhalation hazard zone D) | 30 m | (100 ft) | 0.1 km | (0.1 mi) | 0.1 km | (0.1 mi) | 30 m | (100 ft) | 0.1 km | (0.1 mi) | 0.1 km | (0.1 mi) |
| 3512<br>3512 | **173**<br>**173** | Adsorbed gas, toxic, n.o.s.<br>Adsorbed gas, toxic, n.o.s. (Inhalation hazard zone A) | 30 m | (100 ft) | 0.1 km | (0.1 mi) | 0.2 km | (0.1 mi) | 30 m | (100 ft) | 0.1 km | (0.1 mi) | 0.4 km | (0.2 mi) |
| 3512<br>3512<br>3512 | **173**<br>**173**<br>**173** | Adsorbed gas, toxic, n.o.s. (Inhalation hazard zone B)<br>Adsorbed gas, toxic, n.o.s. (Inhalation hazard zone C)<br>Adsorbed gas, toxic, n.o.s. (Inhalation hazard zone D) | 30 m | (100 ft) | 0.1 km | (0.1 mi) | 0.1 km | (0.1 mi) | 30 m | (100 ft) | 0.1 km | (0.1 mi) | 0.1 km | (0.1 mi) |
| 3514<br>3514 | **173**<br>**173** | Adsorbed gas, poisonous, flammable, n.o.s.<br>Adsorbed gas, poisonous, flammable, n.o.s. (Inhalation hazard zone A) | 30 m | (100 ft) | 0.1 km | (0.1 mi) | 0.2 km | (0.1 mi) | 30 m | (100 ft) | 0.1 km | (0.1 mi) | 0.4 km | (0.2 mi) |
| 3514<br>3514<br>3514 | **173**<br>**173**<br>**173** | Adsorbed gas, poisonous, flammable, n.o.s. (Inhalation hazard zone B)<br>Adsorbed gas, poisonous, flammable, n.o.s. (Inhalation hazard zone C)<br>Adsorbed gas, poisonous, flammable, n.o.s. (Inhalation hazard zone D) | 30 m | (100 ft) | 0.1 km | (0.1 mi) | 0.1 km | (0.1 mi) | 30 m | (100 ft) | 0.1 km | (0.1 mi) | 0.1 km | (0.1 mi) |

**"+" means distance can be larger in certain atmospheric conditions**

## TABLE 1 - INITIAL ISOLATION AND PROTECTIVE ACTION DISTANCES

| ID No. | Guide | NAME OF MATERIAL | SMALL SPILLS (From a small package or small leak from a large package) First ISOLATE in all Directions Meters (Feet) | SMALL SPILLS Then PROTECT persons Downwind during DAY Kilometers (Miles) | SMALL SPILLS Then PROTECT persons Downwind during NIGHT Kilometers (Miles) | LARGE SPILLS (From a large package or from many small packages) First ISOLATE in all Directions Meters (Feet) | LARGE SPILLS Then PROTECT persons Downwind during DAY Kilometers (Miles) | LARGE SPILLS Then PROTECT persons Downwind during NIGHT Kilometers (Miles) |
|---|---|---|---|---|---|---|---|---|
| 3514 | **173** | Adsorbed gas, toxic, flammable, n.o.s. | | | | | | |
| 3514 | **173** | Adsorbed gas, toxic, flammable, n.o.s. (Inhalation hazard zone A) | 30 m (100 ft) | 0.1 km (0.1 mi) | 0.2 km (0.1 mi) | 30 m (100 ft) | 0.1 km (0.1 mi) | 0.4 km (0.2 mi) |
| 3514 | **173** | Adsorbed gas, toxic, flammable, n.o.s. (Inhalation hazard zone B) | | | | | | |
| 3514 | **173** | Adsorbed gas, toxic, flammable, n.o.s. (Inhalation hazard zone C) | 30 m (100 ft) | 0.1 km (0.1 mi) | 0.1 km (0.1 mi) | 30 m (100 ft) | 0.1 km (0.1 mi) | 0.1 km (0.1 mi) |
| 3514 | **173** | Adsorbed gas, toxic, flammable, n.o.s. (Inhalation hazard zone D) | | | | | | |
| 3515 | **173** | Adsorbed gas, poisonous, oxidizing, n.o.s. | | | | | | |
| 3515 | **173** | Adsorbed gas, poisonous, oxidizing, n.o.s. (Inhalation hazard zone A) | 30 m (100 ft) | 0.1 km (0.1 mi) | 0.2 km (0.1 mi) | 30 m (100 ft) | 0.1 km (0.1 mi) | 0.4 km (0.2 mi) |
| 3515 | **173** | Adsorbed gas, poisonous, oxidizing, n.o.s. (Inhalation hazard zone B) | | | | | | |
| 3515 | **173** | Adsorbed gas, poisonous, oxidizing, n.o.s. (Inhalation hazard zone C) | 30 m (100 ft) | 0.1 km (0.1 mi) | 0.1 km (0.1 mi) | 30 m (100 ft) | 0.1 km (0.1 mi) | 0.1 km (0.1 mi) |
| 3515 | **173** | Adsorbed gas, poisonous, oxidizing, n.o.s. (Inhalation hazard zone D) | | | | | | |

| | | | | | | | | | | | | | | |
|---|---|---|---|---|---|---|---|---|---|---|---|---|---|---|
| 3515 | **173** | Adsorbed gas, toxic, oxidizing, n.o.s. | | | | | | | | | | | | |
| 3515 | **173** | Adsorbed gas, toxic, oxidizing, n.o.s. (Inhalation hazard zone A) | 30 m | (100 ft) | 0.1 km | (0.1 mi) | 0.2 km | (0.1 mi) | 30 m | (100 ft) | 0.1 km | (0.1 mi) | 0.4 km | (0.2 mi) |
| 3515 | **173** | Adsorbed gas, toxic, oxidizing, n.o.s. (Inhalation hazard zone B) | | | | | | | | | | | | |
| 3515 | **173** | Adsorbed gas, toxic, oxidizing, n.o.s. (Inhalation hazard zone C) | 30 m | (100 ft) | 0.1 km | (0.1 mi) | 0.1 km | (0.1 mi) | 30 m | (100 ft) | 0.1 km | (0.1 mi) | 0.1 km | (0.1 mi) |
| 3515 | **173** | Adsorbed gas, toxic, oxidizing, n.o.s. (Inhalation hazard zone D) | | | | | | | | | | | | |
| 3516 | **173** | Adsorbed gas, poisonous, corrosive, n.o.s. | | | | | | | | | | | | |
| 3516 | **173** | Adsorbed gas, poisonous, corrosive, n.o.s. (Inhalation hazard zone A) | 30 m | (100 ft) | 0.1 km | (0.1 mi) | 0.2 km | (0.1 mi) | 30 m | (100 ft) | 0.1 km | (0.1 mi) | 0.4 km | (0.2 mi) |
| 3516 | **173** | Adsorbed gas, poisonous, corrosive, n.o.s. (Inhalation hazard zone B) | | | | | | | | | | | | |
| 3516 | **173** | Adsorbed gas, poisonous, corrosive, n.o.s. (Inhalation hazard zone C) | 30 m | (100 ft) | 0.1 km | (0.1 mi) | 0.1 km | (0.1 mi) | 30 m | (100 ft) | 0.1 km | (0.1 mi) | 0.1 km | (0.1 mi) |
| 3516 | **173** | Adsorbed gas, poisonous, corrosive, n.o.s. (Inhalation hazard zone D) | | | | | | | | | | | | |

**"+" means distance can be larger in certain atmospheric conditions**

# TABLE 1 - INITIAL ISOLATION AND PROTECTIVE ACTION DISTANCES

| ID No. | Guide | NAME OF MATERIAL | SMALL SPILLS (From a small package or small leak from a large package) First ISOLATE in all Directions Meters (Feet) | SMALL SPILLS Then PROTECT persons Downwind during DAY Kilometers (Miles) | SMALL SPILLS Then PROTECT persons Downwind during NIGHT Kilometers (Miles) | LARGE SPILLS (From a large package or from many small packages) First ISOLATE in all Directions Meters (Feet) | LARGE SPILLS Then PROTECT persons Downwind during DAY Kilometers (Miles) | LARGE SPILLS Then PROTECT persons Downwind during NIGHT Kilometers (Miles) |
|---|---|---|---|---|---|---|---|---|
| 3516 | **173** | Adsorbed gas, toxic, corrosive, n.o.s. | | | | | | |
| 3516 | **173** | Adsorbed gas, toxic, corrosive, n.o.s. (Inhalation hazard zone A) | 30 m (100 ft) | 0.1 km (0.1 mi) | 0.2 km (0.1 mi) | 30 m (100 ft) | 0.1 km (0.1 mi) | 0.4 km (0.2 mi) |
| 3516 | **173** | Adsorbed gas, toxic, corrosive, n.o.s. (Inhalation hazard zone B) | | | | | | |
| 3516 | **173** | Adsorbed gas, toxic, corrosive, n.o.s. (Inhalation hazard zone C) | 30 m (100 ft) | 0.1 km (0.1 mi) | 0.1 km (0.1 mi) | 30 m (100 ft) | 0.1 km (0.1 mi) | 0.1 km (0.1 mi) |
| 3516 | **173** | Adsorbed gas, toxic, corrosive, n.o.s. (Inhalation hazard zone D) | | | | | | |
| 3517 | **173** | Adsorbed gas, poisonous, flammable, corrosive, n.o.s. | | | | | | |
| 3517 | **173** | Adsorbed gas, poisonous, flammable, corrosive, n.o.s. (Inhalation hazard zone A) | 30 m (100 ft) | 0.1 km (0.1 mi) | 0.2 km (0.1 mi) | 30 m (100 ft) | 0.1 km (0.1 mi) | 0.4 km (0.2 mi) |

| | | | | | | | | | | | | | | |
|---|---|---|---|---|---|---|---|---|---|---|---|---|---|---|
| 3517 | **173** | Adsorbed gas, poisonous, flammable, corrosive, n.o.s. (Inhalation hazard zone B) | | | | | | | | | | | | |
| 3517 | **173** | Adsorbed gas, poisonous, flammable, corrosive, n.o.s. (Inhalation hazard zone C) | 30 m | (100 ft) | 0.1 km | (0.1 mi) | 0.1 km | (0.1 mi) | 30 m | (100 ft) | 0.1 km | (0.1 mi) | 0.1 km | (0.1 mi) |
| 3517 | **173** | Adsorbed gas, poisonous, flammable, corrosive, n.o.s. (Inhalation hazard zone D) | | | | | | | | | | | | |
| 3517 | **173** | Adsorbed gas, toxic, flammable, corrosive, n.o.s | | | | | | | | | | | | |
| 3517 | **173** | Adsorbed gas, toxic, flammable, corrosive, n.o.s. (Inhalation hazard zone A) | 30 m | (100 ft) | 0.1 km | (0.1 mi) | 0.2 km | (0.1 mi) | 30 m | (100 ft) | 0.1 km | (0.1 mi) | 0.4 km | (0.2 mi) |
| 3517 | **173** | Adsorbed gas, toxic, flammable, corrosive, n.o.s. (Inhalation hazard zone B) | | | | | | | | | | | | |
| 3517 | **173** | Adsorbed gas, toxic, flammable, corrosive, n.o.s. (Inhalation hazard zone C) | 30 m | (100 ft) | 0.1 km | (0.1 mi) | 0.1 km | (0.1 mi) | 30 m | (100 ft) | 0.1 km | (0.1 mi) | 0.1 km | (0.1 mi) |
| 3517 | **173** | Adsorbed gas, toxic, flammable, corrosive, n.o.s. (Inhalation hazard zone D) | | | | | | | | | | | | |
| 3518 | **173** | Adsorbed gas, poisonous, oxidizing, corrosive, n.o.s | | | | | | | | | | | | |
| 3518 | **173** | Adsorbed gas, poisonous, oxidizing, corrosive, n.o.s. (Inhalation hazard zone A) | 30 m | (100 ft) | 0.1 km | (0.1 mi) | 0.2 km | (0.1 mi) | 30 m | (100 ft) | 0.1 km | (0.1 mi) | 0.4 km | (0.2 mi) |

**"+" means distance can be larger in certain atmospheric conditions**

# TABLE 1 - INITIAL ISOLATION AND PROTECTIVE ACTION DISTANCES

| ID No. | Guide | NAME OF MATERIAL | SMALL SPILLS (From a small package or small leak from a large package) First ISOLATE in all Directions Meters (Feet) | SMALL SPILLS Then PROTECT persons Downwind during DAY Kilometers (Miles) | SMALL SPILLS Then PROTECT persons Downwind during NIGHT Kilometers (Miles) | LARGE SPILLS (From a large package or from many small packages) First ISOLATE in all Directions Meters (Feet) | LARGE SPILLS Then PROTECT persons Downwind during DAY Kilometers (Miles) | LARGE SPILLS Then PROTECT persons Downwind during NIGHT Kilometers (Miles) |
|---|---|---|---|---|---|---|---|---|
| 3518<br>3518<br>3518 | 173<br>173<br>173 | Adsorbed gas, poisonous, oxidizing, corrosive, n.o.s. (Inhalation hazard zone B)<br>Adsorbed gas, poisonous, oxidizing, corrosive, n.o.s. (Inhalation hazard zone C)<br>Adsorbed gas, poisonous, oxidizing, corrosive, n.o.s. (Inhalation hazard zone D) | 30 m (100 ft) | 0.1 km (0.1 mi) | 0.1 km (0.1 mi) | 30 m (100 ft) | 0.1 km (0.1 mi) | 0.1 km (0.1 mi) |
| 3518<br>3518 | 173<br>173 | Adsorbed gas, toxic, oxidizing, corrosive, n.o.s.<br>Adsorbed gas, toxic, oxidizing, corrosive, n.o.s. (Inhalation hazard zone A) | 30 m (100 ft) | 0.1 km (0.1 mi) | 0.2 km (0.1 mi) | 30 m (100 ft) | 0.1 km (0.1 mi) | 0.4 km (0.2 mi) |
| 3518<br>3518<br>3518 | 173<br>173<br>173 | Adsorbed gas, toxic, oxidizing, corrosive, n.o.s. (Inhalation hazard zone B)<br>Adsorbed gas, toxic, oxidizing, corrosive, n.o.s. (Inhalation hazard zone C)<br>Adsorbed gas, toxic, oxidizing, corrosive, n.o.s. (Inhalation hazard zone D) | 30 m (100 ft) | 0.1 km (0.1 mi) | 0.1 km (0.1 mi) | 30 m (100 ft) | 0.1 km (0.1 mi) | 0.1 km (0.1 mi) |
| 3519 | 173 | Boron trifluoride, adsorbed | 30 m (100 ft) | 0.1 km (0.1 mi) | 0.1 km (0.1 mi) | 30 m (100 ft) | 0.1 km (0.1 mi) | 0.1 km (0.1 mi) |
| 3520 | 173 | Chlorine, adsorbed | 30 m (100 ft) | 0.1 km (0.1 mi) | 0.1 km (0.1 mi) | 30 m (100 ft) | 0.1 km (0.1 mi) | 0.1 km (0.1 mi) |
| 3521 | 173 | Silicon tetrafluoride, adsorbed | 30 m (100 ft) | 0.1 km (0.1 mi) | 0.1 km (0.1 mi) | 30 m (100 ft) | 0.1 km (0.1 mi) | 0.1 km (0.1 mi) |

| ID No. | Guide | Name of Material | | | | | | | | | | | | |
|---|---|---|---|---|---|---|---|---|---|---|---|---|---|---|
| 3523 | **173** | Germane, adsorbed | 30 m | (100 ft) | 0.1 km | (0.1 mi) | 0.2 km | (0.1 mi) | 30 m | (100 ft) | 0.1 km | (0.1 mi) | 0.4 km | (0.2 mi) |
| 3524 | **173** | Phosphorus pentafluoride, adsorbed | 30 m | (100 ft) | 0.1 km | (0.1 mi) | 0.1 km | (0.1 mi) | 30 m | (100 ft) | 0.1 km | (0.1 mi) | 0.1 km | (0.1 mi) |
| 3525 | **173** | Phosphine, adsorbed | 30 m | (100 ft) | 0.1 km | (0.1 mi) | 0.1 km | (0.1 mi) | 30 m | (100 ft) | 0.1 km | (0.1 mi) | 0.2 km | (0.1 mi) |
| 3526 | **173** | Hydrogen selenide, adsorbed | 30 m | (100 ft) | 0.1 km | (0.1 mi) | 0.2 km | (0.1 mi) | 30 m | (100 ft) | 0.1 km | (0.1 mi) | 0.4 km | (0.3 mi) |
| 9191 | **143** | Chlorine dioxide, hydrate, frozen (**when spilled In water**) | 30 m | (100 ft) | 0.1 km | (0.1 mi) | 0.1 km | (0.1 mi) | 30 m | (100 ft) | 0.2 km | (0.1 mi) | 0.5 km | (0.3 mi) |
| 9202 | **168** | Carbon monoxide, refrigerated liquid (cryogenic liquid) | 30 m | (100 ft) | 0.1 km | (0.1 mi) | 0.2 km | (0.1 mi) | 200 m | (600 ft) | 1.2 km | (0.7 mi) | 4.4 km | (2.8 mi) |
| 9206 | **137** | Methyl phosphonic dichloride | 30 m | (100 ft) | 0.1 km | (0.1 mi) | 0.2 km | (0.1 mi) | 30 m | (100 ft) | 0.4 km | (0.2 mi) | 0.5 km | (0.3 mi) |
| 9263 | **156** | Chloropivaloyl chloride | 30 m | (100 ft) | 0.1 km | (0.1 mi) | 0.1 km | (0.1 mi) | 30 m | (100 ft) | 0.2 km | (0.2 mi) | 0.3 km | (0.2 mi) |
| 9264 | **151** | 3,5-Dichloro-2,4,6-trifluoropyridine | 30 m | (100 ft) | 0.1 km | (0.1 mi) | 0.1 km | (0.1 mi) | 30 m | (100 ft) | 0.2 km | (0.2 mi) | 0.3 km | (0.2 mi) |
| 9269 | **132** | Trimethoxysilane | 30 m | (100 ft) | 0.2 km | (0.2 mi) | 0.6 km | (0.4 mi) | 100 m | (300 ft) | 1.3 km | (0.8 mi) | 2.4 km | (1.5 mi) |

**See Next Page for Table of Water-Reactive Materials Which Produce Toxic Gases**

**"+" means distance can be larger in certain atmospheric conditions**

## HOW TO USE TABLE 2 – WATER-REACTIVE MATERIALS WHICH PRODUCE TOXIC GASES

Table 2 lists materials which produce large amounts of Toxic Inhalation Hazard (TIH) (PIH in the US) gases when spilled in water and identifies the TIH gases produced.

The materials are listed by ID number order.

These Water Reactive materials are easily identified in Table 1 as their name is immediately followed by "(**when spilled in water**)".

**Note 1:** Some Water Reactive materials are also TIH materials themselves (e.g., Bromine trifluoride (UN1746), Thionyl chloride (UN1836), etc.). In these instances, two entries are provided in **Table 1** for land-based and water-based spills. If the Water Reactive material **is NOT** a TIH and this material **is NOT** spilled in water, **Table 1** and **Table 2 do NOT** apply and safety distances will be found within the appropriate orange guide.

**Note 2:** Materials classified as a Division 4.3 are substances that, on contact with water, are liable to become spontaneously FLAMMABLE or give off **FLAMMABLE** or sometimes **TOXIC** gases in dangerous quantities. For the purpose of this table, water reactive materials are materials that generate substantial quantities of **TOXIC** gases rapidly after a spill into water. Therefore, a material classified as a Division 4.3 will not always be included in Table 2.

# TABLE 2 - WATER-REACTIVE MATERIALS WHICH PRODUCE TOXIC GASES

**Materials Which Produce Large Amounts of Toxic-by-Inhalation (TIH) (PIH in the US) Gas(es) *When Spilled in Water***

| ID No. | Guide No. | Name of Material | TIH Gas(es) Produced |
|---|---|---|---|
| 1162 | 155 | Dimethyldichlorosilane | HCl |
| 1183 | 139 | Ethyldichlorosilane | HCl |
| 1196 | 155 | Ethyltrichlorosilane | HCl |
| 1242 | 139 | Methyldichlorosilane | HCl |
| 1250 | 155 | Methyltrichlorosilane | HCl |
| 1295 | 139 | Trichlorosilane | HCl |
| 1298 | 155 | Trimethylchlorosilane | HCl |
| 1305 | 155P | Vinyltrichlorosilane | HCl |
| 1305 | 155P | Vinyltrichlorosilane, stabilized | HCl |
| 1340 | 139 | Phosphorus pentasulfide, free from yellow and white Phosphorus | $H_2S$ |
| 1340 | 139 | Phosphorus pentasulphide, free from yellow and white Phosphorus | $H_2S$ |
| 1360 | 139 | Calcium phosphide | $PH_3$ |
| 1384 | 135 | Sodium dithionite | $H_2S$ $SO_2$ |
| 1384 | 135 | Sodium hydrosulfite | $H_2S$ $SO_2$ |
| 1384 | 135 | Sodium hydrosulphite | $H_2S$ $SO_2$ |
| 1397 | 139 | Aluminum phosphide | $PH_3$ |
| 1419 | 139 | Magnesium aluminum phosphide | $PH_3$ |
| 1432 | 139 | Sodium phosphide | $PH_3$ |
| 1541 | 155 | Acetone cyanohydrin, stabilized | HCN |
| 1680 | 157 | Potassium cyanide | HCN |
| 1680 | 157 | Potassium cyanide, solid | HCN |
| 1689 | 157 | Sodium cyanide | HCN |
| 1689 | 157 | Sodium cyanide, solid | HCN |

**Chemical Symbols for TIH (PIH in the US) Gases:**

| Symbol | Name | Symbol | Name | Symbol | Name |
|---|---|---|---|---|---|
| $Br_2$ | Bromine | HF | Hydrogen fluoride | $NO_2$ | Nitrogen dioxide |
| $Cl_2$ | Chlorine | HI | Hydrogen iodide | $PH_3$ | Phosphine |
| HBr | Hydrogen bromide | $H_2S$ | Hydrogen sulfide | $SO_2$ | Sulfur dioxide |
| HCl | Hydrogen chloride | $H_2S$ | Hydrogen sulphide | $SO_2$ | Sulphur dioxide |
| HCN | Hydrogen cyanide | $NH_3$ | Ammonia | | |

# TABLE 2 - WATER-REACTIVE MATERIALS WHICH PRODUCE TOXIC GASES

**Materials Which Produce Large Amounts of Toxic-by-Inhalation (TIH) (PIH in the US) Gas(es) *When Spilled in Water***

| ID No. | Guide No. | Name of Material | TIH Gas(es) Produced |
|---|---|---|---|
| 1716 | 156 | Acetyl bromide | HBr |
| 1717 | 155 | Acetyl chloride | HCl |
| 1724 | 155 | Allyltrichlorosilane, stabilized | HCl |
| 1725 | 137 | Aluminum bromide, anhydrous | HBr |
| 1726 | 137 | Aluminum chloride, anhydrous | HCl |
| 1728 | 155 | Amyltrichlorosilane | HCl |
| 1732 | 157 | Antimony pentafluoride | HF |
| 1741 | 125 | Boron trichloride | HCl |
| 1745 | 144 | Bromine pentafluoride | HF $Br_2$ |
| 1746 | 144 | Bromine trifluoride | HF $Br_2$ |
| 1747 | 155 | Butyltrichlorosilane | HCl |
| 1752 | 156 | Chloroacetyl chloride | HCl |
| 1753 | 156 | Chlorophenyltrichlorosilane | HCl |
| 1754 | 137 | Chlorosulfonic acid (with or without sulfur trioxide mixture) | HCl |
| 1754 | 137 | Chlorosulphonic acid (with or without sulphur trioxide mixture) | HCl |
| 1758 | 137 | Chromium oxychloride | HCl |
| 1762 | 156 | Cyclohexenyltrichlorosilane | HCl |
| 1763 | 156 | Cyclohexyltrichlorosilane | HCl |
| 1765 | 156 | Dichloroacetyl chloride | HCl |
| 1766 | 156 | Dichlorophenyltrichlorosilane | HCl |
| 1767 | 155 | Diethyldichlorosilane | HCl |
| 1769 | 156 | Diphenyldichlorosilane | HCl |
| 1771 | 156 | Dodecyltrichlorosilane | HCl |

**Chemical Symbols for TIH (PIH in the US) Gases:**

| Symbol | Name | Symbol | Name | Symbol | Name |
|---|---|---|---|---|---|
| $Br_2$ | Bromine | HF | Hydrogen fluoride | $NO_2$ | Nitrogen dioxide |
| $Cl_2$ | Chlorine | HI | Hydrogen iodide | $PH_3$ | Phosphine |
| HBr | Hydrogen bromide | $H_2S$ | Hydrogen sulfide | $SO_2$ | Sulfur dioxide |
| HCl | Hydrogen chloride | $H_2S$ | Hydrogen sulphide | $SO_2$ | Sulphur dioxide |
| HCN | Hydrogen cyanide | $NH_3$ | Ammonia | | |

 **Use this list only when material is spilled in water.**

# TABLE 2 - WATER-REACTIVE MATERIALS WHICH PRODUCE TOXIC GASES

**Materials Which Produce Large Amounts of Toxic-by-Inhalation (TIH) (PIH in the US) Gas(es) *When Spilled in Water***

| ID No. | Guide No. | Name of Material | TIH Gas(es) Produced |
|---|---|---|---|
| 1777 | 137 | Fluorosulfonic acid | HF |
| 1777 | 137 | Fluorosulphonic acid | HF |
| 1781 | 156 | Hexadecyltrichlorosilane | HCl |
| 1784 | 156 | Hexyltrichlorosilane | HCl |
| 1799 | 156 | Nonyltrichlorosilane | HCl |
| 1800 | 156 | Octadecyltrichlorosilane | HCl |
| 1801 | 156 | Octyltrichlorosilane | HCl |
| 1804 | 156 | Phenyltrichlorosilane | HCl |
| 1806 | 137 | Phosphorus pentachloride | HCl |
| 1808 | 137 | Phosphorus tribromide | HBr |
| 1809 | 137 | Phosphorus trichloride | HCl |
| 1810 | 137 | Phosphorus oxychloride | HCl |
| 1815 | 132 | Propionyl chloride | HCl |
| 1816 | 155 | Propyltrichlorosilane | HCl |
| 1818 | 157 | Silicon tetrachloride | HCl |
| 1828 | 137 | Sulfur chlorides | HCl $SO_2$ $H_2S$ |
| 1828 | 137 | Sulphur chlorides | HCl $SO_2$ $H_2S$ |
| 1834 | 137 | Sulfuryl chloride | HCl |
| 1834 | 137 | Sulphuryl chloride | HCl |
| 1836 | 137 | Thionyl chloride | HCl $SO_2$ |
| 1838 | 137 | Titanium tetrachloride | HCl |
| 1898 | 156 | Acetyl iodide | HI |
| 1923 | 135 | Calcium dithionite | $H_2S$ $SO_2$ |

**Chemical Symbols for TIH (PIH in the US) Gases:**

| | | | | | |
|---|---|---|---|---|---|
| $Br_2$ | Bromine | HF | Hydrogen fluoride | $NO_2$ | Nitrogen dioxide |
| $Cl_2$ | Chlorine | HI | Hydrogen iodide | $PH_3$ | Phosphine |
| HBr | Hydrogen bromide | $H_2S$ | Hydrogen sulfide | $SO_2$ | Sulfur dioxide |
| HCl | Hydrogen chloride | $H_2S$ | Hydrogen sulphide | $SO_2$ | Sulphur dioxide |
| HCN | Hydrogen cyanide | $NH_3$ | Ammonia | | |

**Use this list only when material is spilled in water.**

## TABLE 2 - WATER-REACTIVE MATERIALS WHICH PRODUCE TOXIC GASES

**Materials Which Produce Large Amounts of Toxic-by-Inhalation (TIH) (PIH in the US) Gas(es) *When Spilled in Water***

| ID No. | Guide No. | Name of Material | TIH Gas(es) Produced |
|---|---|---|---|
| 1923 | 135 | Calcium hydrosulfite | $H_2S$ $SO_2$ |
| 1923 | 135 | Calcium hydrosulphite | $H_2S$ $SO_2$ |
| 1929 | 135 | Potassium dithionite | $H_2S$ $SO_2$ |
| 1929 | 135 | Potassium hydrosulfite | $H_2S$ $SO_2$ |
| 1929 | 135 | Potassium hydrosulphite | $H_2S$ $SO_2$ |
| 1931 | 171 | Zinc dithionite | $H_2S$ $SO_2$ |
| 1931 | 171 | Zinc hydrosulfite | $H_2S$ $SO_2$ |
| 1931 | 171 | Zinc hydrosulphite | $H_2S$ $SO_2$ |
| 2004 | 135 | Magnesium diamide | $NH_3$ |
| 2011 | 139 | Magnesium phosphide | $PH_3$ |
| 2012 | 139 | Potassium phosphide | $PH_3$ |
| 2013 | 139 | Strontium phosphide | $PH_3$ |
| 2308 | 157 | Nitrosylsulfuric acid, liquid | $NO_2$ |
| 2308 | 157 | Nitrosylsulfuric acid, solid | $NO_2$ |
| 2308 | 157 | Nitrosylsulphuric acid, liquid | $NO_2$ |
| 2308 | 157 | Nitrosylsulphuric acid, solid | $NO_2$ |
| 2353 | 132 | Butyryl chloride | HCl |
| 2395 | 132 | Isobutyryl chloride | HCl |
| 2434 | 156 | Dibenzyldichlorosilane | HCl |
| 2435 | 156 | Ethylphenyldichlorosilane | HCl |
| 2437 | 156 | Methylphenyldichlorosilane | HCl |
| 2495 | 144 | Iodine pentafluoride | HF |
| 2691 | 137 | Phosphorus pentabromide | HBr |

**Chemical Symbols for TIH (PIH in the US) Gases:**

| | | | | | |
|---|---|---|---|---|---|
| $Br_2$ | Bromine | HF | Hydrogen fluoride | $NO_2$ | Nitrogen dioxide |
| $Cl_2$ | Chlorine | HI | Hydrogen iodide | $PH_3$ | Phosphine |
| HBr | Hydrogen bromide | $H_2S$ | Hydrogen sulfide | $SO_2$ | Sulfur dioxide |
| HCl | Hydrogen chloride | $H_2S$ | Hydrogen sulphide | $SO_2$ | Sulphur dioxide |
| HCN | Hydrogen cyanide | $NH_3$ | Ammonia | | |



**Use this list only when material is spilled in water.**

# TABLE 2 - WATER-REACTIVE MATERIALS WHICH PRODUCE TOXIC GASES

**Materials Which Produce Large Amounts of Toxic-by-Inhalation (TIH) (PIH in the US) Gas(es) *When Spilled in Water***

| ID No. | Guide No. | Name of Material | TIH Gas(es) Produced |
|---|---|---|---|
| 2692 | 157 | Boron tribromide | HBr |
| 2806 | 138 | Lithium nitride | $NH_3$ |
| 2977 | 166 | Radioactive material, Uranium hexafluoride, fissile | HF |
| 2977 | 166 | Uranium hexafluoride, radioactive material, fissile | HF |
| 2978 | 166 | Radioactive material, Uranium hexafluoride, non fissile or fissile-excepted | HF |
| 2978 | 166 | Uranium hexafluoride, radioactive material, non fissile or fissile-excepted | HF |
| 2985 | 155 | Chlorosilanes, flammable, corrosive, n.o.s | HCl |
| 2986 | 155 | Chlorosilanes, corrosive, flammable, n.o.s | HCl |
| 2987 | 156 | Chlorosilanes, corrosive, n.o.s | HCl |
| 2988 | 139 | Chlorosilanes, water-reactive, flammable, corrosive, n.o.s. | HCl |
| 3048 | 157 | Aluminum phosphide pesticide | $PH_3$ |
| 3049 | 138 | Metal alkyl halides, water-reactive, n.o.s | HCl |
| 3049 | 138 | Metal aryl halides, water-reactive, n.o.s | HCl |
| 3052 | 135 | Aluminum alkyl halides, liquid | HCl |
| 3052 | 135 | Aluminum alkyl halides, solid | HCl |
| 3361 | 156 | Chlorosilanes, poisonous, corrosive, n.o.s. | HCl |
| 3361 | 156 | Chlorosilanes, toxic, corrosive, n.o.s. | HCl |
| 3362 | 155 | Chlorosilanes, poisonous, corrosive, flammable, n.o.s. | HCl |
| 3362 | 155 | Chlorosilanes, toxic, corrosive, flammable, n.o.s. | HCl |
| 3456 | 157 | Nitrosylsulfuric acid, solid | $NO_2$ |
| 3456 | 157 | Nitrosylsulphuric acid, solid | $NO_2$ |

**Chemical Symbols for TIH (PIH in the US) Gases:**

| Symbol | Name | Symbol | Name | Symbol | Name |
|---|---|---|---|---|---|
| $Br_2$ | Bromine | HF | Hydrogen fluoride | $NO_2$ | Nitrogen dioxide |
| $Cl_2$ | Chlorine | HI | Hydrogen iodide | $PH_3$ | Phosphine |
| HBr | Hydrogen bromide | $H_2S$ | Hydrogen sulfide | $SO_2$ | Sulfur dioxide |
| HCl | Hydrogen chloride | $H_2S$ | Hydrogen sulphide | $SO_2$ | Sulphur dioxide |
| HCN | Hydrogen cyanide | $NH_3$ | Ammonia | | |

**Materials Which Produce Large Amounts of Toxic-by-Inhalation (TIH) (PIH in the US) Gas(es) *When Spilled in Water***

| ID No. | Guide No. | Name of Material | TIH Gas(es) Produced |
|---|---|---|---|
| 3461 | 135 | Aluminum alkyl halides, solid | HCl |
| 3507 | 166 | Uranium hexafluoride, radioactive material, excepted package, less than 0.1 kg per package, non-fissile or fissile-excepted | HF |
| 9191 | 143 | Chlorine dioxide, hydrate, frozen | $Cl_2$ |

**Chemical Symbols for TIH (PIH in the US) Gases:**

| Symbol | Name | Symbol | Name | Symbol | Name |
|---|---|---|---|---|---|
| $Br_2$ | Bromine | HF | Hydrogen fluoride | $NO_2$ | Nitrogen dioxide |
| $Cl_2$ | Chlorine | HI | Hydrogen iodide | $PH_3$ | Phosphine |
| HBr | Hydrogen bromide | $H_2S$ | Hydrogen sulfide | $SO_2$ | Sulfur dioxide |
| HCl | Hydrogen chloride | $H_2S$ | Hydrogen sulphide | $SO_2$ | Sulphur dioxide |
| HCN | Hydrogen cyanide | $NH_3$ | Ammonia | | |

 **Use this list only when material is spilled in water.**

## NOTES

## HOW TO USE TABLE 3 – INITIAL ISOLATION AND PROTECTIVE ACTION DISTANCES FOR LARGE SPILLS FOR DIFFERENT QUANTITIES OF SIX COMMON TIH (PIH in the US) GASES

Table 3 lists Toxic Inhalation Hazard materials that may be more commonly encountered.

The selected materials are:

- Ammonia, anhydrous (UN1005)
- Chlorine (UN1017)
- Ethylene oxide (UN1040)
- Hydrogen chloride, anhydrous (UN1050) and Hydrogen chloride, refrigerated liquid (UN2186)
- Hydrogen fluoride, anhydrous (UN1052)
- Sulfur dioxide/Sulphur dioxide (UN1079)

The materials are presented in alphabetical order and provide Initial Isolation and Protective Action Distances **FOR LARGE SPILLS** (more than 208 liters or 55 US gallons) involving different container types (therefore different volume capacities) for day time and night time situations and different wind speeds.

**Estimating Wind Speed from Environmental Clues**

| mph | km/h | Wind Description | Specifications |
|---|---|---|---|
| < 6 | < 10 | Low wind | Wind felt on face; leaves rustle; ordinary vane moved by wind |
| 6 - 12 | 10 - 20 | Moderate wind | Raises dust, loose paper; small branches are moved |
| > 12 | > 20 | High wind | Large branches in motion; whistling heard in telephone wires; umbrellas used with difficulty |

TABLE 3 - INITIAL ISOLATION AND PROTECTIVE ACTION DISTANCES FOR LARGE SPILLS FOR DIFFERENT QUANTITIES OF SIX COMMON TIH (PIH in the US) GASES

| | First ISOLATE in all Directions | | Then **PROTECT** persons Downwind during | | | | | | | | | | | |
|---|---|---|---|---|---|---|---|---|---|---|---|---|---|---|
| | | | DAY | | | | | | NIGHT | | | | | |
| | | | Low wind (< 6 mph = < 10 km/h) | | Moderate wind (6-12 mph = 10 - 20 km/h) | | High wind (> 12 mph = > 20 km/h) | | Low wind (< 6 mph = < 10 km/h) | | Moderate wind (6-12 mph = 10 - 20 km/h) | | High wind (> 12 mph = > 20 km/h) | |
| | Meters | (Feet) | km | (Miles) | km | (Miles) | km | (Miles) | km | (Miles) | km | (Miles) | km | (Miles) |
| **TRANSPORT CONTAINER** | **UN1005 Ammonia, anhydrous: Large Spills** | | | | | | | | | | | | | |
| Rail tank car | 300 | (1000) | 1.7 | (1.1) | 1.3 | (0.8) | 1.0 | (0.6) | 4.3 | (2.7) | 2.3 | (1.4) | 1.3 | (0.8) |
| Highway tank truck or trailer | 150 | (500) | 0.9 | (0.6) | 0.5 | (0.3) | 0.4 | (0.3) | 2.0 | (1.3) | 0.8 | (0.5) | 0.6 | (0.4) |
| Agricultural nurse tank | 60 | (200) | 0.5 | (0.3) | 0.3 | (0.2) | 0.3 | (0.2) | 1.3 | (0.8) | 0.3 | (0.2) | 0.3 | (0.2) |
| Multiple small cylinders | 30 | (100) | 0.3 | (0.2) | 0.2 | (0.1) | 0.1 | (0.1) | 0.7 | (0.5) | 0.3 | (0.2) | 0.2 | (0.1) |
| **TRANSPORT CONTAINER** | **UN1017 Chlorine: Large Spills** | | | | | | | | | | | | | |
| Rail tank car | 1000 | (3000) | 9.9 | (6.2) | 6.4 | (4.0) | 5.1 | (3.2) | 11+ | (7+) | 9.0 | (5.6) | 6.7 | (4.2) |
| Highway tank truck or trailer | 600 | (2000) | 5.8 | (3.6) | 3.4 | (2.1) | 2.9 | (1.8) | 6.7 | (4.3) | 5.0 | (3.1) | 4.1 | (2.5) |
| Multiple ton cylinders | 300 | (1000) | 2.1 | (1.3) | 1.3 | (0.8) | 1.0 | (0.6) | 4.0 | (2.5) | 2.4 | (1.5) | 1.3 | (0.8) |
| Multiple small cylinders or single ton cylinder | 150 | (500) | 1.5 | (0.9) | 0.8 | (0.5) | 0.5 | (0.3) | 2.9 | (1.8) | 1.3 | (0.8) | 0.6 | (0.4) |

"+" means distance can be larger in certain atmospheric conditions

## TABLE 3 - INITIAL ISOLATION AND PROTECTIVE ACTION DISTANCES FOR LARGE SPILLS FOR DIFFERENT QUANTITIES OF SIX COMMON TIH (PIH in the US) GASES

| | First ISOLATE in all Directions | | Then **PROTECT** persons Downwind during | | | | | | | | | | | |
|---|---|---|---|---|---|---|---|---|---|---|---|---|---|---|
| | | | DAY | | | | | | NIGHT | | | | | |
| | | | Low wind (< 6 mph = < 10 km/h) | | Moderate wind (6-12 mph = 10 - 20 km/h) | | High wind (> 12 mph = > 20 km/h) | | Low wind (< 6 mph = < 10 km/h) | | Moderate wind (6-12 mph = 10 - 20 km/h) | | High wind (> 12 mph = > 20 km/h) | |
| | Meters | (Feet) | km | (Miles) | km | (Miles) | km | (Miles) | km | (Miles) | km | (Miles) | km | (Miles) |
| **TRANSPORT CONTAINER** | **UN1040 Ethylene oxide: Large Spills** | | | | | | | | | | | | | |
| Rail tank car | 200 | (600) | 1.6 | (1.0) | 0.8 | (0.5) | 0.7 | (0.5) | 3.3 | (2.1) | 1.4 | (0.9) | 0.8 | (0.5) |
| Highway tank truck or trailer | 100 | (300) | 0.9 | (0.6) | 0.5 | (0.3) | 0.4 | (0.3) | 2.0 | (1.3) | 0.7 | (0.4) | 0.4 | (0.3) |
| Multiple small cylinders or single ton cylinder | 30 | (100) | 0.4 | (0.3) | 0.2 | (0.1) | 0.1 | (0.1) | 0.9 | (0.6) | 0.3 | (0.2) | 0.2 | (0.1) |
| **TRANSPORT CONTAINER** | **UN1050 Hydrogen chloride, anhydrous: Large Spills<br>UN2186 Hydrogen chloride, refrigerated liquid: Large Spills** | | | | | | | | | | | | | |
| Rail tank car | 500 | (1500) | 3.7 | (2.3) | 2.0 | (1.2) | 1.7 | (1.1) | 9.9 | (6.2) | 3.4 | (2.1) | 2.3 | (1.5) |
| Highway tank truck or trailer | 200 | (600) | 1.5 | (0.9) | 0.8 | (0.5) | 0.6 | (0.4) | 3.8 | (2.4) | 1.5 | (0.9) | 0.8 | (0.5) |
| Multiple ton cylinders | 30 | (100) | 0.4 | (0.3) | 0.2 | (0.1) | 0.1 | (0.1) | 1.1 | (0.7) | 0.3 | (0.2) | 0.2 | (0.1) |
| Multiple small cylinders or single ton cylinder | 30 | (100) | 0.3 | (0.2) | 0.2 | (0.1) | 0.1 | (0.1) | 0.9 | (0.6) | 0.3 | (0.2) | 0.2 | (0.1) |

## TABLE 3 - INITIAL ISOLATION AND PROTECTIVE ACTION DISTANCES FOR LARGE SPILLS FOR DIFFERENT QUANTITIES OF SIX COMMON TIH (PIH in the US) GASES

| | First ISOLATE in all Directions | | Then **PROTECT** persons Downwind during | | | | | | | | | | | |
|---|---|---|---|---|---|---|---|---|---|---|---|---|---|---|
| | | | DAY | | | | | | NIGHT | | | | | |
| | | | Low wind (< 6 mph = < 10 km/h) | | Moderate wind (6-12 mph = 10 - 20 km/h) | | High wind (> 12 mph = > 20 km/h) | | Low wind (< 6 mph = < 10 km/h) | | Moderate wind (6-12 mph = 10 - 20 km/h) | | High wind (> 12 mph = > 20 km/h) | |
| | Meters | (Feet) | km | (Miles) | km | (Miles) | km | (Miles) | km | (Miles) | km | (Miles) | km | (Miles) |
| **TRANSPORT CONTAINER** | **UN1052 Hydrogen fluoride, anhydrous: Large Spills** | | | | | | | | | | | | | |
| Rail tank car | 400 | (1250) | 3.1 | (1.9) | 1.9 | (1.2) | 1.6 | (1.0) | 6.1 | (3.8) | 2.9 | (1.8) | 1.9 | (1.2) |
| Highway tank truck or trailer | 200 | (700) | 1.9 | (1.2) | 1.0 | (0.7) | 0.9 | (0.6) | 3.4 | (2.2) | 1.6 | (1.0) | 0.9 | (0.6) |
| Multiple small cylinders or single ton cylinder | 100 | (300) | 0.8 | (0.5) | 0.4 | (0.2) | 0.3 | (0.2) | 1.6 | (1.0) | 0.5 | (0.3) | 0.3 | (0.2) |
| **TRANSPORT CONTAINER** | **UN1079 Sulfur dioxide/Sulphur dioxide: Large Spills** | | | | | | | | | | | | | |
| Rail tank car | 1000 | (3000) | 11+ | (7+) | 11+ | (7+) | 7.0 | (4.4) | 11+ | (7+) | 11+ | (7+) | 9.8 | (6.1) |
| Highway tank truck or trailer | 1000 | (3000) | 11+ | (7+) | 5.8 | (3.6) | 5.0 | (3.1) | 11+ | (7+) | 8.0 | (5.0) | 6.1 | (3.8) |
| Multiple ton cylinders | 500 | (1500) | 5.2 | (3.2) | 2.4 | (1.5) | 1.8 | (1.1) | 7.5 | (4.7) | 4.0 | (2.5) | 2.8 | (1.7) |
| Multiple small cylinders or single ton cylinder | 200 | (600) | 3.1 | (1.9) | 1.5 | (0.9) | 1.1 | (0.7) | 5.6 | (3.5) | 2.4 | (1.5) | 1.5 | (0.9) |

"+" means distance can be larger in certain atmospheric conditions

## ERG2016 USER'S GUIDE

The 2016 Emergency Response Guidebook (ERG2016) was developed jointly by Transport Canada (TC), the U.S. Department of Transportation (DOT), the Secretariat of Communications and Transport of Mexico (SCT) and with the collaboration of CIQUIME (Centro de Información Química para Emergencias) of Argentina, for use by fire fighters, police, and other emergency services personnel who may be the first to arrive at the scene of a transportation incident involving dangerous goods. **It is primarily a guide to aid first responders in quickly identifying the specific or generic hazards of the material(s) involved in the incident, and protecting themselves and the general public during the initial response phase of the incident.** For the purposes of this guidebook, the "initial response phase" is that period following arrival at the scene of an incident during which the presence and/or identification of dangerous goods is confirmed, protective actions and area securement are initiated, and assistance of qualified personnel is requested. It is not intended to provide information on the physical or chemical properties of dangerous goods.

This guidebook will assist responders in making initial decisions upon arriving at the scene of a dangerous goods incident. It should not be considered as a substitute for emergency response training, knowledge or sound judgment. ERG2016 does not address all possible circumstances that may be associated with a dangerous goods incident. It is primarily designed for use at a dangerous goods incident occurring on a highway or railroad. Be mindful that there may be limited value in its application at fixed facility locations.

ERG2016 incorporates dangerous goods lists from the most recent United Nations Recommendations as well as from other international and national regulations. Explosives are not listed individually by either proper shipping name or ID Number. They do, however, appear under the general heading "Explosives" on the first page of the ID Number index (yellow-bordered pages) and alphabetically in the Name of Material index (blue-bordered pages). Also, the letter **(P)** following the guide number in the yellow-bordered and blue-bordered pages identifies those materials which present a polymerization hazard under certain conditions, for example: Acrolein, stabilized **131P.**

First responders at the scene of a dangerous goods incident should seek additional specific information about any material in question as soon as possible. The information received by contacting the appropriate emergency response agency, by calling the emergency response telephone number on the shipping document, or by consulting the information on or accompanying the shipping document, may be more specific and accurate than this guidebook in providing guidance for the materials involved.

**BEFORE AN EMERGENCY – BECOME FAMILIAR WITH THIS GUIDEBOOK!** In the U.S., according to the requirements of the U.S. Department of Labor's Occupational Safety and Health Administration (OSHA, 29 CFR 1910.120), and regulations issued by the U.S. Environmental Protection Agency (EPA, 40 CFR Part 311), first responders must be trained regarding the use of this guidebook.

## Guidebook Contents

**1-Yellow-bordered pages:** Index list of dangerous goods in numerical order of ID number. This section quickly identifies the guide to be consulted from the ID Number of the material involved. This list displays the 4-digit ID number of the material followed by its assigned emergency response guide and the material name.

| For example: | ID No. | GUIDE No. | Name of Material |
|---|---|---|---|
| | 1090 | 127 | Acetone |

**2-Blue-bordered pages:** Index list of dangerous goods in alphabetical order of material name. This section quickly identifies the guide to be consulted from the name of the material involved. This list displays the name of the material followed by its assigned emergency response guide and 4-digit ID number.

| For example: | Name of Material | GUIDE No. | ID No. |
|---|---|---|---|
| | Sulfuric acid | 137 | 1830 |

**3-Orange-bordered pages:** This section is the most important section of the guidebook because it is where all safety recommendations are provided. It comprises a total of 63 individual guides, presented in a two-page format. Each guide provides safety recommendations and emergency response information to protect yourself and the public. The left-hand page provides safety-related information whereas the right-hand page provides emergency response guidance and activities for fire situations, spill or leak incidents and first aid. Each guide is designed to cover a group of materials which possess similar chemical and toxicological characteristics.

The guide title identifies the general hazards of the dangerous goods covered.

**For example:** **GUIDE 124** - Gases-Toxic and/or Corrosive-Oxidizing.

Each guide is divided into three main sections: the first section describes **potential hazards** that the material may display in terms of fire/explosion and health effects upon exposure. The highest potential is listed first. The emergency responder should consult this section first. This allows the responder to make decisions regarding the protection of the emergency response team as well as the surrounding population.

The second section outlines suggested **public safety** measures based on the situation at hand. It provides general information regarding immediate isolation of the incident site, recommended type of protective clothing and respiratory protection. Suggested evacuation distances are listed for small and large spills and for fire situations (fragmentation hazard). It also directs the reader to consult the tables listing Toxic Inhalation Hazard (TIH) (PIH in the US) materials, chemical warfare agents and water-reactive materials (green-bordered pages) when the material is highlighted in the yellow-bordered and blue-bordered pages.

The third section covers **emergency response** actions, including first aid. It outlines special precautions for incidents which involve fire, spill or chemical exposure. Several recommendations are listed under each part which will further assist in the decision making process. The information on first aid is general guidance prior to seeking medical care.

**4-Green-bordered pages:** This section contains three tables.

**Table 1** lists, by ID number order, TIH (PIH in the US) materials, including certain chemical warfare agents, and water-reactive materials which produce toxic gases upon contact with water. This table provides two different types of recommended safe distances which are "Initial isolation distances" and "Protective action distances". The materials are highlighted in green for easy identification in both numeric (yellow-bordered pages) and alphabetic (blue-bordered pages) lists of the guidebook. This table provides distances for both small (approximately 208 liters (55 US gallons) or less for liquids and 300 kilograms (660 pounds) or less for solids when spilled in water) and large spills (more than 208 liters (55 US gallons) for liquids and more than 300 kilograms (660 pounds) for solids when spilled in water) for all highlighted materials. The list is further subdivided into daytime and nighttime situations. This is necessary due to varying atmospheric conditions which greatly affect the size of the hazardous area. The distances change from daytime to nighttime due to different mixing and dispersion conditions in the air. During the night, the air is generally calmer and this causes the material to disperse less and therefore create a toxic zone which is greater than would usually occur during the day. During the day, a more active atmosphere will cause a greater dispersion of the material resulting in a lower concentration of the material in the surrounding air. The actual area where toxic levels are reached will be smaller (due to increased dispersion). In fact, it is the quantity or concentration of the material vapor that poses problems not its mere presence.

The "Initial Isolation Distance" is a distance within which all persons should be considered for evacuation in all directions from the actual spill/leak source. It is a distance (radius) which defines a circle (Initial Isolation Zone) within which persons may be exposed to dangerous concentrations upwind of the source and may be exposed to life-threatening concentrations downwind of the source. For example, in the case of Compressed gas, toxic, n.o.s., UN1955, Inhalation Hazard Zone A, the isolation distance for small spills is 100 meters (300 feet), therefore, representing an evacuation circle of 200 meters (600 feet) in diameter.

For the same material, the "Protective Action Distance" for a small spill is 0.5 kilometers (0.3 miles) for a daytime incident and 2.5 kilometers (1.6 miles) for a nighttime incident, these distances represent a downwind distance from the spill/leak source within which Protective Actions could be implemented. Protective Actions are those steps taken to preserve the health and safety of emergency responders and the public. People in this area could be evacuated and/or sheltered in-place. For more information, consult pages 289 to 295.

## Toxic Inhalation Hazard (TIH) Materials

A TIH (PIH in the US) material is a gas or volatile liquid which is known to be so toxic to humans as to pose a hazard to health during transportation, or in the absence of adequate data on human toxicity, is presumed to be toxic to humans because when tested on laboratory animals it has a Lethal Concentration 50 (LC50) value of not more than 5000 ppm.

It is important to note that even though the term zone is used, the hazard zones do not represent any actual area or distance. The assignment of the zones is strictly a function of their Lethal Concentration 50 (LC50); for example, TIH Zone A is more toxic than Zone D. All distances which are listed in the green-bordered pages are calculated by the use of mathematical models for each TIH material. For the assignment of hazard zones refer to the glossary.

**Table 2** lists, by ID number order, materials that produce large amounts of Toxic Inhalation Hazard (TIH) gases when spilled in water and identifies the TIH gases produced. These Water Reactive materials are easily identified in **Table 1** as their name is immediately followed by (**when spilled in water**). Some Water Reactive materials are also TIH materials themselves (e.g., Bromine trifluoride (UN1746), Thionyl chloride (UN1836), etc.). In these instances, two entries are provided in **Table 1** for land-based and water-based spills. If the Water Reactive material is NOT a TIH, and this material is NOT spilled in water, **Table 1** and **Table 2** do not apply and safety distances will be found within the appropriate orange-bordered guide.

**Table 3** provides, by alphabetical order of material name, initial isolation and protective action distances for six Toxic Inhalation Hazard materials that may be more commonly encountered. The selected materials are:

- Ammonia, anhydrous (UN1005)
- Chlorine (UN1017)
- Ethylene oxide (UN1040)
- Hydrogen chloride, anhydrous (UN1050) and Hydrogen chloride, refrigerated liquid (UN2186)
- Hydrogen fluoride, anhydrous (UN1052)
- Sulfur dioxide/Sulphur dioxide (UN1079)

The table provides Initial Isolation and Protective Action Distances for large spills (more than 208 liters or 55 US gallons) involving different container types (therefore different volume capacities) for day-time and night-time situations and different wind speeds.

## Isolation and Evacuation Distances

Isolation or evacuation distances are shown in the guides (orange-bordered pages) and in the Table 1 - Initial Isolation and Protective Action Distances (green-bordered pages). This may confuse users not thoroughly familiar with ERG2016.

It is important to note that some guides refer only to non-TIH (PIH in the US) materials (37 guides), some refer to both TIH and non-TIH materials (21 guides) and some (5 guides) refer only to TIH or Water-reactive materials (WRM). A guide refers to both TIH and non-TIH materials (for example see GUIDE 131) when the following sentence appears under the title EVACUATION-Spill: "See Table 1 - Initial Isolation and Protective Action Distances for highlighted materials. For non-highlighted materials, increase, in the downwind direction, as necessary, the isolation distance shown under 'PUBLIC SAFETY.'" A guide refers only to TIH or WRM materials (for example see GUIDE 124) when the following sentence appears under the title EVACUATION-Spill: "See Table 1 - Initial Isolation and Protective Action Distances". If the previous sentences do not appear in a guide, then this particular guide refers only to non-TIH materials (for example see GUIDE 128).

In order to identify appropriate isolation and protective action distances, use the following:

If you are dealing with a **TIH/WRM/Chemical warfare** material (highlighted entries in the index lists), the isolation and evacuation distances are found directly in the green-bordered pages. The guides (orange-bordered pages) also remind the user to refer to the green-bordered pages for evacuation-specific information involving highlighted materials.

If you are dealing with a **non-TIH material but the guide refers to both TIH and non-TIH materials,** an immediate isolation distance is provided under the heading PUBLIC SAFETY as a precautionary measure to prevent injuries. It applies to the non-TIH materials only. In addition, for evacuation purposes, the guide informs the user under the title EVACUATION-Spill to increase, for non-highlighted materials, in the downwind direction, if necessary, the immediate isolation distance listed under "PUBLIC SAFETY". For example, GUIDE 131 – Flammable Liquids-Toxic, instructs the user to: "As an immediate precautionary measure, isolate spill or leak area for at least 50 meters (150 feet) in all directions." In case of a large spill, the isolation area could be expanded from 50 meters (150 feet) to a distance deemed as safe by the on-scene commander and emergency responders.

If you are dealing with a **non-TIH material and the guide refers only to non-TIH materials,** the immediate isolation and evacuation distances are specified as actual distances in the guide (orange-bordered pages) and are not referenced in the green-bordered pages.

**Note 1:** If an entry is highlighted in green in either the yellow-bordered or blue-bordered pages AND THERE IS NO FIRE, go directly to Table 1 - Initial Isolation and Protective Action Distances (green-bordered pages) and look up the ID number and name of material to obtain initial isolation and protective action distances. IF A FIRE IS INVOLVED, ALSO CONSULT the assigned guide (orange-bordered pages) and apply as appropriate the evacuation information shown under PUBLIC SAFETY.

**Note 2:** If the name in **Table 1** is shown with "***(when spilled in water)***", these materials produce large amounts of Toxic Inhalation Hazard (TIH) gases when spilled in water. Some Water Reactive materials are also TIH materials themselves (e.g., Bromine trifluoride (UN1746), Thionyl chloride (UN1836), etc.). In these instances, two entries are provided in **Table 1** for land-based and water-based spills. If the Water Reactive material **is NOT** a TIH and this material **is NOT** spilled in water, **Table 1** and **Table 2** do not apply and safety distances will be found within the appropriate orange-bordered guide.

## PROTECTIVE CLOTHING

**Street Clothing and Work Uniforms.** These garments, such as uniforms worn by police and emergency medical services personnel, provide almost no protection from the harmful effects of dangerous goods.

**Structural Fire Fighters' Protective Clothing (SFPC).** This category of clothing, often called turnout or bunker gear, means the protective clothing normally worn by fire fighters during structural fire fighting operations. It includes a helmet, coat, pants, boots, gloves and a hood to cover parts of the head not protected by the helmet and facepiece. This clothing must be used with full-facepiece positive pressure self-contained breathing apparatus (SCBA). This protective clothing should, at a minimum, meet the OSHA Fire Brigades Standard (29 CFR 1910.156). Structural fire fighters' protective clothing provides limited protection from heat and cold, but may not provide adequate protection from the harmful vapors or liquids that are encountered during dangerous goods incidents. Each guide includes a statement about the use of SFPC in incidents involving those materials referenced by that guide. Some guides state that SFPC provides limited protection. In those cases, the responder wearing SFPC and SCBA may be able to perform an expedient, that is, quick "in-and-out", operation. However, this type of operation can place the responder at risk of exposure, injury or death. The incident commander makes the decision to perform this operation only if an overriding benefit can be gained (i.e., perform an immediate rescue, turn off a valve to control a leak, etc.). The coverall-type protective clothing customarily worn to fight fires in forests or wildlands is not SFPC and **is not** recommended nor referred to elsewhere in this guidebook.

**Positive Pressure Self-Contained Breathing Apparatus (SCBA).** This apparatus provides a constant, positive pressure flow of air within the facepiece, even if one inhales deeply while doing heavy work. Use apparatus certified by NIOSH and the Department of Labor/Mine Safety and Health Administration in accordance with 42 CFR Part 84. Use it in accordance with the requirements for respiratory protection specified in OSHA 29 CFR 1910.134 (Respiratory Protection) and/or 29 CFR 1910.156 (f) (Fire Brigades Standard). Chemical-cartridge respirators or other filtering masks are not acceptable substitutes for positive pressure self-contained breathing apparatus. Demand-type SCBA does not meet the OSHA 29 CFR 1910.156 (f)(1)(i) of the Fire Brigades Standard. If it is suspected that a Chemical Warfare Agent (CW) is involved, the use of NIOSH-certified respirators with CBRN protection are highly recommended.

**Respirators.** N95 respirator is the most common of the seven types of particulate filtering facepiece respirators. This product filters at least 95% of airborne particles (0.3 microns) but is not resistant to oil. N95 filtering facepiece respirators do not provide protection against gas and vapor exposures. PAPR (Powered Air-Purifying Respirator) is an air-purifying respirator that uses a blower to force ambient air through the air-purifying cartridge or filter into the facepiece. A PAPR is not a supplied-air respirator. A PAPR does not supply oxygen or air from a separate source (i.e., cylinders).

**Chemical Protective Clothing and Equipment**. Safe use of this type of protective clothing and equipment requires specific skills developed through training and experience. It is generally not available to, or used by, first responders. This type of special clothing may protect against one chemical, yet be readily permeated by chemicals for which it was not designed. Therefore, protective clothing should not be used unless it is compatible with the released material. This type of special clothing offers little or no protection against heat and/or cold. Examples of this type of equipment have been described as (1) Vapor Protective Suits (NFPA 1991), also known as Totally-Encapsulating Chemical Protective (TECP) Suits or Level A* protection (OSHA 29 CFR 1910.120, Appendix A & B), and (2) Liquid-Splash Protective Suits (NFPA 1992), also known as Level B* or C* protection (OSHA 29 CFR 1910.120, Appendix A & B) or suits for chemical/biological terrorism incidents (NFPA 1994), class 1, 2 or 3 Ensembles and Standard CAN/CGSB/CSA-Z1610-11 – Protection of first responders from chemical, biological, radiological, and nuclear (CBRN) events (2011). No single protective clothing material will protect you from all dangerous goods. Do not assume any protective clothing is resistant to cold and/or heat or flame exposure unless it is so certified by the manufacturer (NFPA 1991 5-3 Flammability Resistance Test and 5-6 Cold Temperature Performance Test).

* Consult glossary for additional protection levels under the heading “Protective Clothing”.

## FIRE AND SPILL CONTROL

### FIRE CONTROL

Water is the most common and generally most available fire extinguishing agent. Exercise caution in selecting a fire extinguishing method since there are many factors to be considered in an incident. Water may be ineffective in fighting fires involving some materials; its effectiveness depends greatly on the method of application.

Fires involving a spill of flammable liquids are generally controlled by applying a fire fighting foam to the surface of the burning material. Fighting flammable liquid fires requires foam concentrate which is chemically compatible with the burning material, correct mixing of the foam concentrate with water and air, and careful application and maintenance of the foam blanket. There are two general types of fire fighting foam: regular and alcohol-resistant. Examples of regular foam are protein-base, fluoroprotein, and aqueous film-forming foam (AFFF). Some flammable liquids, including many petroleum products, can be controlled by applying regular foam. Other flammable liquids, including polar solvents (flammable liquids which are water soluble) such as alcohols and ketones, have different chemical properties. A fire involving these materials cannot be easily controlled with regular foam and requires application of alcohol-resistant foam. Polar solvent fires may be difficult to control and require a higher foam application rate than other flammable liquid fires (see NFPA/ANSI Standards 11 and 11A for further information). Refer to the appropriate guide to determine which type of foam is recommended. Although it is impossible to make specific recommendations for flammable liquids which have subsidiary corrosive or toxic hazards, alcohol-resistant foam may be effective for many of these materials. The emergency response telephone number on the shipping document, or the appropriate emergency response agency, should be contacted as soon as possible for guidance on the proper fire extinguishing agent to use. The final selection of the agent and method depends on many factors such as incident location, exposure hazards, size of the fire, environmental concerns, as well as the availability of extinguishing agents and equipment at the scene.

### WATER REACTIVE MATERIALS

Water is sometimes used to flush spills and to reduce or direct vapors in spill situations. Some of the materials covered by the guidebook can react violently or even explosively with water. In these cases, consider letting the fire burn or leaving the spill alone (except to prevent its spreading by diking) until additional technical advice can be obtained. The applicable guides clearly warn you of these potentially dangerous reactions. These materials require technical advice since:

(1) water getting inside a ruptured or leaking container may cause an explosion;

(2) water may be needed to cool adjoining containers to prevent their rupturing (exploding) or further spread of the fires;

(3) water may be effective in mitigating an incident involving a water-reactive material only if it can be applied at a sufficient flooding rate for an extended period; and

(4) the products from the reaction with water may be more toxic, corrosive, or otherwise more undesirable than the product of the fire without water applied.

When responding to an incident involving water-reactive materials, take into account the existing conditions such as wind, precipitation, location and accessibility to the incident, as well as the availability of the agents to control the fire or spill. Because there are variables to consider, the decision to use water on fires or spills involving water-reactive materials should be based on information from an authoritative source; for example, a producer of the material, who can be contacted through the emergency response telephone number or the appropriate emergency response agency.

## VAPOR CONTROL

Limiting the amount of vapor released from a pool of flammable or corrosive liquids is an operational concern. It requires the use of proper protective clothing, specialized equipment, appropriate chemical agents, and skilled personnel. Before engaging in vapor control, get advice from an authoritative source as to the proper tactics.

There are several ways to minimize the amount of vapors escaping from pools of spilled liquids, such as special foams, adsorbing agents, absorbing agents, and neutralizing agents. To be effective, these vapor control methods must be selected for the specific material involved and performed in a manner that will mitigate, not worsen, the incident.

Where specific materials are known, such as at manufacturing or storage facilities, it is desirable for the dangerous goods response team to prearrange with the facility operators to select and stockpile these control agents in advance of a spill. In the field, first responders may not have the most effective vapor control agent for the material available. They are likely to have only water and only one type of fire fighting foam on their vehicles. If the available foam is inappropriate for use, they are likely to use water spray. Because the water is being used to form a vapor seal, care must be taken not to churn or further spread the spill during application. Vapors that do not react with water may be directed away from the site using the air currents surrounding the water spray. Before using water spray or other methods to safely control vapor emission or to suppress ignition, obtain technical advice, based on specific chemical name identification.

## BLEVE (Boiling Liquid Expanding Vapor Explosion)

The following section presents, in a two-page format, background information on BLEVEs and includes a chart that provides important safety-related information to consider when confronted with this type of situation involving Liquefied Petroleum Gases (LPG), UN1075. LPGs include the following flammable gases: Butane, UN1011; Butylene, UN1012; Isobutylene, UN1055; Propylene, UN1077; Isobutane, UN1969; and Propane, UN1978.

**What are the main hazards from a BLEVE?**

The main hazards from a propane or LPG BLEVE are:

- fire
- thermal radiation from the fire
- blast
- projectiles

The danger from these decreases as you move away from the BLEVE centre. The furthest reaching hazard is projectiles.

This information was prepared for Transport Canada, the Canadian Association of Fire Chiefs and the Propane Gas Association of Canada Inc. by Dr. A. M. Birk, Queen's University, Kingston (Ontario) Canada.

For a video with information on critical safety issues concerning BLEVEs, please visit http://www.tc.gc.ca/eng/tdg/publications-menu-1238.html. This video can be viewed directly on the website. To order a DVD copy of the video, contact us by email at: TDG-RD-TMD@tc.gc.ca.

## BLEVE – SAFETY PRECAUTIONS

**Use with caution**. The following table gives a summary of tank properties, critical times, critical distances and cooling water flow rates for various tank sizes. This table is provided to give responders some guidance but it should be used with caution.

**Tank dimensions are approximate** and can vary depending on the tank design and application.

**Minimum time to failure** is based on ***severe torch fire impingement*** on the vapor space of a tank in good condition, and is approximate. Tanks may fail earlier if they are damaged or corroded. Tanks may fail minutes or hours later than these minimum times depending on the conditions. It has been assumed here that the tanks are not equipped with thermal barriers or water spray cooling.

**Minimum time to empty** is based on an engulfing fire with a properly sized pressure relief valve. If the tank is only partially engulfed, then time to empty will increase (i.e., if tank is 50% engulfed, then the tanks will take twice as long to empty). Once again, it has been assumed that the tank is not equipped with a thermal barrier or water spray.

**Tanks equipped with thermal barriers or water spray cooling** significantly increase the times to failure and the times to empty. A thermal barrier can reduce the heat input to a tank by a factor of ten or more. This means it could take ten times as long to empty the tank through the Pressure Relief Valve (PRV).

**Fireball radius and emergency response distance** is based on mathematical equations and is approximate. They assume spherical fireballs and this is not always the case.

**Two safety distances for public evacuation**. The minimum distance is based on tanks that are launched with a small elevation angle (i.e., a few degrees above horizontal). This is most common for horizontal cylinders. The preferred evacuation distance has more margin of safety since it assumes the tanks are launched at a 45 degree angle to the horizontal. This might be more appropriate if a vertical cylinder is involved.

It is understood that these distances are very large and may not be practical in a highly populated area. However, it should be understood that the risks increase rapidly the closer you are to a BLEVE. Keep in mind that the furthest reaching projectiles tend to come off in the zones 45 degrees on each side of the tank ends.

**Water flow rate is based on 5 ( $\sqrt{\text{capacity (USgal)}}$ ) = USgal/min needed to cool tank metal.**

**Warning**: the data given are approximate and should only be used with extreme caution. For example, where times are given for tank failure or tank emptying through the pressure relief valve – these times are typical but they can vary from situation to situation. Therefore, never risk life based on these times.

**WARNING:** The data given are approximate and should only be used with extreme caution. These times can vary from situation to situation. LPG tanks have been known to BLEVE within minutes. Therefore, never risk life based on these times.

## BLEVE (USE WITH CAUTION)

| Capacity | | Diameter | | Length | | Propane Mass | | Minimum time to failure for severe torch | Approximate time to empty for engulfing fire | Fireball radius | | Emergency response distance | | Minimum evacuation distance | | Preferred evacuation distance | | Cooling water flow rate | |
|---|---|---|---|---|---|---|---|---|---|---|---|---|---|---|---|---|---|---|---|
| Litres | (Gallons) | Meters | (Feet) | Meters | (Feet) | Kilograms | (Pounds) | Minutes | Minutes | Meters | (Feet) | Meters | (Feet) | Meters | (Feet) | Meters | (Feet) | Litres/min | USgal/min |
| 100 | (26.4) | 0.3 | (1) | 1.5 | (4.9) | 40 | (88) | 4 | 8 | 10 | (33) | 90 | (295) | 154 | (505) | 307 | (1007) | 94.6 | 25 |
| 400 | (106) | 0.61 | (2) | 1.5 | (4.9) | 160 | (353) | 4 | 12 | 16 | (53) | 90 | (295) | 244 | (801) | 488 | (1601) | 189.3 | 50 |
| 2000 | (528) | 0.96 | (3.2) | 3 | (9.8) | 800 | (1764) | 5 | 18 | 28 | (92) | 111 | (364) | 417 | (1368) | 834 | (2736) | 424 | 112 |
| 4000 | (1057) | 1 | (3.3) | 4.9 | (16.1) | 1600 | (3527) | 5 | 20 | 35 | (115) | 140 | (459) | 525 | (1722) | 1050 | (3445) | 598 | 158 |
| 8000 | (2113) | 1.25 | (4.1) | 6.5 | (21.3) | 3200 | (7055) | 6 | 22 | 44 | (144) | 176 | (577) | 661 | (2169) | 1323 | (4341) | 848 | 224 |
| 22000 | (5812) | 2.1 | (6.9) | 6.7 | (22) | 8800 | (19400) | 7 | 28 | 62 | (203) | 247 | (810) | 926 | (3038) | 1852 | (6076) | 1404 | 371 |
| 42000 | (11095) | 2.1 | (6.9) | 11.8 | (38.7) | 16800 | (37037) | 7 | 32 | 77 | (253) | 306 | (1004) | 1149 | (3770) | 2200 | (7218) | 1938 | 512 |
| 82000 | (21662) | 2.75 | (9) | 13.7 | (45) | 32800 | (72310) | 8 | 40 | 96 | (315) | 383 | (1257) | 1435 | (4708) | 2200 | (7218) | 2710 | 716 |
| 140000 | (36984) | 3.3 | (10.8) | 17.2 | (56.4) | 56000 | (123457) | 9 | 45 | 114 | (374) | 457 | (1499) | 1715 | (5627) | 2200 | (7218) | 3539 | 935 |

## CRIMINAL/TERRORIST USE OF CHEMICAL/BIOLOGICAL/RADIOLOGICAL AGENTS

The following is intended to supply information to first responders for use in making a preliminary assessment of a situation that they suspect involves criminal/terrorist use of chemical, biological agents and/or radioactive materials (CBRN). To aid in the assessment, a list of observable indicators of the use and/or presence of a CB agent or radioactive material is provided in the following paragraphs. This section ends with a Safe Standoff Distance Chart for various threats when Improvised Explosive Devices are involved.

### DIFFERENCES BETWEEN A CHEMICAL, BIOLOGICAL AND RADIOLOGICAL AGENT

Chemical and biological agents as well as radioactive materials can be dispersed in the air we breathe, the water we drink, or on surfaces we physically contact. Dispersion methods may be as simple as opening a container, using conventional (garden) spray devices, or as elaborate as detonating an improvised explosive device.

**Chemical Incidents** are characterized by the rapid onset of medical symptoms (minutes to hours) and easily observed signatures (colored residue, dead foliage, pungent odor, dead insects and animals).

**Biological Incidents** are characterized by the onset of symptoms in hours to days. Typically, there will be no characteristic signatures because biological agents are usually odorless and colorless. Because of the delayed onset of symptoms in a biological incident, the area affected may be greater due to the movement of infected individuals.

**Radiological Incidents** are characterized by the onset of symptoms, if any, in days to weeks or longer. Typically, there will be no characteristic signatures because radioactive materials are usually odorless and colorless. Specialized equipment is required to determine the size of the affected area, and whether the level of radioactivity presents an immediate or long-term health hazard. Because radioactivity is not detectable without special equipment, the affected area may be greater due to the migration of contaminated individuals.

At the levels created by most probable sources, not enough radiation would be generated to kill people or cause severe illness. In a radiological incident generated by a "dirty bomb", or Radiological Dispersal Device (RDD), in which a conventional explosive is detonated to spread radioactive contamination, the primary hazard is from the explosion. However, certain radioactive materials dispersed in the air could contaminate up to several city blocks, creating fear and possibly panic, and requiring potentially costly cleanup.

### INDICATORS OF A POSSIBLE CHEMICAL INCIDENT

**Dead animals/birds/fish** — Not just an occasional road kill, but numerous animals (wild and domestic, small and large), birds, and fish in the same area.

**Lack of insect life** — If normal insect activity (ground, air, and/or water) is missing, check the ground/water surface/shore line for dead insects. If near water, check for dead fish/aquatic birds.

## INDICATORS OF A POSSIBLE CHEMICAL INCIDENT (Continued)

| | |
|---|---|
| **Unexplained odors** | Smells may range from fruity to flowery to sharp/pungent to garlic/horseradish-like to bitter almonds/peach kernels to newly mown hay. It is important to note that the particular odor is completely out of character with its surroundings. |
| **Unusual numbers of dying or sick people (mass casualties)** | Health problems including nausea, disorientation, difficulty in breathing, convulsions, localized sweating, conjunctivitis (reddening of eyes/nerve agent symptoms), erythema (reddening of skin/vesicant symptoms) and death. |
| **Pattern of casualties** | Casualties will likely be distributed downwind, or if indoors, by the air ventilation system. |
| **Blisters/rashes** | Numerous individuals experiencing unexplained water-like blisters, weals (like bee stings), and/or rashes. |
| **Illness in confined area** | Different casualty rates for people working indoors versus outdoors dependent on where the agent was released. |
| **Unusual liquid droplets** | Numerous surfaces exhibit oily droplets/film; numerous water surfaces have an oily film. (No recent rain.) |
| **Different-looking areas** | Not just a patch of dead weeds, but trees, shrubs, bushes, food crops, and/or lawns that are dead, discolored, or withered. (No current drought.) |
| **Low-lying clouds** | Low-lying cloud/fog-like condition that is not consistent with its surroundings. |
| **Unusual metal debris** | Unexplained bomb/munitions-like material, especially if it contains a liquid. |

## INDICATORS OF A POSSIBLE BIOLOGICAL INCIDENT

| | |
|---|---|
| **Unusual numbers of sick or dying people or animals** | Any number of symptoms may occur. Casualties may occur hours to days after an incident has occurred. The time required before symptoms are observed is dependent on the agent used. |
| **Unscheduled and unusual spray being disseminated** | Especially if outdoors during periods of darkness. |
| **Abandoned spray devices** | Devices may not have distinct odors. |

## INDICATORS OF A POSSIBLE RADIOLOGICAL INCIDENT

| | |
|---|---|
| **Radiation Symbols** | Containers may display a "propeller" radiation symbol. |
| **Unusual metal debris** | Unexplained bomb/munitions-like material. |

## INDICATORS OF A POSSIBLE RADIOLOGICAL INCIDENT (continued)

| | |
|---|---|
| **Heat-emitting material** | Material that is hot or seems to emit heat without any sign of an external heat source. |
| **Glowing material** | Strongly radioactive material may emit or cause radioluminescence. |
| **Sick people/animals** | In very improbable scenarios there may be unusual numbers of sick or dying people or animals. Casualties may occur hours to days or weeks after an incident has occurred. The time required before symptoms are observed is dependent on the radioactive material used, and the dose received. Possible symptoms include skin reddening or vomiting. |

## PERSONAL SAFETY CONSIDERATIONS

When approaching a scene that may involve CB agents or radioactive materials, the most critical consideration is the safety of oneself and other responders. Protective clothing and respiratory protection of appropriate level of safety must be used. In incidents where it is suspected that CBRN materials have been used as weapons, NIOSH-certified respirators with CBRN protection are highly recommended. Be aware that the presence and identification of CB agents or radioactive materials may not be verifiable, especially in the case of biological or radiological agents. The following actions/measures to be considered are applicable to either a chemical, biological or radiological incident. The guidance is general in nature, not all encompassing, and its applicability should be evaluated on a case-by-case basis.

**Approach and response strategies.** Protect yourself and use a safe approach (minimize any exposure time, maximize the distance between you and the item that is likely to harm you, use cover as protection and wear appropriate personal protective equipment and respiratory protection). Identify and estimate the hazard by using indicators as provided above. Isolate the area and secure the scene; potentially contaminated people should be isolated and decontaminated as soon as possible. To the extent possible, take measures to limit the spread of contamination. In the event of a chemical incident, the fading of chemical odors is not necessarily an indication of reduced vapor concentrations. Some chemicals deaden the senses giving the false perception that the chemical is no longer present.

If there is any indication that an area may be contaminated with radioactive materials, including the site of any non-accidental explosion, responder personnel should be equipped with radiation detection equipment that would alert them if they are entering a radiologically compromised environment, and should have received adequate training in its use. This equipment should be designed in such a way that it can also alert the responders when an unacceptable ambient dose rate or ambient dose has been reached.

**Initial actions** to consider in a potential CBRN/Hazmat Terrorism Event:

- Avoid using cell phones, radios, etc. within 100 meters (300 feet) of a suspect device
- NOTIFY your local police by calling 911.
- Set up Incident command upwind and uphill of the area.
- Do NOT touch or move suspicious packages/containers.
- Be cautious regarding potential presence of secondary devices (e.g. Improvised Explosive Devices (IEDs)).
- Avoid contamination.
- Limit access to only those responsible for rescue of victims or assessment of unknown materials or devices.
- Evacuate and isolate individuals potentially exposed to dangerous goods/hazardous materials.
- Isolate contaminated areas and secure the scene for analysis of material.

**Decontamination measures.** Emergency responders should follow standard decontamination procedures (flush-strip-flush). Mass casualty decontamination should begin as soon as possible by stripping (all clothing) and flushing (soap and water). **If biological agents are involved or suspected**, careful washing and use of a brush are more effective. **If chemical agents are suspected**, the most important and effective decontamination will be the one done within the first one or two minutes. If possible, further decontamination should be performed using a 0.5% hypochlorite solution (1 part household bleach mixed with 9 parts water). **If biological agents are suspected**, a contact time of 10 to 15 minutes should be allowed before rinsing. The solution can be used on soft tissue wounds, but must not be used in eyes or open wounds of the abdomen, chest, head, or spine. For further information contact the agencies listed in this guidebook.

**For persons contaminated with radioactive material**, remove them to a low radiation area if necessary. Remove their clothing and place it in a clearly marked and sealed receptacle, such as a plastic bag, for later testing. Use decontamination methods described above, but avoid breaking the skin, e.g., from shaving, or overly vigorous brushing. External radiological contamination on intact skin surface rarely causes a high enough dose to be a hazard to either the contaminated person or the first responders. For this reason, except in very unusual circumstances, an injured person who is also radiologically contaminated should be medically stabilized, taking care to minimize the spread of the contamination to the extent possible, before decontamination measures are initiated.

**Note:** The above information was developed in part by the Department of National Defence (Canada), the U.S. Department of the Army, Aberdeen Proving Ground and the Federal Bureau of Investigation (FBI).

## Improvised Explosive Device (IED) SAFE STAND-OFF DISTANCE

| | Threat Description | Explosives Capacity[1] | | Mandatory Evacuation Distance[2] | | Shelter-in-Place Zone | | Preferred Evacuation Distance[3] | |
|---|---|---|---|---|---|---|---|---|---|
| High Explosives (TNT Equivalent) | Pipe Bomb | 5 lbs | 2.3 kg | 70 ft | 21 m | 71 - 1,199 ft | 22 - 365 m | +1,200 ft | 366 m |
| | Suicide Bomber | 20 lbs | 9 kg | 110 ft | 34 m | 111 - 1,699 ft | 35 - 518 m | +1,700 ft | 519 m |
| | Briefcase/Suitcase | 50 lbs | 23 kg | 150 ft | 46 m | 151 - 1,849 ft | 47 - 563 m | +1,850 ft | 564 m |
| | Car | 500 lbs | 227 kg | 320 ft | 98 m | 321 - 1,899 ft | 99 - 579 m | +1,900 ft | 580 m |
| | SUV/Van | 1,000 lbs | 454 kg | 400 ft | 122 m | 401 - 2,399 ft | 123 - 731 m | +2,400 ft | 732 m |
| | Small Delivery Truck | 4,000 lbs | 1,814 kg | 640 ft | 195 m | 641 - 3,799 ft | 196 - 1,158 m | +3,800 ft | 1,159 m |
| | Container/Water Truck | 10,000 lbs | 4,536 kg | 860 ft | 263 m | 861 - 5,099 ft | 264 - 1,554 m | +5,100 ft | 1,555 m |
| | Semi-Trailer | 60,000 lbs | 27,216 kg | 1,570 ft | 475 m | 1,571 - 9,299 ft | 476 - 2,834 m | +9,300 ft | 2,835 m |

[1] Based on the maximum amount of material that could reasonably fit into a container or vehicle. Variations possible.

[2] Governed by the ability of an unreinforced building to withstand severe damage or collapse.

[3] Governed by the greater of fragment throw distance or glass breakage/falling glass hazard distance. These distances can be reduced for personnel wearing ballistic protection. Note that the pipe bomb, suicide bomb, and briefcase/suitcase bomb are assumed to have a fragmentation characteristic that requires greater stand-off distances than an equal amount of explosives in a vehicle.

## Improvised Explosive Device (IED)
## SAFE STAND-OFF DISTANCE

| | Threat Description | LPG Mass / Volume[1] | | Fireball Diameter[2] | | Safe Distance[3] | |
|---|---|---|---|---|---|---|---|
| LPG - Butane or Propane | Small LPG Tank | 20 lbs / 5 gal | 9 kg / 19 L | 40 ft | 12 m | 160 ft | 48 m |
| | Large LPG Tank | 100 lbs / 25 gal | 45 kg / 95 L | 69 ft | 21 m | 276 ft | 84 m |
| | Commercial/Residential LPG Tank | 2,000 lbs / 500 gal | 907 kg / 1,893 L | 184 ft | 56 m | 736 ft | 224 m |
| | Small LPG Truck | 8,000 lbs / 2,000 gal | 3,630 kg / 7,570 L | 292 ft | 89 m | 1,168 ft | 356 m |
| | Semitanker LPG | 40,000 lbs / 10,000 gal | 18,144 kg / 37,850 L | 499 ft | 152 m | 1,996 ft | 608 m |

[1] Based on the maximum amount of material that could reasonably fit into a container or vehicle. Variations possible.

[2] Assuming efficient mixing of the flammable gas with ambient air.

[3] Determined by U.S. firefighting practices wherein safe distances are approximately 4 times the flame height. Note that an LPG tank filled with high explosives would require a significantly greater stand-off distance than if it were filled with LPG.

# GLOSSARY

**Adsorption** In this guidebook, means a process by which a gas adheres to the surface of a solid but does not penetrate it, such as in adsorption of gases by activated carbon (charcoal).

**AEGL(s)** Acute Exposure Guideline Level(s), AEGLs represent threshold exposure limits for the general public after a once-in-a-lifetime, or rare, exposure and are applicable to emergency exposure periods ranging from 10 minutes to 8 hours. Three levels AEGL-1, AEGL-2 and AEGL-3 are developed for each of five exposure periods (10 and 30 minutes, 1 hour, 4 hours, and 8 hours) and are distinguished by varying degrees of severity of toxic effects; see AEGL-1, AEGL-2 and AEGL-3.

**AEGL-1** AEGL-1 is the airborne concentration (expressed as parts per million or milligrams per cubic meter [ppm or $mg/m^3$]) of a substance above which it is predicted that the general population, including susceptible individuals, could experience notable discomfort, irritation, or certain asymptomatic, non-sensory effects. However, the effects are not disabling and are transient and reversible upon cessation of exposure.

**AEGL-2** AEGL-2 is the airborne concentration (expressed as ppm or $mg/m^3$) of a substance above which it is predicted that the general population, including susceptible individuals, could experience irreversible or other serious, long-lasting adverse health effects or an impaired ability to escape.

**AEGL-3** AEGL-3 is the airborne concentration (expressed as ppm or $mg/m^3$) of a substance above which it is predicted that the general population, including susceptible individuals, could experience life-threatening health effects or death.

**Alcohol-resistant foam** A foam that is resistant to "polar" chemicals such as ketones and esters which may break down other types of foam.

**Biological agents** Living organisms that cause disease, sickness and mortality in humans. Anthrax and Ebola are examples of biological agents. **Refer to GUIDE 158.**

**Blister agents (vesicants)** Substances that cause blistering of the skin. Exposure is through liquid or vapor contact with any exposed tissue (eyes, skin, lungs). Mustard (H), Distilled Mustard (HD), Nitrogen Mustard (HN) and Lewisite (L) are blister agents.

**Symptoms:** Red eyes, skin irritation, burning of skin, blisters, upper respiratory damage, cough, hoarseness.

## GLOSSARY

| | |
|---|---|
| **Blood agents** | Substances that injure a person by interfering with cell respiration (the exchange of oxygen and carbon dioxide between blood and tissues). Hydrogen cyanide (AC) and Cyanogen chloride (CK) are blood agents.<br>**Symptoms:** Respiratory distress, headache, unresponsiveness, seizures, coma. |
| **Burn** | Refers to either a chemical or thermal burn, the former may be caused by corrosive substances and the latter by liquefied cryogenic gases, hot molten substances, or flames. |
| **Carcinogen** | A substance or mixture which induces cancer or increases its incidence. |
| **Category A** | An infectious substance that poses a high risk to the health of individuals and/or animals or public health. These substances can cause serious disease and can lead to death. Effective treatment and preventative measures may not be available. |
| **Category B** | An infectious substance that poses a low to moderate risk to individuals and/or animals and/or public health. These substances are unlikely to cause serious disease. Effective treatment and preventative measures are available. |
| **CBRN** | Chemical, biological, radiological or nuclear warfare agent. |
| **Choking agents** | Substances that cause physical injury to the lungs. Exposure is through inhalation. In extreme cases, membranes swell and lungs become filled with liquid (pulmonary edema). Death results from lack of oxygen; hence, the victim is "choked". Phosgene (CG) is a choking agent.<br>**Symptoms:** Irritation to eyes/nose/throat, respiratory distress, nausea and vomiting, burning of exposed skin. |
| **$CO_2$** | Carbon dioxide gas. |
| **Cold zone** | Area where the command post and support functions that are necessary to control the incident are located. This is also referred to as the clean zone, green zone or support zone in other documents. (EPA Standard Operating Safety Guidelines, OSHA 29 CFR 1910.120, NFPA 472). |
| **Combustible liquid** | Liquids which have a flash point greater than 60°C (140°F) and below 93°C (200°F). U.S. regulations permit a flammable liquid with a flash point between 38°C (100°F) and 60°C (140°F) to be reclassed as a combustible liquid. |

## GLOSSARY

**Compatibility Group**

Letters identify explosives that are deemed to be compatible. The definition of these Compatibility Groups in this Glossary are intended to be descriptive. Please consult the transportation of dangerous goods/hazardous materials or explosives regulations of your jurisdiction for the exact wording of the definitions. Class 1 materials are considered to be "compatible" if they can be transported together without significantly increasing either the probability of an incident or, for a given quantity, the magnitude of the effects of such an incident.

A Substances which are expected to mass detonate very soon after fire reaches them.

B Articles which are expected to mass detonate very soon after fire reaches them.

C Substances or articles which may be readily ignited and burn violently without necessarily exploding.

D Substances or articles which may mass detonate (with blast and/or fragment hazard) when exposed to fire.

E&F Articles which may mass detonate in a fire.

G Substances and articles which may mass explode and give off smoke or toxic gases.

H Articles which in a fire may eject hazardous projectiles and dense white smoke.

J Articles which may mass explode.

K Articles which in a fire may eject hazardous projectiles and toxic gases.

L Substances and articles which present a special risk and could be activated by exposure to air or water.

N Articles which contain only extremely insensitive detonating substances and demonstrate a negligible probability of accidental ignition or propagation.

S Packaged substances or articles which, if accidentally initiated, produce effects that are usually confined to the immediate vicinity.

## GLOSSARY

**Control zones** Designated areas at dangerous goods incidents, based on safety and the degree of hazard. Many terms are used to describe control zones; however, in this guidebook, these zones are defined as the hot/exclusion/red/restricted zone, warm/contamination reduction/yellow/limited access zone, and cold/support/green/clean zone. (EPA Standard Operating Safety Guidelines, OSHA 29 CFR 1910.120, NFPA 472).

**Cryogenic liquid** A refrigerated, liquefied gas that has a boiling point colder than -90°C (-130°F) at atmospheric pressure.

**Decomposition products** Products of a chemical or thermal break-down of a substance.

**Decontamination** The removal of dangerous goods from personnel and equipment to the extent necessary to prevent potential adverse health effects. Always avoid direct or indirect contact with dangerous goods; however, if contact occurs, personnel should be decontaminated as soon as possible. Since the methods used to decontaminate personnel and equipment differ from one chemical to another, contact the chemical manufacturer, through the agencies listed on the inside back cover, to determine the appropriate procedure. Contaminated clothing and equipment should be removed after use and stored in a controlled area (warm/contamination reduction/yellow/limited access zone) until cleanup procedures can be initiated. In some cases, protective clothing and equipment cannot be decontaminated and must be disposed of in a proper manner.

**Dry chemical** A preparation designed for fighting fires involving flammable liquids, pyrophoric substances and electrical equipment. Common types contain sodium bicarbonate or potassium bicarbonate.

**Edema** The accumulation of an excessive amount of watery fluid in cells and tissues. Pulmonary edema is an excessive buildup of water in the lungs, for instance, after inhalation of a gas that is corrosive to lung tissue.

**ERPG(s)** Emergency Response Planning Guideline(s). Values intended to provide estimates of concentration ranges above which one could reasonably anticipate observing adverse health effects; see ERPG-1, ERPG-2 and ERPG-3.

# GLOSSARY

**ERPG-1**
The maximum airborne concentration below which it is believed nearly all individuals could be exposed for up to 1 hour without experiencing more than mild, transient adverse health effects or without perceiving a clearly defined objectionable odor.

**ERPG-2**
The maximum airborne concentration below which it is believed nearly all individuals could be exposed for up to 1 hour without experiencing or developing irreversible or other serious health effects or symptoms that could impair an individual's ability to take protective action.

**ERPG-3**
The maximum airborne concentration below which it is believed nearly all individuals could be exposed for up to 1 hour without experiencing or developing life-threatening health effects.

**Flammable liquid**
A liquid that has a flash point of 60°C (140°F) or lower.

**Flash point**
Lowest temperature at which a liquid or solid gives off vapor in such a concentration that, when the vapor combines with air near the surface of the liquid or solid, a flammable mixture is formed. Hence, the lower the flash point, the more flammable the material.

**Hazard zones (Inhalation Hazard Zones)**

**HAZARD ZONE A:** Gases: LC50 of less than or equal to 200 ppm, Liquids: V equal to or greater than 500 LC50 and LC50 less than or equal to 200 ppm,

**HAZARD ZONE B:** Gases: LC50 greater than 200 ppm and less than or equal to 1000 ppm, Liquids: V equal to or greater than 10 LC50; LC50 less than or equal to 1000 ppm and criteria for Hazard Zone A are not met.

**HAZARD ZONE C:** LC50 greater than 1000 ppm and less than or equal to 3000 ppm,

**HAZARD ZONE D:** LC50 greater than 3000 ppm and less than or equal to 5000 ppm.

## GLOSSARY

**Hot zone** Area immediately surrounding a dangerous goods incident which extends far enough to prevent adverse effects from released dangerous goods to personnel outside the zone. This zone is also referred to as exclusion zone, red zone or restricted zone in other documents. (EPA Standard Operating Safety Guidelines, OSHA 29 CFR 1910.120, NFPA 472).

**IED** See "Improvised Explosive Device".

**Immiscible** In this guidebook, means that a material does not mix readily with water.

**Improvised Explosive Device** A bomb that is manufactured from commercial, military or homemade explosives.

**Large spill** A spill that involves quantities that are greater than 208 liters (55 US gallons) for liquids and greater than 300 kilograms (660 pounds) for solids.

**LC50** Lethal concentration 50. The concentration of a material administered by inhalation that is expected to cause the death of 50% of an experimental animal population within a specified time. (Concentration is reported in either ppm or mg/m$^3$).

**Mass explosion** Explosion which affects almost the entire load virtually instantaneously.

**MAWP** Maximum Allowable Working Pressure: The maximum allowable internal pressure that the tank may experience during normal operations

**mg/m$^3$** Milligrams of a material per cubic meter of air.

**Miscible** In this guidebook, means that a material mixes readily with water.

**mL/m$^3$** Milliliters of a material per cubic meter of air. (1 mL/m$^3$ equals 1 ppm).

**Mutagen** An agent giving rise to an increased occurrence of mutations in populations of cells and/or organisms. Mutation means a permanent change in the amount or structure of the genetic material in a cell.

## GLOSSARY

**Narcotic** A substance which acts as a central nervous system depressor producing effects such as drowsiness, narcosis, reduced alertness, loss of reflexes, lack of coordination, and vertigo. These effects can also be manifested as severe headache or nausea, and can lead to reduced judgment, dizziness, irritability, fatigue, impaired memory function, deficit in perception and coordination, reaction time, or sleepiness.

**Nerve agents** Substances that interfere with the central nervous system. Exposure is primarily through contact with the liquid (via skin and eyes) and secondarily through inhalation of the vapor. Tabun (GA), Sarin (GB), Soman (GD) and VX are nerve agents.

**Symptoms:** Pinpoint pupils, extreme headache, severe tightness in the chest, dyspnea, runny nose, coughing, salivation, unresponsiveness, seizures.

**n.o.s.** These letters refer to "not otherwise specified". The entries which use this description are generic names such as "Corrosive liquid, n.o.s." This means that the actual chemical name for that corrosive liquid is not listed in the regulations; therefore, a generic name must be used to describe it on shipping papers.

**Noxious** In this guidebook, means that a material may be harmful or injurious to health or physical well-being.

**Oxidizer** A chemical which supplies its own oxygen and which helps other combustible material burn more readily.

**P** See "Polymerization".

**Packing Group** The Packing Group (PG) is assigned based on the degree of danger presented by the hazardous material:

PG I : Great danger
PG II : Medium danger
PG III : Minor danger

**PG** See "Packing Group".

**pH** pH is a value that represents the acidity or alkalinity of a water solution. Pure water has a pH of 7. A pH value below 7 indicates an acid solution (a pH of 1 is extremely acidic). A pH above 7 indicates an alkaline solution (a pH of 14 is extremely alkaline). Acids and alkalies (bases) are commonly referred to as corrosive materials.

**PIH** — Poison Inhalation Hazard. Term used to describe gases and volatile liquids that are toxic when inhaled. (Same as TIH).

**Polar** — See "Miscible".

**Polymerization** — A chemical reaction that often produces heat and pressure. Once initiated, the reaction is accelerated by the heat that it produces. The uncontrolled buildup of heat and pressure can cause a fire or an explosion, or can rupture closed containers. The letter (**P**) following a guide number in the yellow-bordered and blue-bordered pages identifies a material that may polymerize violently under high temperature conditions or contamination with other products. It is also used to identify materials that have a strong potential for polymerization in the absence of an inhibitor due to depletion of this inhibitor caused by accident conditions.

**ppm** — Parts per million. (1 ppm equals 1 $mL/m^3$).

**Protective clothing** — Includes both respiratory and physical protection. One cannot assign a level of protection to clothing or respiratory devices separately. These levels were accepted and defined by response organizations such as U.S. Coast Guard, NIOSH, and U.S. EPA.

- Level A: SCBA plus totally encapsulating chemical resistant clothing (permeation resistant).
- Level B: SCBA plus hooded chemical resistant clothing (splash suit).
- Level C: Full or half-face respirator plus hooded chemical resistant clothing (splash suit).
- Level D: Coverall with no respiratory protection.

**Pyrophoric** — A material which ignites spontaneously upon exposure to air (or oxygen).

**Radiation Authority** — As referred to in GUIDES 161 through 166 for radioactive materials, the Radiation Authority is either a Federal, state/provincial agency or state/province designated official. The responsibilities of this authority include evaluating radiological hazard conditions during normal operations and during emergencies. If the identity and telephone number of the authority are not known by emergency responders, or included in the local response plan, the information can be obtained from the agencies listed on the inside back cover. They maintain a periodically updated list of radiation authorities.

# GLOSSARY

**Radioactivity** The property of some substances to emit invisible and potentially harmful radiation.

**Refrigerated liquid** See "Cryogenic liquid".

**Respiratory sensitizer** A substance that induces hypersensitivity of the airways following inhalation of the substance.

**Right-of-way** A defined area on a property containing one or more high-pressure natural gas pipelines.

**Shelter in-place** People should seek shelter inside a building and remain inside until the danger passes. **Sheltering in-place is used when evacuating the public would cause greater risk than staying where they are, or when an evacuation cannot be performed**. Direct the people inside to **close all doors and windows** and to **shut off all ventilating, heating and cooling systems**. In-place protection (shelter in-place) may not be the best option if (a) the vapors are flammable; (b) if it will take a long time for the gas to clear the area; or (c) if buildings cannot be closed tightly. Vehicles can offer some protection for a short period if the windows are closed and the ventilating systems are shut off. Vehicles are not as effective as buildings for in-place protection.

**Skin corrosion** The production of irreversible damage to the skin following the application of a test substance for up to 4 hours.

**Skin irritation** The production of reversible damage to the skin following the application of a test substance for up to 4 hours.

**Skin sensitizer** A substance that will induce an allergic response following skin contact.

**Small spill** A spill that involves quantities that are less than 208 liters (55 US gallons) for liquids and less than 300 kilograms (660 pounds) for solids.

**Specific gravity** Weight of a substance compared to the weight of an equal volume of water at a given temperature. Specific gravity less than 1 indicates a substance is lighter than water; specific gravity greater than 1 indicates a substance is heavier than water.

## GLOSSARY

**Straight (solid) stream** Method used to apply or distribute water from the end of a hose. The water is delivered under pressure for penetration. In an efficient straight (solid) stream, approximately 90% of the water passes through an imaginary circle 38 cm (15 inches) in diameter at the breaking point. Hose (solid or straight) streams are frequently used to cool tanks and other equipment exposed to flammable liquid fires, or for washing burning spills away from danger points. However, straight streams will cause a spill fire to spread if improperly used or when directed into open containers of flammable and combustible liquids.

**TIH** Toxic Inhalation Hazard. Term used to describe gases and volatile liquids that are toxic when inhaled. (Same as PIH).

**V** Saturated vapor concentration in air of a material in $mL/m^3$ (volatility) at 20°C and standard atmospheric pressure.

**Vapor density** Weight of a volume of pure vapor or gas (with no air present) compared to the weight of an equal volume of dry air at the same temperature and pressure. A vapor density less than 1 (one) indicates that the vapor is lighter than air and will tend to rise. A vapor density greater than 1 (one) indicates that the vapor is heavier than air and may travel along the ground.

**Vapor pressure** Pressure at which a liquid and its vapor are in equilibrium at a given temperature. Liquids with high vapor pressures evaporate rapidly.

**Viscosity** Measure of a liquid's internal resistance to flow. This property is important because it indicates how fast a material will leak out through holes in containers or tanks.

**Warm zone** Area between Hot and Cold zones where personnel and equipment decontamination and hot zone support take place. It includes control points for the access corridor and thus assists in reducing the spread of contamination. Also referred to as the contamination reduction corridor (CRC), contamination reduction zone (CRZ), yellow zone or limited access zone in other documents. (EPA Standard Operating Safety Guidelines, OSHA 29 CFR 1910.120, NFPA 472).

**Water Reactive Material** For the purpose of this guidebook, produces significant toxic gas when it comes in contact with water.

**Water-sensitive** Substances which may produce flammable and/or toxic decomposition products upon contact with water.

**Water spray (fog)**

Method or way to apply or distribute water. The water is finely divided to provide for high heat absorption. Water spray patterns can range from about 10 to 90 degrees. Water spray streams can be used to extinguish or control the burning of a fire or to provide exposure protection for personnel, equipment, buildings, etc. **(This method can be used to absorb vapors, knock-down vapors or disperse vapors. Direct a water spray (fog), rather than a straight (solid) stream, into the vapor cloud to accomplish any of the above).**

Water spray is particularly effective on fires of flammable liquids and volatile solids having flash points above 37.8°C (100°F).

Regardless of the above, water spray can be used successfully on flammable liquids with low flash points. The effectiveness depends particularly on the method of application. With proper nozzles, even gasoline spill fires of some types have been extinguished when coordinated hose lines were used to sweep the flames off the surface of the liquid. Furthermore, water spray carefully applied has frequently been used with success in extinguishing fires involving flammable liquids with high flash points (or any viscous liquids) by causing frothing to occur only on the surface, and this foaming action blankets and extinguishes the fire.

## PUBLICATION DATA

The 2016 Emergency Response Guidebook (ERG2016) was prepared by the staff of Transport Canada, the U.S. Department of Transportation, and the Secretariat of Communications and Transport of Mexico with the assistance of many interested parties from government and industry including the collaboration of CIQUIME of Argentina. The original authors of the ERG are Transport Canada's Michel Cloutier and U.S. DOT's George Cushmac. Printing and publication services are provided through U.S. DOT's Pipeline and Hazardous Materials Safety Administration (PHMSA), Outreach, Training, and Grants Division.

ERG2016 is based on earlier Transport Canada, U.S. DOT, and Secretariat of Communications and Transport emergency response guidebooks. ERG2016 is published in three languages: English, French and Spanish. The Emergency Response Guidebook has been translated and printed in other languages, including Chinese, German, Hebrew, Japanese, Portuguese, Korean, Hungarian, Polish, Turkish and Thai.

We encourage countries that wish to translate this Guidebook to please contact any of the websites or telephone numbers in the next paragraph.

## DISTRIBUTION OF THIS GUIDEBOOK

The primary objective is to place one copy of the ERG2016 in each publicly owned emergency service vehicle through distribution to Federal, state, provincial and local public safety authorities. The distribution of this guidebook is being accomplished through the voluntary cooperation of a network of key agencies. Emergency service organizations that have not yet received copies of ERG2016 should contact the respective distribution center in their country, state or province. In the U.S., information about the distribution center for your location may be obtained from the Office of Hazardous Materials Safety website at http://phmsa.dot.gov/hazmat/outreach-training/erg or call 202-366-4900. In Canada, contact CANUTEC at 613-992-4624 or via the website at http://www.tc.gc.ca/canutec for information. In Mexico, call SCT at 50-11-92-20, 50-11-92-40 or 50-11-92-70 or via email at iflores@sct.gob.mx. In Argentina, call CIQUIME at 011-4611-2007, or via the website at http://www.ciquime.org.ar, or via email at gre2016@ciquime.org.ar.

## REPRODUCTION AND RESALE

Constructive comments concerning ERG2016 are solicited; in particular, comments concerning its use in handling incidents involving dangerous goods. Comments should be addressed to:

**In Canada:**


Director, CANUTEC
Transport Dangerous Goods
Transport Canada
Ottawa, Ontario
Canada K1A 0N5

Phone: 613-992-4624 (information)
Fax: 613-954-5101
Email: canutec@tc.gc.ca


**In the U.S.:**


U. S. Department of Transportation
Pipeline and Hazardous Materials Safety Administration
Outreach, Training, and Grants Division (PHH-50)
Washington, DC 20590-0001

Phone: 202-366-4900
Fax: 202-366-7342
Email: ERGComments@dot.gov


**In Mexico:**


Secretariat of Communications and Transportation
Federal Motor Carrier General Direction
Deputy General Director for Standards, Technical
Specifications and Motor Carrier Safety
Calz. de las Bombas No. 411 2nd floor
Col. Los Girasoles
Del. Coyoacan
C.P.04920
Mexico D.F.
Phone: (+52) (55) 50-11-92-20, (55) 50-11-92-40 and (55) 50-11-92-70


**In Argentina:**


Centro de Información Química para Emergencias (CIQUIME)
Juan Bautista Alberdi 2986
C1406GSS Buenos Aires, Argentina
Phone: +54-11-4611-2007 Fax +54-11-4613-3707
Email: gre2016@ciquime.org.ar

The Emergency Response Guidebook is normally revised and reissued every four years. However, in the event of a significant mistake, omission or change in the state of knowledge, special instructions to change the guidebook (in pen-and-ink, with paste-over stickers, or with a supplement) may be issued.

Users of this guidebook should check periodically (about every 6 months) to make sure their version is current. Changes should be annotated below. Contact:

**DOT/PHMSA**
http://phmsa.dot.gov/hazmat/outreach-training/erg

**TRANSPORT CANADA**
https://www.tc.gc.ca/eng/canutec/menu.htm

**CIQUIME**
http://www.ciquime.org.ar

*This guidebook incorporates changes dated:*

________________________________________

________________________________________

________________________________________

# CANADA AND UNITED STATES NATIONAL RESPONSE CENTERS

## CANADA

### 1. CANUTEC

**CANUTEC** is the **Canadian Transport Emergency Centre** operated by the Transportation of Dangerous Goods Directorate of Transport Canada.

**CANUTEC** provides a national bilingual (French and English) advisory service and is staffed by professional scientists experienced and trained in interpreting technical information and providing emergency response advice.

**In an emergency, CANUTEC may be called at 1-888-CANUTEC (226-8832)**
**or collect at 613-996-6666 (24 hours)**
***666 cellular (Press Star 666, Canada only)**

In a non-emergency situation, please call the information line at 613-992-4624 (24 hours).

### 2. PROVINCIAL/TERRITORIAL AGENCIES

Although technical information and emergency response assistance can be obtained from **CANUTEC**, there are federal, provincial and territorial regulations requiring the reporting of dangerous goods incidents to certain authorities.

The following list of provincial/territorial agencies is supplied for your convenience.

| Province | Emergency Authority and/or Telephone Number |
|---|---|
| Alberta | Local Police and Provincial Authorities<br>1-800-272-9600 or 780-422-9600 |
| British Columbia | Local Police and Provincial Authorities<br>1-800-663-3456 |
| Manitoba | Provincial Authority 204-945-4888 and<br>Local Police or fire brigade, as appropriate |
| New Brunswick | Local Police or 1-800-565-1633 |
| Newfoundland and Labrador | Local Police and 709-772-2083 |
| Northwest Territories | 867-920-8130 |
| Nova Scotia | Local Police or 1-800-565-1633 |
| Nunavut | Local Police and 867-920-8130 |
| Ontario | Local Police |
| Prince Edward Island | Local Police or 1-800-565-1633 |
| Quebec | Local Police |
| Saskatchewan | Local Police or 1-800-667-7525 |
| Yukon Territory | 867-667-7244 |

**NOTE:**

1. The appropriate federal agency must be notified in the case of rail, air or marine incidents.
2. The nearest police department must be notified in the case of lost, stolen or misplaced explosives, radioactive materials or infectious substances.
3. **CANUTEC must** be notified in the case of:
   a. lost, stolen or unlawfully interfered with dangerous goods (except Class 9);
   b. an incident involving infectious substances;
   c. an accidental release from a cylinder that has suffered a catastrophic failure;
   d. an incident where the shipping documents display CANUTEC's telephone number, 1-888-CANUTEC (226-8832) or 613-996-6666, as the emergency telephone number; or
   e. a dangerous goods incident in which a railway vehicle, a ship, an aircraft, an aerodrome or an air cargo facility is involved.

**3. Emergency Response Assistance Plans (Applies in Canada ONLY)**

An ERAP or Emergency Response Assistance Plan is an approved plan that describes what is to be done in the event of a transportation accident involving certain higher risk dangerous goods. The ERAP is required by the Canadian *Transportation of Dangerous Goods Act* for dangerous goods that require special expertise and response equipment to respond to an incident. The plan is intended to assist local emergency responders by providing them with technical experts and specially trained and equipped emergency response personnel at the scene of a dangerous goods incident.

The ERAP will describe the specialized response capabilities, equipment and procedures that will be used to support a response to incidents involving high risk dangerous goods. The plan will also address emergency preparedness, including personnel training, response exercises and equipment maintenance. The ERAP plans supplement those of the carrier and of the local and provincial authorities, and must be integrated with other organizations to help mitigate the consequences of an accident.

For shipments that require an ERAP, the ERAP number and the phone number to activate the ERAP will be included on the shipping document. If additional information is required, or to determine if the product involved in the emergency requires an ERAP, contact **CANUTEC**.

**CANUTEC may be called at 1-888-CANUTEC (226-8832)**
**or collect at 613-996-6666 (24 hours)**
***666 on cellular phone (Press star 666) *In Canada Only***

**UNITED STATES**

## NATIONAL RESPONSE CENTER (NRC)

The NRC, which is operated by the U.S. Coast Guard, receives reports required when dangerous goods and hazardous substances are spilled. After receiving notification of an incident, the NRC will immediately notify the appropriate Federal On-Scene Coordinator and concerned Federal agencies. Federal law requires that anyone who releases into the environment a reportable quantity of a hazardous substance (including oil when water is, or may be affected) or a material identified as a marine pollutant, must **immediately** notify the NRC. When in doubt as to whether the amount released equals the required reporting levels for these materials, the NRC should be notified.

CALL **NRC** (24 hours)

**1-800-424-8802**

(Toll-free in the U.S., Canada, and the U.S. Virgin Islands)

**202-267-2675** in the District of Columbia

Calling the emergency response telephone number, CHEMTREC®, CHEMTEL, INC., INFOTRAC or 3E COMPANY, does not constitute compliance with regulatory requirements to call the NRC.

# NOTES

# NOTES

## NOTES

# EMERGENCY RESPONSE TELEPHONE NUMBERS

## MEXICO

1. **CENACOM**

**01-800-00-413-00** toll free in the Mexican Republic
For calls originating in Mexico City and the Metropolitan Area: **5128-0000**
For calls originating elsewhere, call: **01-55-5128-0000**
**exts. 36469, 36470, 36471, 36472, 37807, 37808, 37809, 37810, 37811, 37812**

2. **CONASENUSA**

**01-800-11-131-68** toll free in the Mexican Republic
**24 hours, 365 days**

3. **SETIQ**

**01-800-00-214-00** in the Mexican Republic
For calls originating in Mexico City and the Metropolitan Area: **5559-1588**
For calls originating elsewhere, call: **+52-55-5559-1588**

## ARGENTINA

1. **CIQUIME**

**0-800-222-2933** in the Republic of Argentina
For calls originating elsewhere, call: **+54-11-4611-2007**
(Collect calls are accepted)

## BRAZIL

1. **PRÓ-QUÍMICA**

**0-800-118270**
(Toll-free in Brazil)
For calls originating elsewhere, call: **+55-19-3833-5310**
(Collect calls are accepted)

## COLOMBIA

1. **CISPROQUIM**

**01-800-091-6012** in Colombia
For calls originating in Bogotá, Colombia call: **288-6012**
For calls originating elsewhere, call
**+57-1-288-6012**

## CHILE

1. **CITUC QUÍMICO**

**2-2247-3600** in the Republic of Chile
For calls originating elsewhere, call
**+56-2-2247-3600**